The Human Body

An Introduction to Structure and Function

Adolf Faller, M.D.
Former Professor
University of Fribourg
Fribourg, Switzerland

Michael Schünke, M.D., Ph.D.
Professor
Institute of Anatomy CAU Kiel
Kiel, Germany

Gabriele Schünke, M.Sc.
Dipl.-Biol.
Kronshagen, Germany

Translated by Oliver French, M.D.; edited by Ethan Taub, M.D.

316 colored illustrations

Thieme
Stuttgart · New York

Library of Congress Cataloging-in-Publication Data is available from the publisher

This book is an authorized and revised translation of the 13th German edition published and copyrighted 1999 by Georg Thieme Verlag, Stuttgart, Germany. Title of the German edition: Der Körper des Menschen: Einführung in Bau und Funktion

Translator: Oliver French M.D., Brooktondal, NY, USA

Editor: Ethan Taub, M.D., Diplomate of the American Board of Neurological Surgery, Klinik im Park, Zürich, Switzerland

1st Dutch edition 1970
2nd Dutch edition 1974
3rd Dutch edition 1978
4th Dutch edition 1981
1st French edition 1970
2nd French edition 1983
3rd French edition 1988
4th French edition 2000
1st German edition 1966
2nd German edition 1967
3rd German edition 1969
4th German edition 1970
5th German edition 1972
6th German edition 1974
7th German edition 1976
8th German edition 1978
9th German edition 1980
10th German edition 1984
11th German edition 1988
12th German edition 1995
1st Italian edition 1973
1st Japanese edition 1982
2nd Japanese edition 1993
3rd Japanese edition 1998
1st Spanish edition 1968
2nd Spanish edition 1984

© 2004 Georg Thieme Verlag,
Rüdigerstrasse 14, 70469 Stuttgart, Germany
http://www.thieme.de
Thieme New York, 333 Seventh Avenue,
New York, NY 10001 USA
http://www.thieme.com

Cover design: Cyclus, Stuttgart
Typesetting by primustype Hurler GmbH, Notzingen
Printed in Germany by Grammlich, Pliezhausen

ISBN 3-13-129271-7 (GTV)
ISBN 1-58890-122-X (TNY)   1 2 3 4 5

Important note: Medicine is an ever-changing science undergoing continual development. Research and clinical experience are continually expanding our knowledge, in particular our knowledge of proper treatment and drug therapy. Insofar as this book mentions any dosage or application, readers may rest assured that the authors, editors, and publishers have made every effort to ensure that such references are in accordance with **the state of knowledge at the time of production of the book.**

Nevertheless, this does not involve, imply, or express any guarantee or responsibility on the part of the publishers in respect to any dosage instructions and forms of applications stated in the book. **Every user is requested to examine carefully** the manufacturers' leaflets accompanying each drug and to check, if necessary in consultation with a physician or specialist, whether the dosage schedules mentioned therein or the contraindications stated by the manufacturers differ from the statements made in the present book. Such examination is particularly important with drugs that are either rarely used or have been newly released on the market. Every dosage schedule or every form of application used is entirely at the user's own risk and responsibility. The authors and publishers request every user to report to the publishers any discrepancies or inaccuracies noticed.

Some of the product names, patents, and registered designs referred to in this book are in fact registered trademarks or proprietary names even though specific reference to this fact is not always made in the text. Therefore, the appearance of a name without designation as proprietary is not to be construed as a representation by the publisher that it is in the public domain.

This book, including all parts thereof, is legally protected by copyright. Any use, exploitation, or commercialization outside the narrow limits set by copyright legislation, without the publisher's consent, is illegal and liable to prosecution. This applies in particular to photostat reproduction, copying, mimeographing, preparation of microfilms, and electronic data processing and storage.

Preface to the First English Edition

The first German edition of this book, which was later lovingly known as *"The Faller,"* published in 1966. At this time nobody could ever have imagined that *"The Human Body,"* written by Swiss anatomist Adolf Faller, would remain uniquely successful for almost 40 years. Thirteen German editions and several editions in other languages speak for themselves. Fifteen years after Faller's death, the thoroughly and extensively revised 13th German edition published. The current English edition is based upon this German edition.

The new version contains almost 200 more pages than the original. In addition, more than 50 new illustrations have been added to facilitate an easier approach to sometimes difficult information. Where necessary, entire chapters have been rewritten to cover the latest developments in human biology and medicine. All these changes have been made with the reader in mind. In fact, many of the changes were suggestions from the readers which we have happily incorporated. These include a brief summary at the end of each chapter, a fold-out depicting the complete human skeleton, and a table of contents at the beginning of each chapter. We therefore thank our readers for their many helpful suggestions and hope that readers of the English edition will follow suit.

Many thanks go to our translator Oliver French MD, who not only skilfully translated the text but also adapted it to American medical practice. Due to his expertise this book is far more than a simple translation of a German textbook; it has really become an international textbook in its own right. Many helpful suggestions from Ethan Taub MD, a New York-trained neurosurgeon, were also incorporated into the text.

Preparing this English edition was a rewarding experience and we hope that the reader will share our enthusiam when studying the fascinating fabric of the human body. This work has been made particularly enjoyable by the help of the experienced Thieme staff. We would like to express our appreciation to Ms G Kuhn, Mr R Zepf, and Dr C Bergman. Mr

Markus Voll professionally and skillfully prepared all the new illustrations. Many thanks to them all!

Finally a note on the chapter Evolution. We are aware that many American educational institutions do not teach the theory of evolution and many Americans believe in creationism. However, the theory of evolution is widely accepted in Europe and its application forms the basis of many observations on which medical practice is founded. Its inclusion in this text should therefore not be regarded as *"Weltanschauung"* but as a rather neutral statement about current biological theory.

Kiel, Spring 2004   *Gabriele and Michael Schünke*

Contents

A more detailed table of contents can be found at the beginning of each chapter

1

Biology of the Cell

Contents

■ Introduction

The basic building block of the human body as well as of all animals and plants is the cell. It is the smallest independent living entity and can live independently as a single-celled (*unicellular*) organism (e.g., flagellates, amebas). In *multicellular organisms* (metazoa) the cells organize in large units and become functional entities within an overarching framework. In unicellular organisms, such as bacteria and fungi, all the cells exhibit an identical basic structure. Multicellular organisms, such as plants, animals, and humans, also exhibit a fundamentally uniform organization. Here, however, there are great differences in the variety of tasks, and each type of cell specializes in the execution of a specific task within the organism. For instance, red blood cells (erythrocytes) transport oxygen, while other cells serve as conduits for stimuli (nerve cells) or serve reproduction (germ cells).

The actions of each individual cell in an organism depend on *specific genetic information*. In the cell this information is stored in certain sections of the substance termed *deoxyribonucleic acid* (*DNA*) in the genes. It consists of programs to direct cell reproduction as well as the synthesis of proteins. Both functions are essential to ensure that a fertilized ovum can develop into a multicellular organism and that cells differentiated in various ways, such as brain, lung, muscle, or liver cells, can develop from common precursor cells.

■ Number, Size, Shape, and Properties of Cells

Number, Size, and Shape

The human body is composed of roughly **75×10^{12} cells** (= 75 000 billion cells), of which as many as 25×10^{12} (25 000 billion) occur as erythrocytes in the blood and which therefore constitute the commonest type of cell. Of the remaining cells, 100×10^9 (= 100 billion) are part of the nervous system. Since the number of cells is so great, each individual building block must be microscopically small. The size of each cell varies in the human body between 5 μm (e.g., single connective tissue cells) and 150 μm (the ovum of the female). When cell processes are included, however, some cells can reach considerable lengths; for example, nerve cells that run from the brain to the spinal cord attain lengths of up to 1 m. The shapes of the various cells also vary considerably. Ova are round, connective tissue cells form processes, and other cells are spindle-shaped (muscle cells), flat, cuboid, or highly prismatic (epithelial cells). Size and shape are often closely linked to a cell's specific properties.

Properties

All cells have a number of *basic properties* in common, even if they are differentiated to carry out specific tasks.

■ **Metabolism and the Generation of Energy.** Every cell possesses a metabolism, by which absorbed substances are changed into compounds that serve the organization of the cell and are discharged in the form of end products. Therefore, in order to maintain the normal functions necessary for life, cells require nutrients from which they acquire the energy for their tasks. The chemical processes that take place during the transformation of nutrients (fats, proteins, and carbohydrates) to generate energy are basically the same in all cells, as also is the release of end products into the fluids surrounding the cells.

■ **Reproduction and Life Expectancy.** With few exceptions, almost all cells have the capacity to reproduce themselves by dividing. This property is often retained throughout life and is the prerequisite for the replacement of dead cells and the regeneration (restoration) of tissues and organs after injury. The human bone marrow, for instance, creates about 160 million red blood cells per minute, and in the male the testes create about 85 million sperm cells daily. Another instance of a high rate of cell division is given by the cells of the mucous membrane of the small intestine, which have an average life expectancy of only a few days (30–100 hours). Yet other cells divide only in certain phases of development and subsequently survive for life, e. g., nerve and muscle cells.

■ **Sensitivity to Stimulation and Response to Stimulation.** Almost all cells are connected to their immediate environment by specific structures on their surfaces (e. g., receptors) and can sense, evaluate, and respond to distinct stimuli.

Besides these basic properties, certain cells possess specific properties. These may include *mobility* (e. g., histiocytes in connective tissue; male sperm in the female genital tract), the *assimilation and elimination of substances* (e. g., assimilation of cell debris by defense cells; secretion by glandular cells), or the development of *specific surface differentiations* (e. g., cilia on the mucous membrane cells of the respiratory tract; brush border of the mucous membrane cells of the small intestine).

■ Structure of the Cell and Cell Organelles

Basic Structure

Examination of a cell by light microscopy shows a fluid **cell body** (**cytoplasm**), a **cell nucleus** and the surrounding **cell membrane** (**plasmalemma**) (Fig. 1.**1**). The cytoplasm contains a number of highly organized small bodies, called **cell organelles**, that can often only be seen by electron microscopy. It also contains certain supportive structures (parts of the cytoskeleton) and numerous cell inclusions (e. g., metabolic substrates and end products).

Cell Membrane

The surrounding cell membrane (plasmalemma) contains the fluid cell body (protoplasm). An electron-microscopic section demonstrates a three-layered structure (Fig. 1.**2**): this includes a double layer of lipids in which two layers of lipid molecules (phospholipids, cholesterol), are arranged so that their lipid-soluble parts (fatty acids) oppose each other (light middle line) while the water-soluble ends form the outer and inner boundaries of the cell membrane (dark outer and inner lines). The double lipid layer is infiltrated with proteins in a more or less mosaic-like fashion. These protein molecules have multiple functions. They may form pores that serve the transmission of water and salts, or they may take part in regulatory functions as receptor proteins. The membrane proteins abutting on the outer side of the cell, and in part the water-soluble ends of the phospholipids, are covered with a thin film of sugar molecules (carbohydrates). This film is called the *glycocalyx*. The chemi-

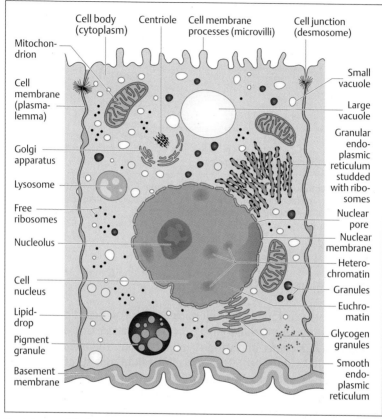

Fig. 1.**1** **Simplified image of a cell representing electron-microscopic findings** (see also Fig. 1.**7**)

cal structure of the glycocalyx is laid down genetically and it is specific for each cell. By this structure cells can "recognize" each other as self and non-self (see Chapter 6: The Immune System, Specific Immunity).

This so-called *elementary membrane* has a thickness of 7.5 nm (1 μm = 1000 nm) and forms a barrier between the cell interior and the extracellular space. The cell organelles are also surrounded by elementary membranes.

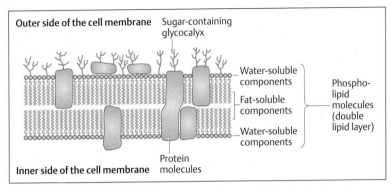

Fig. 1.**2 Schematic cross-section of a cell membrane.** The three-layered structure seen in the electron-microscopic image is produced by the two water-soluble inner and outer components of the double lipid layer, and the fat soluble components between them. (After Leonhardt)

Cytoplasm and Cell Organelles

The cytoplasm surrounds the cell nucleus. It is composed of the *hyaloplasm* or *cytosol* (*intracellular fluid*), *the cell organelles* that perform certain cellular functions, and various cell inclusions, the *metaplasm* (metabolic products of the cell). The intracellular fluid consists of an aqueous saline solution and proteins (microtubules, microfilaments, intermediate filaments) that determine the shape and mechanical solidity of the cell (the so-called cytoskeleton). The organelles vary in number according to the type and function of the cell containing them. The following essential cell organelles may be differentiated:

- Endoplasmic reticulum
- Ribosomes
- Golgi apparatus
- Lysosomes
- Centrioles
- Mitochondria

Endoplasmic Reticulum (ER)

The endoplasmic reticulum (Fig. 1.**1**) criss-crosses the cytoplasm in the form of tubular and vesicular structures surrounded by elementary membranes. It subdivides the interior of the cell into compartments and facilitates the *intracellular transport of substances* along its channels. Its large surface makes possible the rapid completion of specific metabolic processes (e. g., the synthesis of proteins and lipids) and serves as a depot for membranes, i.e., it originates other membranes. In many places the endoplasmic reticulum is dotted with small granular structures, the ribosomes (granular ER), that serve especially for the synthesis of proteins (see below). Granular endoplasmic reticulum is especially prominent in cells such as those of the pancreas. The endoplasmic reticulum is called smooth ER when ribosomes are absent, predominating especially in hormone-secreting cells. All cells except red blood cells contain endoplasmic reticulum.

Ribosomes

Ribosomes (Fig. 1.**1**) serve protein synthesis (see also The Cell Nucleus, Protein Synthesis below) and occur either separately in the form of free ribosomes or in combination with endoplasmic reticulum (granular ER). They are not surrounded by elementary membrane. In the granular ER they are responsible for the production of exported proteins (e. g., glandular secretions), whereas free ribosomes produce intracellular proteins (e. g., enzymes, structural proteins). Ribosomes contain complexes made up of several enzymes consisting of proteins and RNA molecules (ribosomal RNA, rRNA). These create the amino acid chains for protein synthesis. rRNA is also a structural element of ribosomes.

Golgi Apparatus

The Golgi apparatus (Fig. 1.**1**) is composed of several Golgi bodies and also represents a system of internal channels taking part in the ingestion and excretion of substances in the form of *membrane-bounded secretory vesicles*. Lysosomes are also formed by this mechanism. The Golgi bodies have one side for *uptake* and one for *discharge*. Precursors of protein secretions migrate from the granular endoplasmic reticulum to the intake side of the Golgi body, where they are loaded into transport vesicles and flushed out of the cell through the discharge side. During this process, the membrane of the vesicle fuses with the cell membrane. Hence the renewal of the cell membrane is an important task of the Golgi apparatus.

Lysosomes

The more or less spherical lysosomes (Fig. 1.**1**) are the digestive organs of the cell. They contain large quantities of enzymes, especially acid hydrolases and phosphatases, with the aid of which they can degrade ingested foreign material or the cell's own decaying organelles and return them in the form of metabolites for cellular metabolism (recycling). The lysosome's membrane protects intact cells from uncontrolled activity of the lysosomal enzymes. In damaged cells, the liberated enzymes can contribute to tissue autolysis (e. g., in purulent abscesses).

Centrioles

Centrioles (Fig. 1.**1**) are hollow, open-ended cylinders. Their walls are composed of *microtubules*, which are rigid, filamentous proteins. Centrioles play a major role in cell division, when they build threadlike spindle structures that are connected with the movement of the chromosomes. Evidently this process determines the polarity of the cell for the direction of a cell division.

Mitochondria

Mitochondria (Fig. 1.**1**) are small filiform structures, 2–6 µm long that are present in varying numbers (a few to more than a thousand) in all cells with the exception of red blood corpuscles. Their walls consist of an inner and an outer elementary membrane. The inner has multiple folds, and so possesses a large surface area. Mitochondria are the "*power plants*" of the cell, as they provide the energy necessary for all metabolic processes in the form of a universal biological fuel, *adenosine triphosphate (ATP)*. The manufacture of ATP from the three basic materials—proteins, fats, and carbohydrates—takes place almost exclusively in the mitochondria (Fig. 1.**3**), where the energy liberated as part of a process of

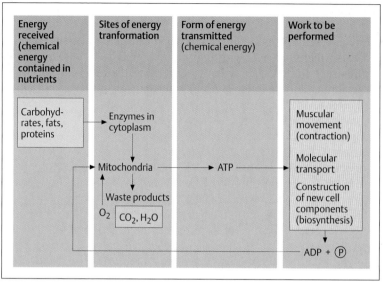

Fig. 1.**3** **Schematic representation of the energy transformation processes in a cell.** (After Beske)

ATP	adenosine triphosphate	CO_2	carbon dioxide
ADP	adenosine diphosphate	O_2	oxygen
P	phosphate	H_2O	water

oxidative combustion (*mitochondrial respiratory sequence*) is not dissipated as heat but is stored in the form of high-energy compounds (ATP).

ATP consists of three chemical substances linked to each other by high-energy bonds: a nitrogen-containing *adenine*, the sugar *ribose*, and three *phosphate* molecules (adenosine triphosphate). When one phosphate molecule is split off, energy is liberated and ATP becomes ADP (adenosine diphosphate), which, with added energy, can revert to adenosine triphosphate in the mitochondria.

From the mitochondria, ATP reaches the sites in the cell where energy is utilized. It is needed among other uses for the transport of materials through the cell membrane, for the synthesis of proteins and other cell components, and for muscle movement (contraction).

The Cell Nucleus

Every cell with the exception of red blood cells has a nucleus (Fig. 1.1). However, there are cells with two nuclei (some liver cells) or greater numbers of nuclei, e. g., osteoclasts in bony tissue (5–20 nuclei) or skeletal muscle cells (more than 1000 nuclei). Cells without nuclei can no longer divide. The nuclei are separated from the surrounding cytoplasm by two elementary membranes (nuclear membranes, nuclear envelope) but are connected to the endoplasmic reticulum by so-called *nuclear pores*. The nucleus usually contains a clearly defined round structure, the *nucleolus*. Its task is the production of ribosomal RNA (rRNA) (see Fig. 1.7). It is therefore inconspicuous in inactive cells, but is well-defined in metabolically active cells with increased protein synthesis. Multiple nucleoli may occur in such cells. The size and shape of the nucleus vary from cell to cell: its form may be round, lobulated, or extended. Its shape and structure also depend at any one time on the current phase of the cell's cycle. For instance, in the phase of cell division, filiform structures—the *chromosomes*—become apparent, while these are invisible in the phase between divisions, the so-called *interphase*.

Chromosomes and Genes

Chromosomes are the carriers of hereditary characteristics called *genes* (see also Chapter 2: Genetics). The human cell nucleus contains 46 chromosomes (diploidy) in the form of 23 chromosome pairs (23 male, 23 female chromosomes). The individual chromosomes can be distinguished by their total length, the lengths of their arms, and the position of their segmentations. By these means, individual chromosomal pairs can be assigned to specific groups (*karyotyping*)and numbered in decreasing size from 1 to 22, with the 23rd pair determining sex (Fig. 1.**4a**, **b**). With the exception of the sex chromosomes (*heterochromosomes = allosomes*), male and female chromosomes (*homologous chromosomes = autosomes*) correspond to each other in their hereditary characteristics. Whereas the female human has two sex chromosomes of equal size, the male human has one large and one small sex chromosome.

In humans the 23 chromosome pairs contain about twice 30 000–40 000 hereditary markers or genes. Each of their genes occurs twice in each cell of the body, namely one male and one female (*diploidy*). In con-

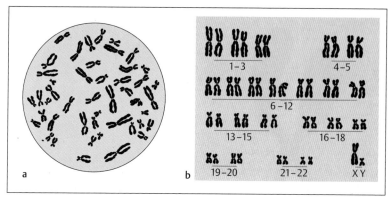

Fig. 1.**4 a, b   Chromosome set of a normal human cell.** (After Langman)

a The chromosomes are prepared and viewed by cultivating the cells in an artificial medium. This is followed by treatment with a colchicine solution, which blocks the mitoses in metaphase. The cells are then fixed, spread on a slide, and stained

b The chromosomes shown in **a** are arranged in a karyotype by total length and position of the centrosome. The two sex chromosomes (XY) determine the sex (male in this case)

trast, the germ cells (egg and sperm cells) each have only a single set of chromosomes (*haploidy*). With 23 chromosomes and a total complement of 30 000–40 000, each chromosome therefore contains about 1300–1700 genes.

■ **Structure of a Chromosome.** Two chromosome arms, connected by a *constriction* (*centromere*) can be distinguished on each chromosome (Fig. 1.**5a, b**). During cell division, two spirally coiled *chromatids* can be seen in the chromosome arms. These uncoil between cell divisions (interphase) and so cannot be seen. Each chromatid consists of a single giant molecule, folded and wound in a complicated double strand in the shape of a double helix of *deoxyribonucleic acid* (DNA). It consists of two threads, only about two one-millionths of a millimeter (2 nm) thick, the length of which is determined by the amount of information stored in it. If, for instance, one were to place all the chromosomes of one cell end to end, they would extend 1 millimeter in a bacterium but more than 2 meters in a human. The two threads run in parallel but counter to each other (in opposite directions) and correspond to each other like a photographic

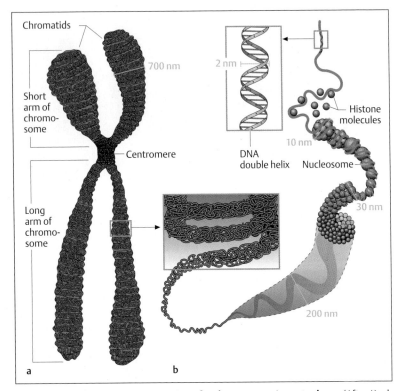

Fig. 1.**5 a, b** **Schematic representation of a chromosome in metaphase.** (After Koolman and Röhm)

a The centromere (primary constriction) is located between the two arms of the chromosome, which are uneven in length and each of which consist of two chromatids

b Section from **a**: DNA, together with basic histone proteins, forms tightly coiled complexes arranged like strings of pearls—the nucleosomes

negative to its print. They wind around an imaginary axis and can be compared to a twisted rope ladder (a double helix) (Fig. 1.**6**). The DNA forms complexes with basic proteins (histones) to form *chromatin*. Chromatin is coiled (condensed) into chromosomes, which are visible in optical microscopes only during cell division. During the interphase, it mostly becomes amorphous (euchromatin) apart from a few regions that do not uncoil (heterochromatin) (Fig. 1.**7**). Euchromatin is the genetically active chromatin (see Protein Synthesis), while heterochromatin is genetically inactive.

Those histones that are intimately associated with DNA form about one half of the chromatin. The DNA is curled around the histone particles, so that a chromatin fiber is structured like a string of pearls (Fig. 1.**5**). A histone particle with a DNA segment curled around it (~180 base pairs, see below) is called a *nucleosome*. Each histone particle consists of eight histone molecules (an octamere).

At the ends of the chromosome arms there are heterochromatin segments (telomeres, satellites) that determine the lifespan of the cell. During each cell division a small segment of chromatin separates until the satellite is used up. At that point the cell dies.

The building blocks of DNA are the *nucleotides* (Fig. 1.**6**). They each consist of a *base* (*adenine, cytosine, guanine, or thymine*), a *sugar* (*deoxyribose*), and an acid phosphate radical. The phosphate radicals of two successive nucleotides form phosphate bridges that connect the nucleotides. Two opposing nucleotides are connected by hydrogen bonds between their bases. When viewed as a rope ladder, the sugar and phosphate units form the sides (the ropes) and the base pairs the rungs of the ladder. The opposing bases are joined in a tongue-and-groove fashion. Because of chemical affinity, adenine always forms a *base pair* with thymine, and guanine forms a base pair with cytosine.

The total human hereditary material is contained in 23 chromosome pairs in the form of deoxyribonucleic acid. The DNA can be subdivided into three separate segments, genes or hereditary factors, and has three important functions:

- **The storing of genetic information** (the genetic code)
- **The transmission of information for protein biosynthesis**
- **The identical duplication (replication) of genetic information during cell division**

The Genetic Code

The genetic information required for the construction of proteins follows from the type and arrangement of amino acids in the protein. The encoding of this information in DNA, the genetic code, is determined by the arrangement of the four bases (contituting the four different nucleotides)

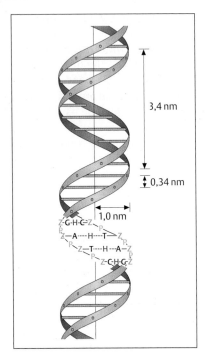

Fig. 1.**6** **Structure of a DNA molecule.**
The double helix consists of the bases
adenine (A), cytosine (C), guanine (G),
and thymine (T), and the sugar deoxyribose (Z), and phosphate bridges formed
by acid phosphate radicals. Each base
combines with a sugar and a phosphate
radical to form a nucleotide. Using the
analogy of a rope ladder, the sugar and
phosphate units form the sides (ropes),
and the bases the rungs of the ladder.
By chemical affinity adenine always
forms a base pair with thymine, and
guanine with cytosine, connected to
each other by bridges of hydrogen
bonds (H). The distances between rungs
and the radius of the double helix are
given in nanometers (1 nm = 10^{-9} m =
one billionth of a meter). (After Beske)

3,4 nm

0,34 nm

1,0 nm

within the DNA and is the same in all living things. The variable sequence
of the various bases determines the specific informational content of the
genes that forms the blueprint for millions of different protein
molecules, just as the placing of the letters of the alphabet in an intel-
ligent sequence determines the informational content of a book (see
Chapter 2: Genetics).

Three bases at a time in varying combinations define one informational unit, a "word"—also called a *triplet* or a *codon*—that must be
translated into one of the 20 amino acids present in proteins. For instance, the combination of the bases guanine (G), adenine (A), and thymine (T)—GAT in abbreviated form—contains the information for the
amino acid asparagine; and the triplet AAG is the code for lysine. The
amino acids present in the cytoplasm are combined according to the
sequence of the base triplets, to form the corresponding protein

molecules (see below). Consequently, the four building blocks provide a total of 4^3 ($4 \times 4 \times 4 = 64$) possible combinations (*informational units* = "words"). Of these, 61 are used in the instructions to build proteins. The remaining triplets indicate the beginning and end of a protein molecule or a gene. The program for the construction of a protein consisting of, say, 340 amino acids therefore includes 340 such base triplets (or codons). The complete set of these triplets is called a *gene* (*factor*).

Thus, a gene determines how many amino acids constitute a protein, and in what sequence these must be arranged. One gene contains on average 300–3000 base triplets. It may take several genes to determine a single characteristic.

Protein Synthesis

Proteins accomplish tasks necessary for life in all organisms. They are some of the most important structural and energizing components of a cell. Some of them, for instance *collagen* in connective and supporting tissue, take on important structural tasks and provide the organism's architecture. Others, such as the *myosin* and *actin* of muscle cells, enable the shortening (contraction) of muscles, and hence movement. Yet other proteins transport oxygen (the *hemoglobin* of the red blood cells) or serve as protective and defensive agents in the immune system (*antibodies*). Of special importance are the proteins that are the catalysts for the metabolism of the organism (*enzymes*). Enzyme proteins synthesize everything the cell needs to survive (proteins, fats, and carbohydrates).

If genetic information is seen as *biological data storage*, then that information must be available at any time. When needed, it must be transported within the cell from the nucleus to the site of protein synthesis (the ribosomes) by a biochemical mechanism. For this purpose, the genetic code is copied within the nucleus to *ribonucleic acid* (RNA), which has a structure similar to that of DNA but contains only a single strand (Fig. 1.**8**). This process is known as *transcription*. Protein synthesis takes place during the interphase of cell division. Chromatin must be uncoiled to allow transcription to take place. Hence only euchromatin is active in transcription (Fig. 1.**7a**). RNA is synthesized from free elements in the nucleus and is linked together into an RNA chain with the help of the enzyme RNA polymerase (Fig. 1.**7a**). RNA brings this message to the ribosomes of the endoplasmic reticulum, and is therefore also known as

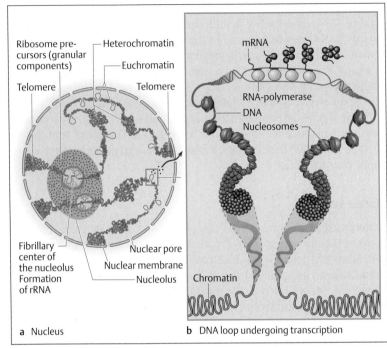

Ribosome pre-cursors (granular components)
Heterochromatin
Euchromatin
Telomere
Telomere
mRNA
RNA-polymerase
DNA
Nucleosomes
Fibrillary center of the nucleolus
Formation of rRNA
Nuclear pore
Nuclear membrane
Nucleolus
Chromatin

a Nucleus

b DNA loop undergoing transcription

Fig. 1.**7 a, b**   **Schematic representation of a nucleus with two chromosomes in inter-phase.** (After Benninghoff)

a Inside the largely uncoiled chromo-somes, amorphous DNA segments (euchromatin) undergoing transcrip-tion alternate with genetically inactive,

not uncoiled DNA segments (hetero-chromatin)

b Section from **a**: DNA loop undergoing transcription

messenger RNA or mRNA (Fig. 1.**8**). Like DNA it is composed of nu-cleotides, but instead of the base thymine it contains the base uracil, and contains the sugar ribose instead of the sugar deoxyribose. The mRNA bonds to the ribosome by base coupling with transfer RNA molecules.

Other relatively short RNA molecules, similarly synthesized from free elements in the nucleus, bond to the amino acids present in the cyto-plasm one-on-one and transport them to the ribosomes, where the mRNA is attached with its copies of the base triplets. These short RNA molecules are therefore also known as tRNA (transport or transfer RNA). Each tRNA is specific for one amino acid and the corresponding triplet on the mRNA (Fig. 1.**8**). In this way, with the aid of ribosomal enzymes, the

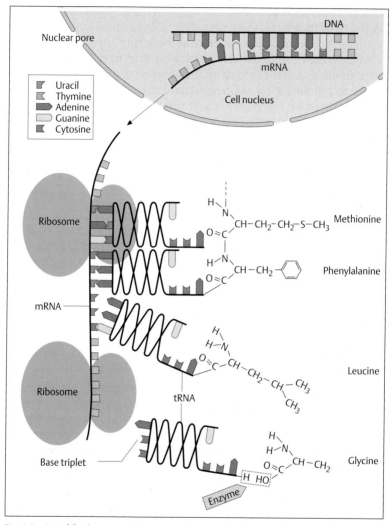

Fig. 1.**8** **Simplified representation of protein synthesis in a cell.** Transfer of the instructions for the manufacture of a protein by copying (transcription) of a single strand of DNA by means of mRNA (in mRNA the base thymine is replaced by the base uracil). This is followed by the manufacture of the protein molecule (translation) on the surface of the ribosome with the help of tRNA molecules. These bind in the cytoplasm specifically to the individual amino acids, e. g. leucine, glycine, or methionine, that correspond to their base triplets and transport them to the ribosomes. With the aid of enzymes and ATP, the individual amino acids are combined into a protein molecule (polypeptide chain) (After Nultsch)

various amino acids are linked into a protein chain, corresponding to the sequence of triplets on the mRNA. The rRNA produced in the nucleus provides the information needed to manufacture these enzymes. The tRNA molecules liberated in this reaction can then be recharged with the same amino acid in the cytoplasm. This process of protein building, also known as *translation*, continues until the complete protein molecule has been synthesized. The protein chain varies in length according to the type of protein (from a few up to several hundred amino acids), and by chemical reactions it can be folded into a three-dimensional functional protein molecule.

Duplication of Genetic Material (Replication)

Because of the structure of the individual strands of DNA, they can make *identical copies* of themselves. During this process the base pairs of the double helix separate in the middle like a zipper (Fig. 1.**9**) and for each single strand an exact *complementary strand* is synthesized. In this way, the two single strands of the original molecule are copied. Through the making of these identical copies of DNA, called *replication*, hereditary information is passed to offspring.

■ Cell Division (Mitosis)

Duplication (replication) of DNA and the transmission of genetic information to the two daughter cells connected with it precede every cell division and take place during the so-called interphase. The interphase is the stage between mitoses and is the *working phase of the cell*. **Chromosomes with two chromatids are formed by duplication of the genetic material during interphase**. This establishes the precondition for mitotic cell division. Chromosomes demonstrate evidence of their duplication by a longitudinal split visible in the microscopic image. The chromosomes become shorter and thicker through increased coiling. After cell division is complete, the chromosomes uncoil and, during the ensuing interphase, replicate again.

Mitotic cell divisions permit a fertilized ovum to develop into an organism. They are the preconditions for physiological renewal of cells and lead to regeneration of tissues after injury. With the exception of a few

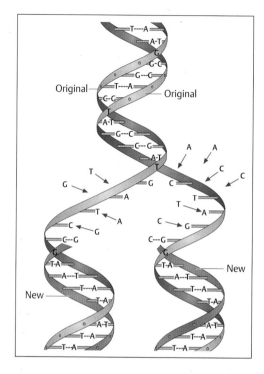

Fig. 1.**9   Double helix of DNA and its duplication (replication).** The double strand of DNA splits like a zipper and forms two new, completely identical DNA molecules. The original strands are shown in blue, the new ones in pink (the sugar–acid phosphate chain is shown as a band; A = adenine, C = cytosine, G = guanine, T = thymine; free nucleotide groups are marked by arrows) (After Hadorn and Wehner)

cells (nerve cells, and cardiac and skeletal muscle cells), the ability to divide is maintained throughout the life cycle, though it varies among cells. As a rule, mitoses are less common in highly differentiated tissues.

■ **Course of a Mitosis.** A number of mitotic stages can be distinguished in the course of the cell division that follows interphase (Fig. 1.**10a–f**):

- Prophase (pro = before)
- Metaphase (meta = between, next)
- Anaphase (ana = upward)
- Telophase (telos = end, goal)

At the beginning of *prophase* the cell becomes round and the chromosomes appear in the nucleus as convoluted threadlike structures. Simul-

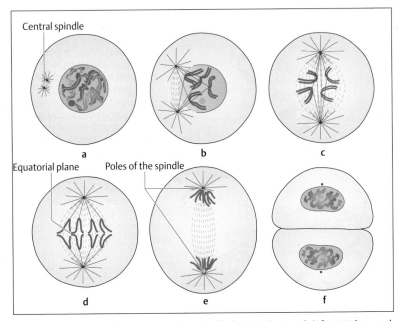

Fig. 1.**10 a–f Schematic representation of cell division (mitosis)** (After Hadorn and Wehner)

a Prophase: Chromosomes in the nucleus become visible by coiling and the nuclear spindle apparatus develops the central spindle;

b Early metaphase: the central spindle stretches and the chromosomes migrate toward the equatorial plane;

c Late metaphase: The division of each chromosome into two chromatids is clearly visible and arrangement along the spindle's equator is complete;

d, e Anaphase: the daughter chromosomes are moving away from each other in the direction of the spindle's pole;

f Telophase: the chromosomes have uncoiled, a nuclear membrane has formed and the cell body is constricted.

taneously, the nuclear membrane disappears and the two centrioles move apart. They migrate toward the poles of the cell and form the so-called *central spindle*. In *metaphase*, which follows, the chromosomes become shorter and thicker, the two chromatids become visible and can be distinguished clearly by their size and shape. As the process continues, the chromosomes arrange themselves in the so-called *equatorial plane* between the two poles.

At the end of metaphase the chromosomes have arranged themselves in the equatorial plane in such a way that each of their constrictions (*centromere*) is oriented toward the central axis. Because the arrangement looks star-shaped when viewed from the two poles, it is called a "*monaster*" (Greek for single star). As *anaphase* begins, the chromatids (chromosome halves) of each chromosome separate, forming two star-shaped figures called "*diasters*" (double star). Since each of the halves of a chromosome (daughter chromatids) migrates to one or other of the two opposite poles, all of the genetic material is divided equally between the two daughter cells.

In the ensuing *telophase* the chromatids, which now form the chromosomes of the two daughter cells, collect near the centrioles, uncoil, and again become invisible. As a new nuclear membrane forms, two new interphase nuclei have been created. There follows a complete division of the cell body, resulting essentially in two equal, independent daughter cells.

On average one mitosis takes about 60 minutes to complete. Anaphase is the shortest phase, lasting about 3 minutes.

■ Reduction or Maturation Division (Meiosis)

Reduction or maturation division (*meiosis*) is a special form of cell division. In preparation for later fertilization, the male and female germ cells must halve their set of chromosomes (to form a *haploid set*), so that when ovum and sperm join, a normal double (*diploid*) set of chromosomes is formed. This process is known as meiosis, a cell division that comprises two steps: **first and second maturation divisions** (Fig. 1.**11**).

Shortly before the first maturation division, the male and female sex cells duplicate their DNA as in mitosis, with each chromosome containing two identical chromatids. In meiosis, the prophase of the first maturation division lasts a good deal longer than the prophase of mitosis. As a rule it takes 24 days in male germ cells, while in the female it may at times take decades, because of an interpolated resting phase (*dictyotene*) (see Chapter 11: Development of the Ovum (Oogenesis) and Follicle Maturation). Prophase is divided into five phases: *leptotene*, *zygotene*, *pachytene*, *diplotene*, and *diakinesis*.

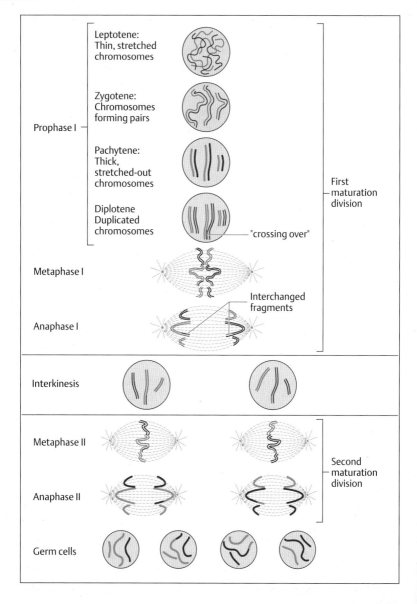

Prophase I

Leptotene:
Thin, stretched
chromosomes

Zygotene:
Chromosomes
forming pairs

Pachytene:
Thick,
stretched-out
chromosomes

Diplotene
Duplicated
chromosomes

"crossing over"

Metaphase I

Anaphase I

Interchanged
fragments

First
maturation
division

Interkinesis

Metaphase II

Anaphase II

Second
maturation
division

Germ cells

First maturation division. During the leptotene of the prophase, the chromosomes become visible as fine threads; in the ensuing zygotene, they arrange themselves side by side in pairs (chromosome pairing). During this process, the corresponding (homologous) paternal and maternal chromosomes are always arranged next to each other. Since each single chromosome contains two chromatids (*sister chromatids*), the chromosome pairs contain four chromatids, two maternal and two paternal, the so-called tetrad, which is especially conspicuous during the diplotene of prophase. At this point the homologous chromosomes begin to separate. During this process, homologous paternal and maternal chromatids lying in parallel next to each other can interchange homologous fragments by so-called *crossing-over* (forming a *chiasma*) and reattachment of the fragments.

In the metaphase which follows, the chromosomes arrange themselves in the equatorial plane, similarly to a mitosis. During anaphase, the separation of the homologous chromosomes by a spindle is completed. Telophase completes the first maturation division. The two daughter cells each now have only half the number of chromosomes of the initial cell, though each chromosome still consists of two chromatids.

Second maturation division. After a brief phase (interkinesis) during which the DNA is not duplicated, the second maturation division begins. This maturation division proceeds entirely like a normal mitosis, that is, during anaphase the two chromatids of each chromosome divide and are distributed to two daughter cells. Consequently, the haploid daughter

◁ Fig. 1.**11   Schematic representation of maturation division (meiosis).** In order to provide a better overview, the course of the two maturation divisions is exemplified in a germ cell with three pairs of chromosomes (red chromosomes = paternal, blue chromosomes = maternal). During the pachytene of the prophase of the first maturation division, the chromatids become visible. The maternal and paternal chromosomes arrange themselves next to each other and form a tetrad (two chromosomes each with two chromatids). During this process the paternal and maternal chromatids partly overlap and when they separate there is an interchange of fragments ("crossing-over"). During the metaphase of the first maturation division, the homologous (paternal and maternal) chromosomes separate, and are randomly distributed to the two daughter cells. This process creates two haploid daughter cells each with a single set of chromosomes. During the second maturation division, the two daughter chromatids separate by mitotic cell division, so that the first and second maturation divisions result in the creation of four haploid sex cells. (After Beske)

cells that originated when the double set of chromosomes was halved during the first maturation division, once again halve their DNA content during the second maturation division.

■ **The result of the two maturation divisions = mature sex cells.** Thus four *daughter cells* (mature sex cells) result from the two-step division of meiosis. In each of these, the number of chromosomes and the DNA content have been reduced to half the original. In addition, the chromosomes have been **restructured** as a result of the crossing-over, and **recombined** as a result of the random distribution of the two homologous chromosomes into the daughter cells. The real biological significance of meiosis lies in this shuffling of genetic material.

■ Exchange of Materials between the Cell and Its Environment

Billions of years ago, life developed in the form of small, single-celled organisms in a large primal ocean (Fig. 1.**12**). Their aqueous (watery) environment was marked by a milieu of constant composition. Nutrients were plentiful, and waste products were instantly diluted effectively to infinity. In a similar way, the cells of a multicellular organism live in an aqueous environment that contains all the salts and nutrients required for the sustenance of the cell. Compared to the primal ocean, however, this fluid has a much smaller volume, and there is a much greater danger of short-term changes in its composition.

Of all the chemical compounds in the organism, water (H_2O) forms the largest percentage part. Thus the body of an adult contains about 60% water, which is distributed in two distinct compartments: the intracellular space (total volume enclosed in all the cells) and the extracellular space (total volume present outside the cells). About two-thirds of the total body fluids are located inside the cells (intracellular fluid) and the remaining third (about 14 liters in a person weighing 70 kg) bathes the exterior of the cells. Of the 14 liters of extracellular (interstitial) fluid, three-quarter are contained in the tiny spaces that separate the cells from each other, and one-quarter in the vascular systems (arteries, veins, capillaries, and lymphatic vessels), where it forms the aqueous part of the plasma and the lymphatic fluid (Fig. 1.**12b**).

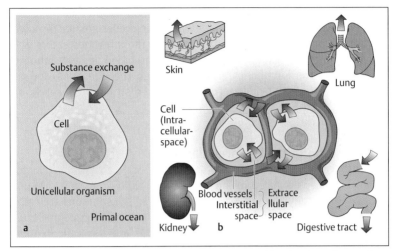

Fig. 1.**12 a, b   The environment (milieu) in which the cell lives.** (After Silbernagel)
a Unicellular organism: Interaction between the first cells and their environment—the primal ocean, a milieu distinguished by its constant composition
b Human: Cells in a multicellular organism are bathed in extracellular fluid, the volume of which is distinctly smaller than that of the fluid inside the cell. This "internal milieu" would change its composition very quickly if the space between the cells (interstitial space, intercellular space) were not connected to organs such as the lung, the kidney, or the digestive tract by the vascular bed, which take up fresh nutrients and eliminate metabolic waste products.

The water content of the body is kept constant with great precision. This is necessary in order not to endanger the equilibrium of the numerous substances dissolved in the body fluids. For instance, physiological water losses (e. g., the production of urine, the secretion of sweat, and loss by humidification of expired air) must be balanced by fluid intake.

Keeping the "internal milieu" constant (*homeostasis*) is a life-preserving precondition for the optimal functioning of every cell in the body. Since the most diverse substances reach the extracellular space as a result of respiration, the intake of nutrients, and the metabolic activity of cells, maintaining homeostasis is one of the most important tasks of the organism. Besides the activity of the lungs, the intestines, and the kidneys, certain specific transport processes are of importance; these processes (e. g., diffusion, osmosis, active transport) serve to exchange solids and fluids between the cell and its environment (see Solid and Fluid Transport below). Transport of substances over greater distances within the body (e. g., nutrients taken up in the intestines and oxygen taken up in the lungs) is accomplished in the blood vessels. Similarly, transport by the lymphatics, passage through the intestines, and the emptying of the gallbladder accomplish rapid distribution of solids and fluids (Fig. 1.**12b**).

Composition of the Extracellular Fluid

The substances dissolved in the extracellular fluid (e. g., salts) are present as electrically charged particles (ions) and the solutions are called electrolytes. Because of their electric charge, ions can migrate in electric fields. For this reason, positively charged ions are also called *cations* (they migrate to the negative pole, the *cathode*) and negatively charged ions are called *anions* (they migrate to the positive pole, the *anode*). The salt present in the largest amount is common table salt (NaCl), consisting of a positively charged sodium ion (Na^+) and a negatively charged chloride ion (Cl^-) dissolved in a concentration of about 9 g/l. Other cations and anions are also present, though in distinctly smaller quantities: e. g., potassium (K^+), calcium (Ca_2^+) and magnesium (Mg_2^+), as well as bicarbonate (HCO_3^-) and negatively charged proteins. The three compartments of the extracellular space—the interstitial fluid, the blood plasma, and the lymph—differ mainly in the amount of protein dissolved in each. For instance, the walls of the blood and lymph capillaries are permeable only to small ions and smaller organic particles, while large proteins are retained within the lumina of these vessels.

Composition of the Intracellular Fluid

In contrast to the extracellular fluid, where sodium predominates, the quantitatively dominant intracellular cation is potassium (K^+). The sodium concentration inside the cell is about 10 times smaller than that outside it. The major portion of the intracellular anions consists of proteins, while phosphates ($HPO_4^-/H_2PO_4^-$) are present in lower concentrations.

■ Membrane or Resting Potential of a Cell

Because the ions are distributed unevenly between the intracellular and extracellular spaces, a potential difference, known as the membrane potential, is created at the cell membrane. This creates a negative charge in the interior of the cell relative to the extracellular space, the so-called resting potential. This potential difference can be measured with sensitive instruments and is about 60–80 mV.

The reason for the negative potential inside the cell with respect to its surroundings lies in the differential distribution of ions between the intracellular and extracellular spaces. Thus, the intracellular potassium concentration is about 35 times greater than the extracellular concentration, while proteins are the preponderant anions inside the cell. Sodium ions dominate in the extracellular space, balanced on the negative side by chloride anions (see the table in Fig. 1.**13**). The accumulation of potassium ions inside the cell is a specific activity of almost every cell and represents one of its most important active transport processes. This "ion pump" transports potassium ions into the cells and, to balance this, transports sodium ions out. It is therefore also called the sodium–potassium (Na^+–K^+) pump. It includes an ATP-splitting enzyme (sodium–potassium ATPase, Na^+,K^+-ATPase). This reaction liberates the energy required for ion transport (Fig. 1.**13**). The cell membrane is impermeable to ions, so there are membrane pores (channels) for Na^+, K^+, and Cl^-, but not for protein anions. During resting potential, the K^+ channels are often open, but the Na^+ and Cl^- channels are mostly closed. Because of the concentration difference, the K^+ ions have a tendency to diffuse outward. However, the diffusion of positively charged potassium ions out of the cell is limited by the negatively charged protein anions, which cannot cross the membrane because of their size. The diffusion of even a few potassium ions out of the cell leaves anions with the opposite (negative) charge (protein anions) on the inside of the cell membrane, so that the interior of the cell is negatively charged with respect to its surroundings. The resting potential is therefore also known as the diffusion potential. **The diffusion of ions outward through the membrane pores is independent of the Na^+–K^+ pump**.

The energy-consuming ion pumps can be impeded or blocked by lack of oxygen (failure of ATP production) or by metabolic poisons (e. g., cyanide), leading to severe disturbances in the specific performance of a cell. The initiation and propagation of nerve or muscle cell excitation de-

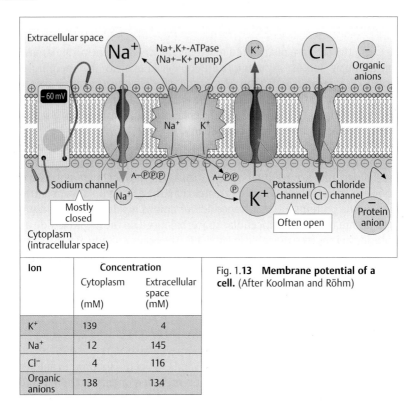

Fig. 1.**13** **Membrane potential of a cell.** (After Koolman and Röhm)

Ion	Concentration	
	Cytoplasm (mM)	Extracellular space (mM)
K$^+$	139	4
Na$^+$	12	145
Cl$^-$	4	116
Organic anions	138	134

pends on brief membrane potential changes (action potentials) (see Chapter 3: Nerve Tissue).

■ Solid and Fluid Transport

The specific transport processes that take place in the microscopic realm, e. g., between the cells on the one hand and the blood capillaries and their surrounding cells on the other, can be divided into essentially passive (diffusion, osmosis, and filtration) and active (energy-dependent) transport processes (active transport, endocytosis, exocytosis).

Diffusion

The simplest interchange process for solids is diffusion. Because of their thermal kinetic energy, atoms and molecules move freely in aqueous solutions or in gases, and differences in concentration equilibrate by diffusion. In this process, molecules diffuse toward the lower concentration until the concentrations even out. The driving force of this process is a concentration or potential gradient, comprehensively called the electrochemical gradient. For instance, a large part of the transport of solids (salts, respiratory gases, nutrients) in the interstitial (intercellular) space and into and out of the cell depends on diffusion processes. Small molecules, such as the respiratory gases O_2 and CO_2 as well as water pass through the cell membrane unimpeded (*free diffusion*). Pores through the membrane (channel proteins, membrane pores) or mobile transport proteins (carriers) facilitate the passage (*facilitated diffusion*) of nutrients (e. g., glucose and amino acids in the cells of the intestinal mucosa) and ions (Fig. 1.**14**).

Osmosis and Osmotic Pressure

When two solutions containing different concentrations of the same solute are separated by a partly permeable membrane, a so-called *semipermeable membrane*, osmosis can take place. In *osmosis* the semipermeable membrane allows the solvent, but not the solute, to pass. Water diffuses through the membrane toward the solution of higher concentration, until equilibrium is attained. During this process the volume of the side that initially contained the higher concentration increases (Fig. 1.**15**). The pressure that must be applied to this side to reverse the process of osmosis is called the *osmotic pressure*. It is expressed in mmHg or in the SI units of pascals (Pa) or kilopascals (kPa). When such a measurement is applied, it is found that the osmotic pressure depends only on the number of dissolved particles in a defined volume, and not on their size or charge.

The cell membranes are more or less semipermeable membranes, since the lipid layer is less permeable to charged molecules such as ions and proteins. The osmotic pressure of the extracellular fluid depends on its content of protein and salts and corresponds approximately to that of a 0.9 % solution of NaCl. Such a *physiological salt solution* is isotonic (that

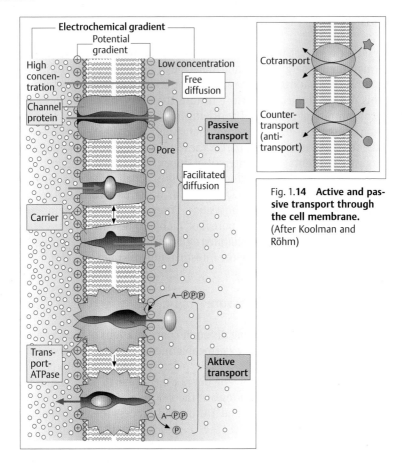

Fig. 1.14 Active and passive transport through the cell membrane. (After Koolman and Röhm)

is, it is in osmotic equilibrium with the cell). Consequently, cells bathed in hypertonic (more concentrated) solutions lose water and shrink, while in hypotonic (less concentrated) solutions they take up water and swell. The organism therefore endeavors by special regulatory mecha nisms to keep the osmotic pressure of the extracellular fluid as constant as possible. Because of the good permeability of cell membranes to water, these mechanisms lead to a more or less constant osmotic pressure in the cell interior.

Fig. 1.**15   Development of osmotic pressure in a semipermeable membrane**

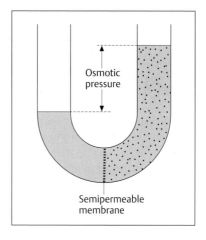

The term **colloid osmotic pressure** is used when, for instance, proteins for which the capillary wall is impermeable are dissolved in the blood plasma and not in the interstitial fluid. They create an osmotic pressure difference of about 25 mmHg (3.3 kPa) between the interstitial fluid and the capillary space. This would lead to a movement of fluid into the vessels if the hydrostatic blood pressure active inside the blood vessels were not opposed to it. Since the blood pressure at the beginning of the capillaries (37 mmHg) is greater than the colloid osmotic pressure, fluid is actually filtered into the interstitial space (see Chapter 5: Capillary Circulation).

Filtration

Filtration occurs when water and any dissolved particles are pushed through cell membranes or pore systems by a hydrostatic pressure difference. Pores occur, for instance, when there are small spaces between endothelial cells (intercellular clefts) or holes (fenestrations) in the cell membranes. Such a process is found in the capillaries of the tissues. The term ultrafiltration is used when, in the course of filtration processes such as that in the capillaries of the renal corpuscles, larger blood components are retained or dissolved molecules are separated out because of their size or charge.

Combined Solid and Water Transport

See Chapter 10: Renal Tubules and Collecting Ducts.

Active Transport

Active transport is the transport of substances through the cell membrane by means of an *energy-consuming transport system* (transport ATPase). Here, again, *ATP* serves as *universal fuel*. Such a transport process can move a substance through the membrane against a concentration gradient (Fig. 1.**14**). Thus cells have the ability to maintain in their interior stable *ion concentrations*, for example, that are clearly different from their concentrations in the extracellular fluid. These active transport processes are served by specialized proteins in the cell membrane that can move several ions simultaneously. In this process, the coupled transport of substances can occur in the same direction (cotransport) or in opposite directions (countertransport) (Fig. 1.**14**). For instance, in the kidney the transport of amino acids is coupled with an active Na^+ transport. Additionally, active ion transport through cell membranes is necessary for the formation of membrane or resting potentials.

Endocytosis and Exocytosis

Large molecules, such as proteins, enter (*endocytosis*) or exit (*exocytosis*) through the cell membrane by so-called *vesicular transport* (Fig. 1.**16**). During this process, substances are attached in part to the outside of the cell by membrane-bound receptors, enclosed by a part of the plasma membrane, and moved into the interior of the cell as a membrane-wrapped vesicle (*receptor-mediated endocytosis*). Depending on the size of the absorbed particle, this process may also be called *pinocytosis* or *phagocytosis.*

In exocytosis, products synthesized in the cell are enclosed in membranous vesicles and, by coalescence of these vesicles with the inside of the plasma membrane, reach the extracellular space. In this way, the transmitter substances in the endings of nerve cell processes are liber-

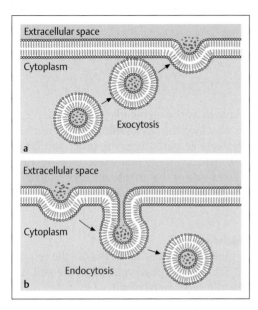

Fig. 1.**16 a, b Exocytosis and endocytosis**

ated at the synapses. The secretory products of most glandular cells leave the cell interior in similar fashion. Endocytosis and exocytosis are dependent on the action of ATP.

Summary **Biology of the Cell**

The smallest living entity of an organism is the cell. In contrast to single-celled organisms that are independent entities, the cells of higher organisms form functional units. In accordance with their function, the cells are differentiated by size, shape, and the degree of definition of certain characteristics.

For all cells of the body there are a certain basic structure and numerous basic properties. The basic properties include the ability to divide and to sense and respond to stimuli.

■ Basic Cell Structure

By and large, the cell consists of the cytoplasm containing the cell organelles, the nucleus, and the cell membrane surrounding the whole structure.

■ Cell Membrane

The cell membrane, also known as the elementary membrane, consists of a double lipid layer, in which the fat-soluble components face each other while the water-soluble parts form the inner and outer boundaries (a three-layered structure). The lipid molecules are infiltrated with proteins. The outer side of the membrane is covered by a glycocalyx. An elementary membrane also surrounds the cell organelles and the nucleus.

■ Cytoplasm and Cell Organelles

The cytoplasm consists of the intracellular fluid (cytosol), the cell organelles, and various cell inclusions (phakeroplasm). The cell organelles are responsible for the cell's metabolism.

Endoplasmic Reticulum (ER)

Present in all cells except erythrocytes; serves intracellular material transport; protein synthesis (granular ER); lipid and hormone synthesis (smooth ER).

Ribosomes

No elementary membrane; multienzyme complexes made up of proteins and rRNA molecules that link amino acid chains for protein synthesis.

Free ribosomes: intracellular proteins (enzymes, etc.). Ribosomes in the ER (granular ER): exported proteins (glandular secretions, etc.).

Golgi Apparatus

Present in all cells except erythrocytes; uptake and discharge products of synthesis in the form of membrane-bounded transport vesicles that are flushed from the cell (secretory vesicles) and serve the renewal of the cell membrane or take part in intracellular digestion as primary lysosomes.

Lysosomes

"Digestive organs" of the cell; with the aid of enzymes they degrade cell-alien structures and the cell's own decaying organelles.

Centrioles

Build the spindle fibers during cell division.

Mitochondria

"Power stations" of the cell; here nutrients (proteins, fats, carbohydrates) are metabolized essentially to CO_2 and H_2O, generating the energy necessary for metabolism (e. g., muscle contraction, synthesis of structural substances), which is then stored in the form of ATP.

■ Cell Nucleus

Present in all cells except erythrocytes; the nucleus contains the nucleolus (production of rRNA ⇒ protein biosynthesis) and the chromosomes, carriers of the hereditary factors (genes). Human nuclei contain 23 chromosome pairs (23 paternal, 23 maternal ⇒ diploid chromosome set); the 23rd pair determines sex.

The appearance of the nucleus and of the chromosomes changes with the individual phases of cell division.

During the interphase (working phase of the cell) between two cell divisions (mitoses) the genetic material is duplicated and chromosomes form, each with two chromatids joined by a constriction (centromere). Each chromatid consists of one molecule of DNA (deoxyribonucleic acid). The basic units contained in DNA, the nucleotides, are each composed of one base (adenine, cytosine, , guanine, or thymine), a sugar (deoxyribose), and an acid phosphate radical. DNA contains the complete hereditary matter in the form of genes.

Each unit of information comprises three bases (triplet, codon) in varying combinations. Each triplet represents the information for one amino acid. One gene consists of about 300–3000 base triplets and provides the information for one protein. This genetic code is the same for all living things and contains the information for the biosynthesis of proteins, the most important structural and energizing substances in all organisms.

Protein Biosynthesis

Single-stranded RNA synthesized in the nucleus copies the genetic code (transcription) and brings the message to the ribosomes, the site of protein biosynthesis. Each copied triplet represents one amino acid in the final protein. tRNA molecules, also synthesized in the nucleus, bind amino acids in accordance with the genetic code (according to the sequence of triplets) and transport them to ribosomes, where they are linked into proteins with the aid of enzymes. Each tRNA is specific for one amino acid.

Cell Division (Mitosis)

Chromosomes containing two chromatids are created by the duplication of genetic material during interphase. This process is necessary for the transmission of genetic information to the daughter cells. Mitotic division of cells makes possible growth and the renewal of cells.

Reduction or Maturation Division (Meiosis)

Two successive cell divisions lead to the creation of male or female sex cells with half the chromosome complement (haploid cells)

First maturation division: The (homologous) paternal and maternal chromosomes lying next to each other separate, which leads to the exchange of homologous fragments by "crossing-over." This results in two daughter cells with haploid chromosome sets.

Second maturation division: Corresponds to a normal mitosis. The chromatids of the chromosomes separate again. The two daughter cells create four mature sex cells with a haploid set of chromosomes.

Fertilization creates a new diploid set of chromosomes. The actual reason for meiosis is the restructuring and recombination of the chromosomes, that is, the shuffling of genetic material.

■ Intracellular and Extracellular Fluid

The body of an adult person consists of 60% water, two-thirds of which is intracellular, one-third extracellular. Of the 14 liters of extracellular fluid, three-quarters occupy the interstitial spaces and one-quarter the vascular system.

■ Membrane Potential

In the extracellular fluid, sodium is the predominant cation and chloride is the predominant anion; in the intracellular fluid, the predominant cation is potassium and proteins are the predominant anions. By the differential distribution of ions in the intracellular and extracellular spaces, a potential difference is created across cell membranes (membrane or resting potential). This is caused by the active accumulation of potassium inside the cell (ATP-dependent Na^+–K^+ pump).

■ Solid and Fluid Transport

Transport processes between the cells and their environment play an important role in the maintenance of the "internal milieu" (homeostasis). A distinction is made between passive and active (energy-dependent) transport processes. Passive processes include free diffusion (e.g., of O_2, CO_2, H_2O), facilitated diffusion (e.g., of glucose and amino acids in the cells of the intestinal mucosa), osmosis, and filtration (e.g., of glucose and amino acids in the capillaries of the tissue). Active processes include active transport (e.g., of ions) as well as endocytosis and exocytosis (e.g., of proteins).

2

Genetics and Evolution

■ Genetics (The Science of Heredity)

Genes, Chromosomes, and the Genome

Genetics is the science of heredity; it deals with the structure and function of the genes. The cells of all living things contain a program that guides their functioning. This program is genetically determined, i.e., it is transmitted to both newly formed cells during every cell division. The transmission must be precise, since otherwise it leads to disturbances in function (mutations, see below). The genetic program consists of individual information units, the *genes* (= hereditary characters), with each gene determining a specific function. The sum total of all genes is the *genome* (the human inheritance includes within a single set of chromosomes approximately 30 000–40 000 genes; see Chapter 1: The Cell Nucleus), which is contained in the sum of chromosomes in each cell nucleus. Genes are arranged along the chromosomes in a linear fashion and have a definite location and structure. They represent the smallest functional genetic unit; each comprises on an average 1000–10 000 base pairs (300–3000 base triplets), a comparatively short chromosome segment (a single set of chromosomes, that is, 23 chromosomes, contains a double strand of DNA with a total length of around 3 billion base pairs). A single gene might, for instance, contain the information for one protein (i.e., how many amino acids it contains and how they are arranged). A single character, on the other hand, may be determined by several genes.

The Allele

With the exception of the sex cells, human cells contain 46 chromosomes: 23 maternal and 23 paternal. In this way, every gene is present on the corresponding paired homologous chromosome in identical or slightly modified form. The genes that are localized at the same site on both the maternal and paternal chromosomes are called *alleles*. If both alleles are completely identical in their genetic information, the carrier of such a character is called *homozygous*; if they differ, the carrier for that character is *heterozygoous*.

Dominance, Recessiveness, and Codominance

When an allele in a heterozygote always prevails over the other allele, so that it is solely responsible for the expression of a character, it is called *dominant*. The allele that is not expressed in the phenotype (see below), that is, is not in evidence, is called *recessive* (suppressed). When in a heterozygote both alleles are expressed in the phenotype, the alleles are called codominant.

Phenotype and Genotype

The two concepts genotype and phenotype refer to the genetic information of a character at the site of each gene (*gene locus*). The observed character, the appearance, is called the *phenotype*; this might be a hair color, a certain blood group, or the color of the flower of a plant. The *genotype* is the genetic information on which the phenotype is based.

The Mendelian Rules

If the transmission of individual hereditary factors (genes) is followed from generation to generation, the distribution of chromosomes during maturation division (meiosis; see Chapter 1) will be seen to follow certain laws. These pertain to the random distribution of the homologous chromosomes during meiosis and the combinatory possibilities when a sperm cell meets an ovum. The Augustinian monk Gregor Johann Mendel (1822–1884) recognized these laws in 1866 during cross-breeding studies with garden peas, even though he did not know about the processes that occur during meiotic maturation division.

To discover the rules for the distribution of hereditary characters, certain conditions must be met: the crossbreeding experiments must be performed with purebred (homozygous) organisms, so that all germ cells receive the same hereditary characters; the hereditary characters studied must be visible externally (genes were unknown at the time); and the factors or genes that determine these characters must be located on different chromosomes. For crossbreeding studies, the first generation is known as the *parental generation* (*P generation*), the first offspring as the *first filial generation* (*F₁ generation*), and the next offspring as the *second filial generation* (*F₂ generation*).

- Mendel's first law: the law of uniformity (dominance) (phenotypic uniformity of the F_1 generation)
- Mendel's second law: the law of segregation (phenotypic segregation in the F_2 generation after dominant–recessive or intermediate hereditary transmission
- Mendel's third law: the law of independence (independent transmission of nonlinked genes)

The Rule of Uniformity (Dominance)

When two different homozygous lines that differ in one or more alleles are crossbred, the result is a heterozygous F_1 generation with a *uniform* (i.e., *dominant*) *phenotype.* If, for instance, a red-flowered homozygous pea plant (RR[1]) is crossed with a white-flowered (rr) homozygous pea plant in generation P, the F_1 heterozygote will be uniformly red (Rr) like the red parent (Fig. 2.**1**). The character of the white parent is suppressed and so cannot become expressed. Hence the white flower character is suppressed in the F_1 generation and so cannot be expressed. Hence the phenotypic character appearing in the F_1 generation (red in this case) is called dominant, while the other is the recessive (suppressed) character.

Dominant–recessive hereditary transmission is by far the commonest form of heredity. Thus, in Mendel's studies of peas not only did red flowers predominate over white, but yellow seed color predominated over green, smooth seeds predominated over wrinkled seeds, and tall plants predominate over short ones.

However, when a purebred red four o'clock plant is crossed with a purebred white, the heterozygous generation's flowers are uniformly pink (Fig. 2.**2**). Such a case, in which the heterozygous F_1 generation differs in phenotype from the two homozygous parents is called *intermediate inheritance.* In the F_1 generation the pink coloration of the flower is

---

[1] Upper-case letters are used for dominant alleles, lower-case for recessives: RR = dominant homozygote, rr = recessive homozygote, Rr = heterozygote with a dominant–recessive hereditary transmission.

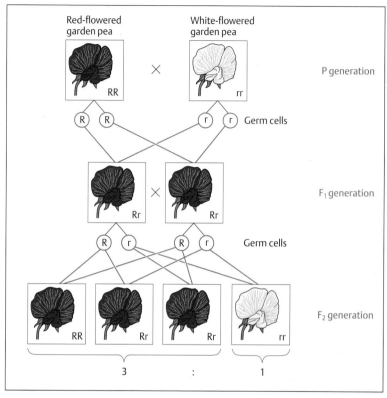

Fig. 2.**1 Dominant–recessive hereditary transmission.** A homozygous red-flowered (RR) garden pea is crossed with a homozygous white (rr) one. The heterozygous F₁ generation is uniformly red, since the flower color red is dominant over white. The F₂ generation splits in the ratio 3 : 1, that is 3 offspring are red-flowered (RR, Rr, and rR) while one offspring is white-flowered (rr)

produced by a blending of the two genes inherited from the P generation (white and red coloration of the flower).

On the other hand, when both alleles are of equal weight and both characters appear in the heterozygote side by side, the condition is called *codominance*. An example is given by the A and B blood groups. If a child receives the blood group A allele from the father and the blood group B allele from the mother, the child will have the blood group AB.

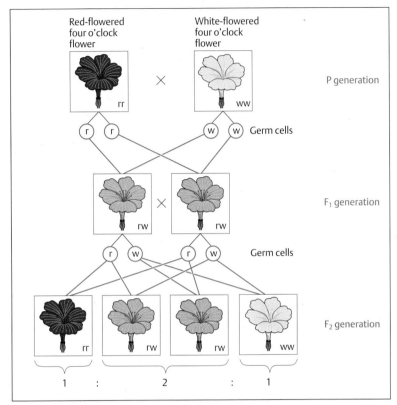

Fig 2.**2 Intermediate hereditary transmission.** Crossing of a homozygous red-flowered (rr) four o'clock flower with a homozygous white-flowered one (ww). The F_1 generation is uniformly pink-flowered (rw) as both flower colors are expressed in the phenotype. The F_2 generation splits in a ratio of 1 : 2 : 1, i.e., one plant is red-flowered (rr), one white-flowered (ww) and two more are pink-flowered (rw, wr)

Rule of Segregation

When the peas plants of the F_1 generation are crossed with each other (Rr × Rr), the next generation (F_2 generation) will show three-quarters red-flowered and one-quarter white-flowered plants (Fig. 2.**1**). The 3 : 1 numerical ratio becomes more exact the more offspring are examined. The phenotypic segregation ratio depends on whether a gene (allele) is dominant or recessive. The dominance of the red-flowered gene of the pea over the white-flowered gene results in a red (R) to white (r) ratio close to 3 : 1 because the combinations RR and Rr both result in the phenotype R.

When the heterozygotes of the F_1 generation of four o'clock flower (rw) differ in phenotype from the rr as well as the ww parents (owing to the intermediate inheritance of the four o'clock flower), then the F_2 generation will show a segregation ratio of 1 : 2 : 1 in phenotype as well as genotype (Fig. 2.**2**). Thus in each case one plant is purebred red (rr) and one white (ww), while two more plants are pink and of mixed inheritance for flower color (rw).

This segregation can be explained by the separation of homologous chromosomes during the first meiotic maturation division, for the germ cells, being haploid, can contain only one of the two alleles: the one for red-colored flowers (r) or the one for white-colored flowers (w). Consequently the zygote may contain one of the gene combinations red/red (rr), red/white (rw), white/red (wr) or white/white (ww). If the genes for red and white are both dominant (or both recessive), all the heterozygotes will be pink and the homozygotes red or white. The segregation ratio must therefore be 1 : 2 : 1. If the inheritance is not intermediate but dominant–recessive the segregation ratio is also 1 : 2 : 1, but only in the genotype. The phenotype has a ratio of 3 : 1, since the heterozygotes show the phenotype of the dominant allele.

Rule of Independence

If two homozygous organisms differing in two alleles are crossed (AAbb × aaBB) (Fig. 2.**3**), the individual genes are inherited independently in the next generation. In fact, this is only valid for genes located on different chromosomes. The rule is not valid for genes located on the same chromosome, since as a rule they remain linked when they are inherited. However, the linkage of all the genes on one chromosome is not necessarily absolute, since, for example, "crossing-over" between homologous chromosomes can take place during meiosis (see Chapter 1: Reduction or Maturation Division). Thus the number of possible gene combinations is increased, a fact that can be of great significance from the point of view of possible genetic variations.

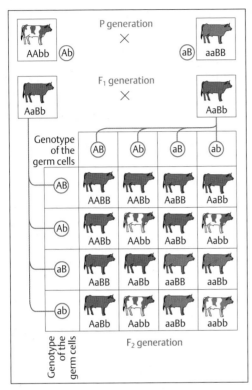

(AA) is dominant over reddish-brown (aa) and solid color (BB) over spotted (bb). The animals of the F_1 generation are all black and solid color (AaBb). If the two alleles for skin color and color distribution are located on different chromosomes, and if the two pairs of alleles can combine independently in forming sex cells, theoretically four egg or sperm cells should be distinguishable genotypically: AB, Ab, aB, and ab. Combination of the sex cells therefore results with equal probability in 16 possible combinations. Crossing the individuals of the F_1 generation with each other results in four distinct phenotypically expressed forms: black solid, black spotted, reddish-brown solid, and reddish-brown spotted in a numerical ratio of $9:3:3:1$.

Fig. 2.**3**   **Independent inheritance of two characters.** Crossing of two strains of cattle, distinguishable by skin color and distribution of skin color (black and spotted or reddish-brown and solid). Black

Autosomal Dominant Hereditary Transmission

One type of dominant–recessive inheritance is autosomal dominant hereditary transmission. Autosomal dominant hereditary transmission of a characteristic occurs when the phenotype is determined by the dominant allele and the gene is located on an autosome (see Chapter 1: Chromosomes and Genes). In humans this transmission occurs with

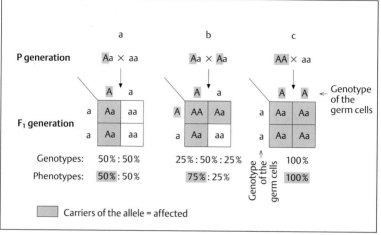

Fig. 2.**4 a–c** **Autosomal dominant hereditary transmission (genotypes and phenotypes).** A= dominant inherited allele (character); *A*= recessive inherited allele (character); AA = homozygous affected; Aa = heterozygous affected; aa = homozygous healthy
a One parent is heterozygous affected, one parent is homozygous healthy = 50% of children are affected
b Both parents are heterozygous affected = 75% of children are affected
c One parent is homozygous affected, one parent is homozygous healthy = 100% of children are affected

many normal characteristics (e. g., dominance of blood groups A and B over blood group O), and also with numerous hereditary diseases, such as polydactyly (more than the normal number of fingers), familial hypercholesteremia (excess cholesterol content in the blood), Huntington chorea (a neurological disease), and Marfan syndrome (disturbance of collagen synthesis).

In autosomal dominant hereditary transmission usually only one parent shows the affected dominant allele on one chromosome (A), while the corresponding allele on the other chromosome is healthy (a). The other parent, by contrast, has two healthy intact alleles (aa) (Fig. 2.**4a**). Thus the constellation that usually creates hereditary transmission occurs when a heterozygous carrier of the disease pairs with a healthy partner. Consequently, for each child, independently of its sex, the probability of hereditary transmission of an autosomal dominant disease is 50%. In this situation it does not matter which parent carries the affected dominant allele. On the other hand, if both parents are affected heterozygotes (Fig. 2.**4b**), 75% of the children will be affected (25% homozygous, 50% heterozygous) and 25% will be healthy homozygotes.

In the rare case when one parent is homozygous and affected with a hereditary autosomal dominant disease, while the other parent is healthy, all children will be heterozygotic carriers (Fig. 2.**4c**).

Autosomal Recessive Hereditary Transmission

Another type of dominant–recessive inheritance is autosomal recessive hereditary transmission. When a recessive allele carries the genetic information on an autosome, autosomal recessive characteristics are expressed phenotypically only in homozygotic carriers in the F_1 generation (Fig. 2.**5a**–c). Heterozygous carriers of the allele do not differ from healthy homozygotes. A phenotypic character is therefore only expressed in affected homozygotes. With all severe autosomal recessive hereditary diseases, those affected will as a rule derive from healthy parents who do not express the allele of the disease phenotypically. If one parent is heterozygous, and the other a healthy homozygote, all the children will be healthy (50% homozygotes, 50% heterozygotes) (Fig. 2.**5a**). If both parents are healthy heterozygotes, the risk of the children being affected is 25% (Fig. 2.**5b**). Half of the children are again healthy heterozygotes and are carriers and transmitters of the tendency inherent in the recessive allele. Finally, 25% are healthy homozygotes. Thus in families with a small number of children, autosomal recessive diseases occur only sporadically. If one parent is an affected homozygote and the other is a healthy homozygote, all the children will be healthy heterozygotes (Fig. 2.**5c**).

Almost all metabolic defects that are caused the absence of an enzyme are transmitted by autosomal recessive inheritance. These include phenylketonuria (a congenital deficiency leading to mental retardation, see below), albinism (lack of tyrosine hydroxylase interferes with the metabolic pathway from tyrosine to the skin pigment melatonin), and cystic fibrosis (mucoviscidosis; thickened secretions from secretory glands lead to severe complications in the respiratory and gastrointestinal tracts). In these conditions, affected heterozygotes as a rule exhibit a 50% diminution in enzyme activity; however, the residual actiivity is

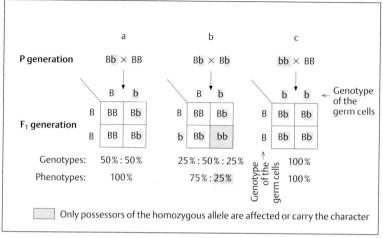

Fig. 2.**5 a–c Autosomal recessive hereditary transmission (genotypes and pheno-types).** B = dominant inherited allele (character); b = recessive inherited allele (character); BB = healthy homozygote; Bb = healthy heterozygote; bb = affected homozygote
a One parent is healthy heterozygote, one parent is healthy homozygote = 100 % of children will be healthy
b Both parents are healthy heterozygotes = 25 % of children will be affected
c One parent is affected homozygote, one parent is healthy homozygote = 100 % of children will be healthy

sufficient for the intact functioning of the relevant enzyme under normal metabolic conditions. Only an affected homozygote shows signs of the illness. Often dominant–recessive inheritance shows a transition to intermediate inheritance, because the recessive hereditary tendency is not fully suppressed in the heterozygote.

In phenylketonuria (incidence 1 : 10 000) the absence of the enzyme phenylalanine hydroxylase interferes with the breakdown of phenylalanine to tyrosine. This results in the metabolic product phenylpyruvic acid, which is excreted as a ketone body in the urine. If this condition is not treated from birth, it leads to mental retardation, delayed physical development and neurological symptoms (seizures). If the illness is recognized in time, essentially normal development can be achieved by eliminating phenylalanine from the diet. The diet must, however, be maintained strictly until the tenth year of life, when the brain is fully developed.

Sex-linked Inheritance

Sex-linked inheritance affects characters that are located on the X chromosome. The X chromosomes are carriers of multiple genes for which there are no homologous alleles on the Y chromosome. Hereditary transmission may be X chromosomal recessive or X chromosomal dominant. This type of hereditary transmission is important because male offspring inherit their X chromosome exclusively from their mother and never pass it on to their sons. While a woman may be homozygous or heterozygous for an X chromosomal allele, a man possesses only one allele of all the genes on the X chromosome, and is thus hemizygous for these.

X Chromosome-linked Dominant Inheritance

It is characteristic for X chromosome-linked dominant inheritance that all daughters of an affected father are carriers of the corresponding factor, since his X chromosomes are always passed on to his daughters (Fig. 2.**6a**). On the other hand, the sons of an affected father are always healthy, since they receive his Y chromosome (Fig. 2.**6a**). The children of a heterozygous affected mother have a 50 % risk of being affected (Fig. 2.**6b**). X chromosomal dominant hereditary diseases are very rare. One example is vitamin D-resistant rickets, in which a low blood phosphate level leads to underdevelopment of dental enamel and anomalous hair follicles.

X Chromosome-linked Recessive Inheritance

In X chromosome-linked recessive inheritance, men are mainly affected since they carry the defective allele on their X chromosome (Fig. 2.**7a**). Women, on the other hand, are only affected when they are homozygous carriers of the gene (very rare) (Fig. 2.**7c**). When they are heterozygous they are phenotypically healthy and only transfer the disease-causing gene to their offspring (so-called carriers) (Fig. 2.**7b**). It follows that 50 % of their sons are affected (show the trait) and 50 % of their daughters are again carriers.

Examples of X-linked recessive hereditary conditions include red–green color blindness (frequency 1 : 15), hemophilia A and B (bleeding disease, frequency 1 : 10 000) and Duchenne muscular dystrophy (frequency 1 : 3000).

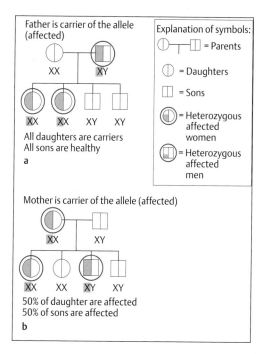

Father is carrier of the allele (affected)

XX XY

XX XX XY XY

All daughters are carriers
All sons are healthy

a

Explanation of symbols:

○—□ = Parents

○ = Daughters

□ = Sons

◐ = Heterozygous affected women

◐ = Heterozygous affected men

Mother is carrier of the allele (affected)

XX XY

XX XX XY XY

50% of daughter are affected
50% of sons are affected

b

Fig. 2.**6 a, b   X chromosome-linked dominant inheritance.** X = X chromosome, Y = Y chromosome; XX = female sex; XY = male sex

a Father is carrier of the X chromosome-linked dominant allele and is an affected heterozygote

b Mother is carrier of the X chromosome-linked dominant allele and is an affected heterozygote

Mutations

As a rule, chromosomes transmit the genes located on them unchanged from generation to generation. However, spontaneous changes in the gene complement, called mutations, may occur in somatic cells (somatic mutations) or in the germ cells (germ cell or germline mutations). In addition to spontaneous mutations, there occur induced mutations, as a result of, for example, ionizing radiation or chemical substances (so-called mutagens). The frequency of mutation in, e. g., a gene is on average between 1 : 10 000 and 1 : 100 000. There are several types of mutations:

- Gene mutations
- Chromosome mutations (structural aberrations in the chromosomes)
- Genome mutations (numerical aberrations in the chromosomes)

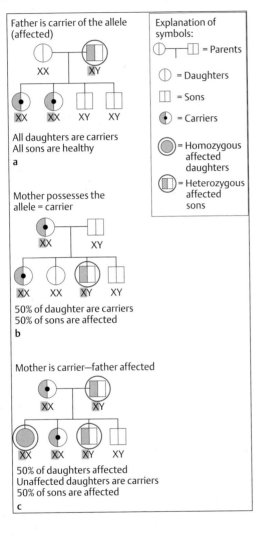

Fig. 2.**7 a–c   X chromosome-linked recessive inheritance.** X = X chromosome; Y = Y chromosome; XX = female sex; XY = male sex

a   Father has the X chromosome-linked recessive allele and is an affected heterozygote

b   Mother has the X chromosome-linked allele and is a healthy heterozygote and a carrier

c   Mother is a carrier and father is affected

Gene Mutations

Gene mutations are the most important and commonest causes of change in the gene complement. They arise through *errors in the identical replication of genes*, when errors that occur during replication of the strands of DNA induce changes in the base sequence. This in turn leads to changes in the frequency of amino acids in the protein coded by the affected DNA molecule. The consequence is a change in the function of the protein, which may show itself in the phenotype of the individual concerned.

Chromosome Mutations

In chromosome mutations, changes in the structure of the chromosome can be seen by light microscopy (structural chromosome aberrations). These may occur through crossing-over, that is, the interchange of chromosome fragments (see Chapter 1: Reduction or Maturation Division) or they may occur when chromosomes break and reunite in a different configuration. Structural chromosome aberrations have an incidence of 1 : 200 newborns, and so are rarer than numerical aberrations (genome mutations). Chromosome mutations include:

- Deletion (loss of a chromosome fragment
- Duplication (duplication of a segment of the same chromosome)
- Inversion (reversal of a chromosome segment)
- Translocation (exchange of segments between two nonhomologous chromosomes).

Genome Mutations

In genome mutations, the number of chromosomes is changed (*numerical chromosome aberration*). This is caused by irregularities during cell divisions following maldistribution during meiosis and mitosis. As a result, chromosome numbers deviate from the normal karyotype (see Chapter 1: Chromosomes and Genes). If, for instance, the first maturation division leads to a lack of separation between homologous chromosomes, the result is termed *nondisjunction* (failure to separate). This can affect the autosomes as well as the sex chromosomes. Possible causes of a numerical chromosome aberration include the loss of the centromere region of one chromosome, or the malformation of the spindle during cell division.

Maldistribution of autosomes can be observed especially in small chromosomes. Live births show trisomies almost exclusively, most commonly on chromosome 21 (trisomy 21 or Down syndrome). It is noteworthy that autosomal trisomies show a marked relationship to age. While the risk of bearing a child with trisomy 21 is about 1 : 2500 in young women, Down syndrome cases increase to 1 : 50 in mothers over 40 years of age. The affected children show mental retardation to a varying degree, as well as typical physical stigmata such as an oblique axis of the eyelids, marked palmar crease, short round skull, flat bridge of the nose, and thick-set body build. Among the internal malformations the commonest affected is the heart.

Maldistributions of sex chromosomes do not in general lead to a nonviable embryo. An extra sex chromosome (*gonosomal trisomy*) or a missing sex chromosome (*gonosomal monosomy*) does not normally lead to severe retardation, as the mental development is usually completely normal. Only reproductive capacity is lost. The only viable monosomy of the sex chromosomes affects the X chromosome (Turner syndrome: karyotype 45, X0[2] with an incidence of 1 : 2500). Women with Turner syndrome have a feminine phenotype and are unable to conceive. Notable physical attributes include short stature, loose skin folds at the neck (pterygium colli), and malformations of inner organs (e. g., cardiac malformations). Klinefelter syndrome consists of a trisomy of a sex chromosome (karyotype: 47, XXY[3] with an incidence of 1 : 900). Those affected have a male phenotype, eunochoid tall stature, and underdeveloped testes (hypogonadism).

---

[2] 45, X0 means 44 autosomes + 1 sex chromosome (X) = 45 chromosomes; one sex chromosome is missing.
[3] 47, XXY means 44 autosomes + 3 sex chromosomes (XXY); one sex chromosome is supernumerary

■ Evolution (The Science of Development; Phylogeny)

The Concept of Evolution

Life on earth is enormously diversified. More than 1.5 million animal species and almost 500000 species of plants have been described to date, and new species are discovered daily (on the other hand, species are destroyed by humans almost daily!). Until the end of the eighteenth century, biology accepted the prevalent teaching derived from the biblical story of creation, that of the "*constancy of species*." The Swedish naturalist Carl von Linné (1707–1778), for instance, subscribed to the belief that all the species found on earth had existed since the beginning of life on earth. His achievement was to describe all the animal and plant species known in his time and to order them into a uniform system based on their structural similarities. It was only at the beginning of the nineteenth century that a resemblance in form began to be seen as an aspect of kinship, that is, related species were ascribed to common ancestors. Eventually it was Charles Darwin (1809–1882) who captured these ideas and completed them with an abundance of observations from comparative anatomy, paleontology, and the distribution of animals and plants. This was the birth of what today is recognized everywhere as the science of evolution. In his book *On the Origin of Species by Means of Natural Selection*, published in 1859, he described the descent of current life forms from primitive simple forms and at the same time provided a convincing explanation of the causes of the evolution of organisms.

Factors in Evolution

Selection

The theory of evolution states that the infinite variety of living things on earth has developed from a few simple forms—perhaps only a single one—in the course of billions of years. In the course of earth's history, living forms underwent change that generally went hand in hand with an increase in structural complexity and enhanced capabilities. An important question in the study of evolution was and remains how evolution came about; that is, to apprehend the factors causing and enabling evolution (the causal study of evolution). Here, too, Darwin provided a remarkably simple explanation to the problem of causality (see below): his theory of *natural selection* (*survival of the fittest*). Darwin based his solution on the following observations:

- Living organisms generate far more offspring than is necessary for the survival of the species. Although two offspring per parental pair would suffice to ensure survival of a species, often thousands or even millions of offspring are generated. Nevertheless, the number of individuals in any one habitat remains constant over long periods of time if the environment does not change.
- Offspring of a single parental pair are not alike but differ in hereditary characteristics.
- Finally, organisms are constantly competing among each other to gain advntageous conditions for items such as food, space, and mates.

From these facts, Darwin concluded that in the struggle for survival only those individuals that are best adapted to their environment survive (survival of the fittest). Such competition is not limited to one species; organisms of different species may compete among each other if, for instance, they occupy similar ecological niches.[4] The result of competition is that often only one species can survive in one ecological niche over the long run. Species that are not as well adapted die out or are crowded into other niches. In this way *natural selection* leads, through a continuously improving adaptation to the environment, to a gradual reshaping of the species. The fitness of an organism is therefore most easily determined by the number of the surviving offspring.

However, Darwin's theory of natural selection was fully validated only when it became possible in the twentieth century to fit the findings of the science of heredity into his theories. Today the following evolutionary factors are recognized:

---

[4] This is not a physical space, but the totality of the environmental factors used by a species in its ecosystem. By using the same ecosystem differently (i.e., by occupying different ecological niches), numerous species can coexist in the same ecosystem without competing with each other.

- Selection
- Mutation
- Recombination
- Gene drift
- Isolation

The Concept of Species

Of foremost significance for the understanding of the effect of these factors on evolution are the concepts of species and population. All organisms that share their essential characteristics and are able to
generate fertile offspring together comprise one species. The individuals
of a species living and reproducing at the same time and in a defined
territory constitute a population.

The sum total of genes, each of which may be represented in many
different alleles (i.e., structural variations), constitutes the so-called *gene
pool* of a population. The frequency with which alleles (genes altered by
mutations) are represented in a population is called the *gene frequency.*
As well as rare genes or alleles with low frequency, such as those only recently developed by mutation, there are genes or alleles with high
frequency. Evolution therefore occurs when the gene frequency of a
population changes in the course of the succession of generations.
Sexual reproduction constantly leads to new gene combinations in the
individuals of a species. This constant change in the combination of
genes is called *genetic variability,* which increases through the occur-
rence of new alleles following mutation in the genes.

Mutation

If evolution is considered a process during which offspring in a succession of generations differ from their ancestors, the *mutability* of genes
has an important function. Mutations—changes in the genetic substance—occur randomly and are the driving force of evolution.

The various kinds of mutations (see earlier) of necessity expand the
genetic variety of a population; the sum of these changes in a defined
time is known as the *mutation pressure.* This is opposed by the *selection
pressure,* which is determined by natural selection and in turn eradicates
unfavorable mutations.

Recombination

New combinations of alleles (*genotypes*) are constantly generated through the recombination of hereditary characters during the formation of the germ cells. This leads to great variability and so to new phenotypes. Hence, conditions are created such that suitable phenotypes with favorable gene combinations will have increased chances of randomly enhanced adaptability. This, then, is the fundamental significance of bisexual reproduction. Genetic recombination is only possible with sexual reproduction, for it is the consequence of random distribution of paternal and maternal chromosomes, as well as crossing-over during meiosis. Since organisms generally possess a large number of genes, there are abundant possibilities for recombination in the offspring. Consequently, the several offspring of the same set of parents are for practical purposes never genetically exactly the same (with the exception of monozygotic twins).

Gene Drift

The term gene drift is applied to *random changes in the gene pool.* Such changes may occur without mutations or selection. Thus a group of organisms affected with a certain character within a population may suddenly become extinct through disease, adverse weather conditions, wildfires, or other conditions. In its stead, the surviving part of the population may expand by means of a different genetic makeup. In this way, fortuitous death or fortuitous survival of those with certain characters (and their genes) can influence the composition of a population decisively.

Isolation

Groups of individuals of one species, i.e., populations, may develop in different ways when they are separated and no longer form a common gene pool. Among the various mechanisms of isolation, so-called *geographic separation* has the most widely distributed and most persistent effect. Geographic separation may occur when the climate changes and different parts of a population are forced in different directions from their habitat, e. g., by the development of deserts, swamps, or glaciers. In this way the original uniform habitat of a species is severely split. The development without exchange of genes between the groups that follows the split creates a division of the species. The first forms that appear differ from each other in only a few characteristics. Such a course creates subspecies or races that are still capable of coupling and creating fertile offspring. If the differences in characteristics continue to increase over time, a reproductive barrier forms and coupling is no longer possible. In this way the two gene pools are conclusively separated, with the formation of two mutually independent species.

Evidence for Evolution

Embryological factors

Embryos of a variety of vertebrate classes are almost indistinguishable by their shape or by the formation of their head and eyes, their trunk, their limbs, and their tail (Fig. 2.**8**). For instance, during development, the germ cells of almost all vertebrates, including humans, go through an embryonic stage in which they bear a remarkable resemblance to a fish embryo. They form gill arches, even though they never develop a complete gill apparatus. This observation serves as evidence that the evolution of vertebrates began with forms that lived in water and breathed through gills. The functional and morphological similarities of early stages of development suggest kinship; that is, the development of the breed (phylogeny[5]) is mirrored in the development of the individual germ cell (ontogeny). The German naturalist Ernst Haeckel (1834–1919) formulated the so-called "*biogenetic law*" (*Haeckel's law, recapitulation theory*), which states that *the development of the embryo (ontogeny) of a vertebrate organism is the brief and rapid recapitulation of the development of the race (phylogeny)*.

---

[5] The history of all living things over millions of years of development of all species from a few simple (unicellular) forms to the variously complex organization of the animals and plants existing today

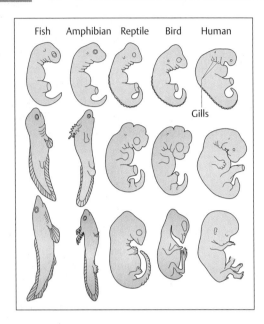

Fig 2.**8** **Different developmental stages of vertebrates during embryonic development.** The early developmental stages (upper row) of human, bird, reptile, amphibian, and fish are very similar, showing a remarkable resemblance in form and the development of gills. During the 5th to 7th week, human embryos resemble the embryos of fishes, evidence for the descent of humans from primitive forms

Homologous Organs

Organs are homologous when they occupy the same location in the structure of organisms and can be traced back to the same morphological structures in their development from ancestral forms. In this sense the wings of a bat, the fossorial (digging) leg of a mole, the fin of a whale, and the arm of a human are homologous organs. Despite the differences in shape, each contains the same subdivisions of upper arm, lower arm, wrist and palmar (metacarpal) bones, and digital phalanges; moreover, despite the very different shapes of these limbs, every single part occupies the same relative location in the whole.

Rudimentary organs

In the course of evolution, organisms continually change their ways of living. This requires a change in the functioning of their organs. Hence, one of the most convincing pieces of evidence for the theory of evolution is the existence of rudimentary organs, that is, involuted forms that in general have largely lost their function. Examples of such involuted forms (organ rudiments) include the dense hair covering of the embryo; the coccyx as a residue of tail vertebrae present in the embryo; the appendix, a wormlike rudiment of a formerly larger attachment to the intestines in which nutrients were broken down; and the muscles of the external ear, which have lost their function. Another example is the so-called Darwinian tubercle of the ear, present in some people and said to correspond to the point of a mammalian ear, reshaped in the course of development.

Atavism

Atavism (reversion) is a condition in which characteristics that have previously disappeared in the course of evolution suddenly recur. For instance, some people can move their ears quite well. Newborns sometimes bear a small tail stump. The appearance of supernumerary nipples arranged along a mammary ridge directed toward the abdomen recalls the abdominal mammary papillae customarily found in mammals with a greater number of offspring per litter. The appearance of atavisms representing a reversal to earlier evolutionary stages suggests that in such cases the corresponding genes continue to exist in the genome but are either blocked or become active at the wrong point in time during ontogeny.

Summary — Genetics and Evolution

■ Genetics

Genes and Alleles

The genetic program is stored in the form of information units, the genes (hereditary characteristics) of the chromosomes in the nucleus of each cell. One gene extends over 1000–10000 base pairs (300–3000 base triplets) in the DNA and contains the information for one protein. One characteristic can be determined by several genes. The DNA of the whole set of chromosomes (23 chromosomes = haploid set of chromosomes) contains 3 billion base pairs.

Twenty-three pairs of chromosomes (= diploid set of chromosomes) contain the whole inheritance (genome) comprising about

100 000 genes. Each of the genes occurs twice, as paternal gene and a maternal gene on the corresponding (homologous) chromosomes. These genes are called alleles. If their information is identical, the carrier for that characteristic is purebred (homozygous); if not, they are of mixed inheritance (heterozygous).

In heterozygotes, an allele is dominant when it is solely responsible for the expression of a characteristic, the phenotype (genotype = the corresponding genetic information). The allele that is not expressed is repressed; it is recessive. When both alleles determine the phenotype, the result is codominance (that is, both characteristics occur simultaneously). In intermediate inheritance, the expressed characteristic is the result of a blending of both alleles.

The Mendelian Rules

The rules for the distribution of individual hereditary characteristics during their transmission from generation to generation. These rules were formulated before genes were discovered. Conditions: (1) the study must be done with purebred organisms (with respect to external observable characters); (2) the observed characteristics or the genes determining them must be located on different chromosomes:

- *Mendel's first law* (*rule of uniformity*): Crossing two purebred organisms that differ in one or more characteristics (alleles) results in phenotypic uniformity in the heterozygous F_1 generation in dominant–recessive inheritance (dominant allele determines phenotype) and in intermediate inheritance.
- *Mendel's second law* (*rule of segregation*): in the F_2 generation the phenotype is segregated $3 : 1$ = dominant : recessive characteristic; the genotype is segregated $1 : 2 : 1$ = purebred for the dominant characteristic : mixed inheritance for the dominant character : purebred for the recessive character. For intermediate inheritance segregation is $1 : 2 : 1$ for genotype as well as phenotype.
- *Mendel's third law* (*the rule of independence*): When two purebred organisms that differ in two characteristics (alleles) are crossed, the genes are inherited independently of each other. Condition: the genes must be located on different chromosomes. This results in 16 different genotypes and 4 phenotypes in the F_2 generation (segregation ratio $9 : 3 : 3 : 1$).

Autosomal Inheritance (Dominant–Recessive)

- *Autosomal-dominant inheritance* (in the phenotype the characteristic is determined by the dominant gene located on an autosome).
- *Autosomal-recessive inheritance* (the gene for the characteristic is located on an autosome, but the character is only expressed in homozygotes).

Sex-linked Inheritance

The genetic information for a specific character is located on the X chromosome. Since no homologous allele is located on the Y chromosome, a man always possesses only a single allele of all the genes on the X chromosome; he is therefore hemizygous. In sex chromosome-linked hereditary diseases, sons are more often affected when the inheritance is X chromosomal recessive, while daughters are more often carriers. In the rare X chromosomal dominant inheritance, daughters are more often affected than sons, because in affected fathers the sons never receive the X chromosome of the father, but the daughters always do.

Mutations

Changes in the gene complement of somatic cells (somatic mutations) or germ cells (germ cell or germline mutations) occurring either spontaneously or by the action of mutagenic substances:

- *Gene mutations:* incidence 1 : 10000 to 1 : 100000; alteration in the base sequence due to errors during replication.
- *Chromosome mutations:* incidence 1 : 200; structural chromosome aberration = alteration in the structure of a chromosome, e. g., by interchange of chromosome fragments during crossing-over or when chromosomes fragment and reunite in a different configuration (deletion, duplication, inversion, translocation).
- *Genome mutations:* change in the number of chromosomes by errors during mitosis or meiosis = numerical chromosome aberrations affecting autosomes as well as sex chromosomes. In autosomes, small chromosomes are mostly affected (trisomies: trisomy 21 with an age-dependent incidence of 1 : 50 to 1 : 2500); sex cells are affected by trisomies in the sex chromosomes (e. g., XXY = Klinefelter syndrome) that, apart from a few physical weaknesses, are primarily infertile, and monosomies that, apart from X0 (= Turner syndrome), are not viable.

■ **Evolution**

Charles Darwin was one of the originators of the theory of evolution, which teaches that today's more complex life forms developed over millions of years from earlier primitive forms. The following factors are today considered to be the driving forces of evolution:

- *Selection:* Darwin's theory of natural selection is based on the principle of the "survival of the fittest." As a consequence of intraspecies (within the species) and interspecies (between species) competition, the weakest offspring will die by natural selection before they have reached sexual maturity. Through this mechanism only those organisms reproduce that are best adapted to the dominant environment. Consequently, a change in the environment brings about a gradual alteration of the species.

- *Mutations:* The various mutations increase the genetic variety of the population.

- *Recombination:* New genotypes and phenotypes are created by recombination during sexual reproduction (random distribution of maternal and paternal chromosomes during meiosis; crossing-over) (increased variability).

- *Gene drift:* Randomly generated changes of the gene pool without mutation or selection, e. g., during natural catastrophes.

- *Isolation:* Interchange of genes between parts of a population is prevented by geographic separation. The consequence is the segregation of the species and the definitive separation of the gene pool. Different environmental conditions favor different characteristics. Once a reproductive barrier is created, two species independent of each other have evolved.

Species = all life forms that correspond in their essential characteristics and that can have fertile offspring with each other.

Population = individuals of one species, who live and reproduce at the same time and in the same territory.

Gene pool = the total stock of genes in a population.

Evidence for Evolution

- *Embryological factors:* "Development of the embryo (ontogeny) is a brief and rapid recapitulation of the development of the race (phylogeny)."

- *Homologous organs:* Organs that can be traced back to the same morphological structures in ancestral forms.
- *Rudimentary organs:* Organs that have lost their function by changes in the way of life of a breed during the course of its development.
- *Atavism:* characteristics that had disappeared in the course of a breed's development suddenly reappear.

3

Tissues

Contents

Tissues are *combinations of similarly differentiated cells and their deriva-tives*, the intercellular substances. They fulfill one or more specific func-tions. By convention tissues are divided into four types:

- Epithelial tissue
- Connective and supporting tissue
- Muscle tissue
- Nerve tissue

■ Epithelial Tissue

Epithelial tissues are divided according to their primary function into **surface epithelia, glandular epithelia**, and **sensory epithelia**.

All epithelia are applied to a thin *basement membrane (basal lamina, hyaline membrane, glassy membrane)*, that provides mechanical support for the epithelium. In the form of surface epithelia they cover the exter-nal and internal surfaces in the body, provide its protection, and by the processes of *secretion (extrusion of substances)* and *resorption (uptake of substances)* connect it to the environment. As glandular epithelia they produce secretions that are deposited on the internal or external sur-faces of the body by glandular ducts (*exocrine glands*), or that reach the bloodstream directly, without any ducts, as with hormones (*endocrine glands, ductless glands*). As sensory epithelia they are part of the struc-ture of sense organs and transmit *sensory impressions* (e. g., the retina of the eye) (Fig. 3.**1a–d**).

Surface Epithelia

Shape and Arrangement

Surface epithelia are divided according to the shape of their cells into *squamous epithelium, cuboid epithelium, columnar epithelium*, and, ac-cording to their layering, into *simple, stratified (more than one layer), and pseudostratified* epithelia (Fig. 3.**2**). In stratified epithelia, the epithelium is named according to the cells on its surface, e. g., stratified squamous epithelium. In pseudostratified epithelium, all the epithelial cells reach the basement membrane, but not all reach the free surface (e. g., the

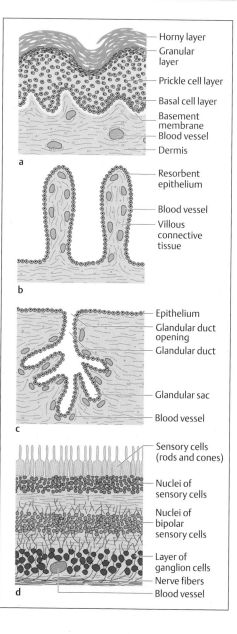

Horny layer
Granular layer
Prickle cell layer
Basal cell layer
Basement membrane
Blood vessel
Dermis

a

Resorbent epithelium
Blood vessel
Villous connective tissue

b

Epithelium
Glandular duct opening
Glandular duct
Glandular sac
Blood vessel

c

Sensory cells (rods and cones)
Nuclei of sensory cells
Nuclei of bipolar sensory cells
Layer of ganglion cells
Nerve fibers
Blood vessel

d

Fig. 3.**1 a–d Examples of different epithelial functions.**
a Epidermis of the skin
b Villi in the small intestine
c Exocrine gland
d Retina in the eye

Fig. 3.**2** Shape and arrangement of epithelial cells

Cell boundaries
Cell nucleus
Basement membrane

Simple squamous epithelium
(e.g., vascular endothelium)

Basement membrane

Simple cuboid epithelium
(e.g., epithelium of the renal tubules)

Microvilli

Basement membrane

Simple columnar epithelium
(e.g. mucous membrane of the small intestine)

Horny layer

Basal cell layer
Basement membrane

Stratified corneal squamous epithelium
(e.g., epidermis of skin)

Cilia

Mucous-forming
goblet cell

Basement membrane

Stratified ciliary epithelium
(e.g., tracheal epithelium)

Contracted
(empty bladder)

Stretched
(full bladder)

Protective layer
(Crusta)

Basement membrane

Transitional epithelium
(e.g., epithelium of the urinary bladder)

double layer of ciliated epithelium in the respiratory tract). A special form of pseudostratified epithelium is the *transitional epithelium of the lower urinary tract*, which can adapt to considerable surface changes, e. g., in the bladder.

Surface Differentiation

Special differentiation of individual epithelial cells at the surface closely relates to function. Absorbent or secretory cells often show on their surface characteristic fingerlike projections of the plasma membrane (*microvilli*), leading to a considerable increase in their surface (Fig. 3.**2**). This so-called brush border speeds the absorption of nutrients from the small intestine and, for example, in the gall bladder serves to thicken the bile by resorbing fluid. *Stereocilia* (nonmotile cilia) form a special type of cell projections. These are thinner than the microvilli and are often arranged in dense clusters on the cell surface. Located in the epididymis, they serve secretory and resorptive processes like other microvilli.

When the processes are motile, they are called cilia. They occur, for example, in the respiratory epithelium of the airways (Fig. 3.**2**). Each cell carries 200–300 cilia. These cilia move in coordinated waves (ca. 20 beats/second) that distribute mucus over the epithelial surface and so can produce unidirectional flow. In the stratified squamous epithelium of the skin, the outer cell layers are dead and so form a horny layer that protects against external agencies. In the transitional epithelium of the urinary bladder, the cell membranes nearest the surface are also protected against the noxious effects of urine by the increased density of certain proteins (crusta) (Fig. 3.**2**).

Cell Junctions

Neighboring cells form junctions in all tissues, not only in epithelia. These assume various forms, including *tight junctions*, *gap junctions*, and *desmosomes*. These three types of junction differ mainly in their functions. Tight junctions, for instance, are found between the columnar epithelial cells of the intestines, where they make the intercellular space between neighboring cells completely impermeable to substances contained in the intestines. Gap junctions form connections between neighboring cells and serve the transport of materials between cells (e.g., heart muscle cells or bone cells). Desmosomes, on the other hand, have an exclusively mechanical significance and serve, for instance, to anchor cells to each other within a squamous epithelium.

Glandular and Sensory Epithelia

The epithelia of glands and sense organs represent distinctively specialized forms of epithelia (Figs. 3.**1c**, **d**). Glandular cells may occur singly among other epithelial cells (e.g., goblet cells in the intestines) or in the form of epithelial organs (sweat glands, salivary glands, tear glands, pancreas). The substances secreted by glands (secretions) are often not used locally; in the case of *exocrine glands* they are transported by way of special secretory ducts to their site of action. In the absence of a specific duct, for instance in the case of hormone-producing glands (thyroid, pituitary), the substances are secreted into the blood, which transports them to their destination (*endocrine glands*).

Sensory cells in epithelial tissues function as *stimulus receptors* (sensory function). They transform arriving stimuli (light, chemical substances, mechanical pressure, pain) into electrical signals and then transmit them in the form of impulses along nerve fibers (Fig. 3.**1d**).

■ Connective and Supporting Tissues

Connective and supporting tissues look distinctly different, yet they are closely related because they are of common origin. They arise from the *mesenchyme*, an embryonic connective tissue. Whereas epithelial, muscular, and nervous tissues are mainly composed of cellular structures, connective and supporting tissues contain both *cellular* and *intercellular substances* (*extracellular matrix, ground substance*), which may be liquid, semisolid, or solid. Both take part in connective and supporting structures in ways that differ qualitatively and quantitatively. The less they serve as support, the more prominent becomes their metabolic function, for connective tissue is well perfused with blood. As its name implies, it connects, among other things, organs with blood vessels.

Supporting tissue includes the harder tissues, bone, and cartilage, in which the supporting function predominates. Of these, bone receives a good blood supply (confined to bone).

Connective Tissue

Functions

■ **Connective Function.** In general, connective tissue forms the sheaths of organs, vessels, and nerves and connects all the components with each other. In the form of ligaments it stabilizes the joints and, in the form of tendons, serves to transmit force from muscles to bones.

■ **Metabolic Function.** Whereas the fibroblasts are the primary site of metabolism, the exchange of metabolic substances takes place in the intercellular substance. The nutrients leaving the blood diffuse through the intercellular substance into the cells. The function of connective tissue is therefore the distribution of nutrients. Correspondingly, excreted substances travel from the cells by way of the connective tissue to be drained away by the blood capillaries and the lymphatic vessels.

■ **Water Balance.** A large part of the extracellular fluid is located in the intercellular spaces of the areolar (loose) connective tissue, which can store large quantities of water. In kidney and heart disease, for instance, abnormal collections of water in the tissues can lead to edema.

■ **Wound Healing.** Wounds heal by the formation of connective tissue (*granulation tissue*) that later becomes indurated scar tissue.

■ **Defense.** Some specialized "free" connective tissue cells (the various kinds of leukocyte, see Chapter 6: The Cells of the Blood) are responsible for the body's defense against pathogenic germs and foreign materials. They have the capacity for *phagocytosis* (taking up solid particles into the cell) and support the body's defenses by the formation of antibodies.

■ **Storage Function.** E.g., fatty (adipose) tissue serves to store calories.

Connective Tissue Cells

One type of cell found in the space occupied by connective tissue is the tissue-specific *fibroblast* (sometimes called the *fibrocyte*, especially when inactive), which produces the intercellular substances (ground substance and connective tissue fibers). Cells of another type found here are cells that have left the blood vascular system and are mostly a part of the immune system. These "*free connective tissue cells*" are not fixed, but can move within the connective tissue by ameboid motion. The current belief is that free connective tissue cells originate in the embryonic mesenchyme, and almost all represent types of white blood cells (*leukocytes*) that have migrated from the blood vessels into connective tissue (cf. Chap. 6: The Cells of the Blood).

Intercellular Matrix (Ground Substance)

Because the intercellular substance develops in two different ways, the connective tissue space functions both as a *conduit between blood vessels and organs* (*ground substance*) and as *actual connective tissue* (*connective tissue fibers*). The ground substance consists essentially of interstitial fluid, protein, polysaccharides, and glycoproteins. Protein polysaccharides add viscosity or solidity to the interstitial fluid. Because of their *property of binding water* they are responsible, for example, for the elastic stability of cartilage in joints and the transparency of the cornea. Glycoproteins occur among other sites at the cell boundary in the form of the glycocalyx and as components of the basement membrane. Part of their function is mechanical (adhesion of the cell to the extracellular matrix) and they probably form a barrier regulating the exchange of substances between the interstitial spaces and the adjoining cells.

Connective tissue fibers are divided into three major kinds: *collagen fibers*, *elastic fibers*, and *reticular fibers.* Collagen fibers are nondistensible and are generated where there is tension (tendons, ligaments); reticular fibers are flexibly elastic and their extended networks form the basic structure of, e. g., lymph nodes and the spleen; elastic fibers are distensible and can be stretched reversibly over $1^1/_2$ times their length (blood vessels).

Loose Areolar (Interstitial) Tissue

The loose areolar (interstitial) connective tissue (Fig. 3.**3**) forms the stroma that connects the specific tissues of organs; it also holds nerves and vessels in place, forming sheaths in which they traverse their surroundings. In addition it stores water and allows other tissues room to shift.

Dense Fibrous White Connective Tissue

In dense white fibrous connective tissue, fibers predominate and there are few cells. The two types are *dense irregular* and *dense regular white fibrous connective tissue* (Fig. 3.**4**). In irregular connective tissue, collagen fibers are arranged in bundles that form a felt-like weave (e. g., capsules of organs, dermis, sclera, dura mater covering of the brain). In regular connective tissue, the collagen fibers are subjected to directional forces (transfer of force from muscle to bone) that induce the formation of parallel-oriented bundles that are visible to the naked eye (Fig. 3.**5a**, **b**) (e. g., tendons and aponeuroses = flattened tendons).

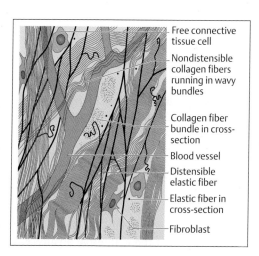

Free connective tissue cell

Nondistensible collagen fibers running in wavy bundles

Collagen fiber bundle in cross-section

Blood vessel

Distensible elastic fiber

Elastic fiber in cross-section

Fibroblast

Fig. 3.**3**   **Loose areolar tissue**

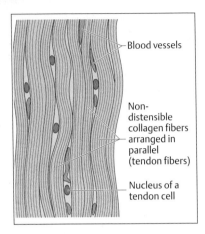

Fig. 3.**4** **Dense regular white connective tissue in a tendon**

Blood vessels

Non-distensible collagen fibers arranged in parallel (tendon fibers)

Nucleus of a tendon cell

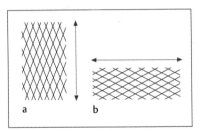

Fig. 3.**5 a, b** **Lattice structure of non-distensible collagen fibers in dense regular white connective tissue**
a In the stretched and
b in the relaxed state

a   b

Reticular Connective Tissue

In its form, reticular connective tissue is closely related to the embryonic connective tissue, the mesenchyme. It is made up of special connective tissue fibers, the *reticular cells*, and a lattice of *reticular fibers* (Fig. 3.**6**). The reticular connective tissue forms among other structures the framework for the lymphatic organs (spleen, lymph nodes), in which the interstices are filled with "free cells" (immune cells, e. g., lymphocytes). In the bone marrow, the interval between the spatially organized reticulum fibers is filled with blood-forming cells. In this way the reticular connective tissue forms a functional unit with the "free cells." However, reticular fibers can also be found in areolar tissue and in internal organs (e. g.,

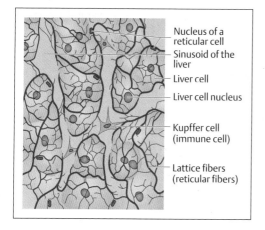

Fig. 3.**6** **Reticular fibers in the liver**

Nucleus of a
reticular cell

Sinusoid of the
liver

Liver cell

Liver cell nucleus

Kupffer cell
(immune cell)

Lattice fibers
(reticular fibers)

liver, kidney), where they are not part of an actual reticular connective tissue. For instance, reticular fibers form a sheath around smooth and striped muscle fibers and unite them into organized structures.

Adipose (Fatty) Tissue

Adipose tissue can be regarded as a specialized form of reticular connective tissue. Fat cells (lipocytes, adipose cells) store fatty substances that are removed from the blood by *pinocytosis* or built up in the cells directly from carbohydrates (sugars). The fat shifts the severely flattened nucleus to the periphery of the cell into a thin rim of cytoplasm (Fig. 3.**7**). Fatty tissue serves a mechanical function, stores energy, and protects against cold.

■ **Storage Fat.** Fat is an outstanding medium for the storage of energy, with a caloric value twice that of carbohydrates or proteins. The areolar connective tissue enveloping blood vessels in subcutaneous connective tissue, for instance, stores excess fat, which can be broken down during periods of starvation. The cells themselves survive and are available for renewed fat deposition. The current view is that the number of fat cells formed in early childhood remains constant through life as a potential fat repository.

■ **Structural Fat.** In contrast to storage fat, structural fat serves as cushioning (e. g., sole of the foot, palm of the hand, buttocks, orbital fat, and

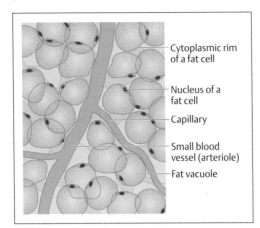

Fig. 3.**7** **Adipose tissue**

Cytoplasmic rim of a fat cell

Nucleus of a fat cell

Capillary

Small blood vessel (arteriole)

Fat vacuole

the buccal pad of the cheek) and is a necessary normal part of the body. It melts down and becomes available for providing energy only in advanced starvation (evidenced as sunken eyes or hollow cheeks).

■ **Brown Adipose Tissue.** Brown adipose tissue (brown fatty tissue, multilocular tissue) is a special kind of fatty tissue that contains numerous mitochondria with a high cytochrome content, which make it look dark. It is found in the newborn, especially in the interscapular region (between the shoulder blades). In the first months of life it serves as an important *heat reservoir*. It is rarely seen in the adult, but regularly persists in rodents (where it raises the temperature after hibernation).

Supporting Tissue

The representative supporting tissues are cartilage and bone tissues. To this must be added *chordate tissue* and *dental tissue*, a highly specialized and extra-hard bone tissue (see Chapter 9: The Oral Cavity). These contain predominantly collagen fibers and so possess the nondistensible character of connective tissue structures. The resistance to pressure is heightened in cartilage by the special development of the extracellular matrix and in bone by the deposition of calcium salts.

Chordate Tissue

The structure of chordate tissue is similar to that of adipose tissue, but the cell is filled with fluid instead of fat. It is found in vertebrates, including man, as the *notochord* (*chorda dorsalis*), the primal embryonic axial organ. The tightly filled cells give it an *elastic solidity*, similar to an inflated tire under pressure. Parts of the intervertebral disks (nucleus pulposus) may represent residual chordate tissue in the adult.

Cartilaginous Tissue

Cartilaginous tissue occurs predominantly in the skeleton and in the airways. The characteristic cells of cartilaginous tissue are *cartilage cells* (*chondrocytes*). They lie in the *cartilaginous ground substance* (*extracellular matrix*) as more or less rounded structures in small groups (*chondrones*) that do not adjoin each other (Fig. 3.**8a–c**). Three types of cartilage can be distinguished: *hyaline cartilage, elastic cartilage and fibrocartilage*, according to the type and density of fibers. None of the three types contain blood vessels in the adult. They are fed by diffusion either from a vascular membrane, the *perichondrium*, or, in the case of the hyaline cartilage of joints, directly by the joint fluid (synovia). The development of cartilage proceeds from the perichondrium, but the ability of cartilage to regenerate is generally insignificant. Without a perichondrium, as in hyaline cartilage, regeneration cannot occur. Cartilage is distinguished by *high resistance to pressure*, is capable of *viscoelastic deformation* and has a high resistance to shear force.

■ **Hyaline Cartilage.** When fresh, hyaline cartilage looks milky-blue and, because of its translucent character, is said to have a ground-glass appearance (Fig. 3.**8a**). It covers the joint surfaces as joint cartilage, forms the cartilage of the ribs, part of the nasal septum, the skeleton of the larynx, the rings of the trachea, and the large bronchi. During the embryonic period, the greater part of the later bony skeleton is laid down in cartilage. During growth, the *epiphyseal joints* (growing end of bone) of the long bones consist of hyaline cartilage (see Fig. 3.**10**), which is only replaced at the conclusion of the growth phase. The hyaline cartilage of joints is the only cartilage without a perichondrium. Hence, after its destruction (by inflammatory or degenerative joint disease) no new functional cartilage can be generated.

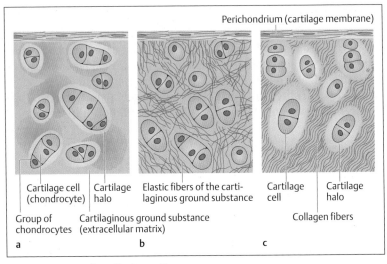

Fig. 3.**8a–c Types of cartilaginous tissue**
a Hyaline cartilage; **b** elastic cartilage; **c** fibrocartilage

■ **Elastic Cartilage.** In addition to the structures contained in hyaline cartilage, elastic cartilage contains elastic fiber networks (Fig. 3.**8b**) that form a latticework structure around the chondrocytes and radiate into the adjacent perichondrium. Because of the elastic fibers, elastic cartilage has a yellowish appearance. In humans it occurs only in the auricle of the ear, parts of the larynx, the epiglottis, and the external auditory meatus (canal of the ear).

■ **Fibrocartilage.** As opposed to hyaline cartilage, fibrous or connective tissue cartilage contains significantly more collagen fibers (Fig. 3.**8c**). It can be found wherever tendons or ligaments exert pressure, as in the *intervertebral disks* (annulus fibrosus) and the *interarticular disks* (*disks and menisces*).

Bone Tissue

Bone tissue is the main supporting tissue, being the structural material of bone, i.e., the skeleton,. A fully differentiated bone is, with the exception of dental material, the hardest substance in the body. It is very *stable under compression* and *tension*, and is extraordinarily resistant to *deformation*. With few exceptions (over the joint cartilage), bone is covered with a *membrane (periosteum)*, from which healing can take place, e. g., after a fracture.

■ **Bone Cells and Intercellular Substance.** *Bone cells (osteocytes)* are connected with each other by a network of long processes. They are enclosed on all sides by a bony ground substance (extracellular matrix), which has some unusual characteristics in its composition and arrangement. The extracellular matrix is rich in collagen fibers, arranged in a ground substance enriched with *inorganic salts* (calcium salts, especially calcium phosphate and calcium carbonate). It is made up of (20–25%) water, (25–30%) organic substances, and (50%) inorganic substances. The minerals are deposited in crystalline form and lend bone its *great physical hardness.* Its excellent blood supply, which facilitates an intensive metabolic exchange, gives bone its *biologic plasticity*. The rigid, extremely hard, bony material is a living substance, which can easily adapt to altered static circumstances in the body such as changes in the direction of stresses. The organic and inorganic components interpenetrate and can only be distinguished by microscopic examination.

If a bone is singed, only the inorganic mineral skeleton remains and the bone becomes brittle. If the bone is placed in acid, only the organic part remains and the bone becomes flexible like rubber.

■ **The Structure of Cancellous Bone.** The structure of bone can be observed especially clearly in the cross-section of a long bone. An *outer compact layer (substantia compacta, compacta* in brief) can be distinguished from an *inner trabeculated (spongy cancellous,)* layer *(substantia spongiosa, spongiosa)* (Fig. 3.**9a**). While the compact layer is present throughout the outer layer of a long bone and is especially developed in the *shaft (diaphysis)*, the spongy bone is especially prominent in the ends *(epiphyses)* of a long bone. Through this "lightweight" construction, bone attains a maximum of strength with a minimum of material. Through the orientation of its trabeculae, the bone can adapt to its function. The trabeculae develop in the form of compression and tension trabeculae under the influence of deformation stresses (Fig. 3.**9d**). In the spaces between the trabeculae of spongy bone is found the red, blood-forming

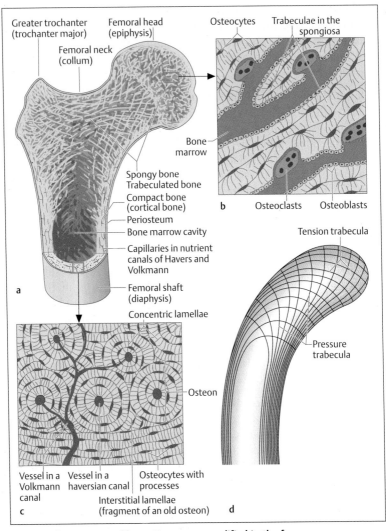

Fig. 3.**9 a–d** **Structure of bony tissue as exemplified in the femur**
a Sagittal section through femoral head, neck, greater trochanter and proximal shaft
b Section from **a**: microscopic section of spongy bone
c Section from **a**: microscopic section of compact bone
d Simplified representation of the tension and compression trabeculae of spongy bone

bone marrow. Yellow bone marrow (fatty marrow) is found especially in the marrow cavity of the diaphysis.

Lamellar bone is named after the lamellar structure of the compact layer of a long bone. The distribution of the lamellar systems (*osteons* or *haversian systems*) is especially clear when seen in cross-section (Fig. 3.**9c**). The center of an osteon consists of a nutrient blood vessel, around which the *osteocytes* and the extracellular matrix are arranged. The osteocytes always lie between the lamellae, in which the collagen fibers are arranged in spirals. The cells are connected to each other by cellular processes running in tiny bone canals, the *canaliculi,* by which nutrients from the inner blood vessel can pass outwards. During the development of an osteon, *bone-building cells* (*osteoblasts*) collect in large numbers from the inside and lay down a layer of bony substance like wallpaper. The collagen fibers are laid down in parallel and in a spiral fashion in this tubular structure. The crystalline inorganic salts are organized in a specific spatial arrangement between these fibers. Another lamella is then laid down from the inside, with collagen fibers running crosswise to the last layer, until there is only little room left in the so-called haversian canal (Fig. 3.**9c**) for some scanty connective tissue and the blood vessels needed for nutrition. A complete osteon is about 1 cm long and consists of 10–20 tubular lamellae fitted inside each other. The bone cells are practically immured between the bony lamellae, and connected to neighboring cells by fine cytoplasmic processes. The osteons are connected with each other by canals (*Volkmann's canals*), in which arterial branches run to junctions with the vessels in the haversian canals.

Spongy bone is also a lamellar structure, but the lamellae are built up in layers as in plywood (Fig. 3.**9b**). Since the bone cells in spongy bone also have a high metabolic rate and require nutrients, the spongy trabeculae are limited in their thickness (ca. 0.5 mm) because the exchange of substances is achieved strictly by diffusion from the surrounding bone marrow.

The osteons of the compact layer and the bony lamellae of spongy bone are rearranged throughout life and can adapt very well to altered static conditions (e. g., fractures). In this way, old lamellar systems are constantly being broken down (Fig. 3.**9c**) and new ones are constructed both in compact and spongy bone. Lamellae are broken down by special *bone-removing* cells called *osteoclasts*, while osteones that are in the process of being rebuilt are called *interstitial lamellae.*

■ **Development of Bone Tissue.** Lamellar bone is not the first stage in the formation of the fully differentiated human bone. Initially, *reticular bone* (*woven bone*) is formed in the embryonic period and also, for example, during healing of a fracture. In reticular bone, blood vessels and collagen fibers are arranged irregularly. Reticular bone corresponds to a hardened connective tissue rich in fibers and can originate in two different ways:

1. A so-called *membrane bone* develops directly from the mesenchyme. This type of ossification is called *membranous or desmal ossification.*
2. A cartilaginous bone precursor first forms in the mesenchyme and is then rebuilt into bone (*endochondral bone*). This process is called *endochondral* or *indirect ossification.*

To adapt to the needs of the growing organism, the developing bone is constantly being shaped, growing by absorption in one place and deposition in another. Greater functional demand, such as increasing body weight, later leads to restructuring of lamellar bones.

■ **Development of a Long Bone.** Most bones develop indirectly by way of a cartilaginous precursor. Only a few bones (some bones in the skull, the clavicle) develop directly by membranous ossification. However, parts of a long bone can develop directly by membranous ossification even where it has been laid down in cartilage, e. g., the perichondral bone cuff that originates in the diaphysis and that provides the base from which the bone grows in thickness (*perichondral ossification*) (Fig. 3.**10**). In the interior of the bone, bony tissue is laid down indirectly, in that the cartilage is first removed by cartilage-absorbing cells (*chondroclasts*) and then replaced by chondral ossification. Where the diaphysis meets the epiphysis, an *epiphyseal plate* develops, where growth in length takes place and in which the cartilage cells divide until growth stops (Fig. 3.**10**). The epiphyseal plate is visible in the radiograph by its lack of calcification. Bone formation within the epiphyses (*ossific centers*) begins only at the time of birth. Many ossific centers develop only in the first years of life. Special ossific centers that develop on bone for the attachment of muscles are called apophyses.

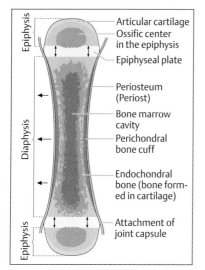

Fig. 3.**10 Simplified representation of the development of a long bone**
← = growth in thickness
↕ = growth in length

Labels in figure:
- Articular cartilage
- Ossific center in the epiphysis
- Epiphyseal plate
- Periosteum (Periost)
- Bone marrow cavity
- Perichondral bone cuff
- Endochondral bone (bone formed in cartilage)
- Attachment of joint capsule
- Epiphysis
- Diaphysis
- Epiphysis

Contrasting Bone and Cartilage

Avascular bone, in which the cells form a dense substance-transport system, regenerates well and adapts to changing static conditions by constant rebuilding. Avascular cartilage, in which the cells are isolated from each other and far from the sources of nutrition, regenerates less well and demonstrates only slight biological adaptability.

■ Muscle Tissue

The cells of muscle tissue can be excited by chemical and electrical stimuli, similarly to nerve cells. The muscle cell, however, has the ability to *shorten* (*contract*), which is triggered by a stimulus and is tied to the presence of certain protein structures (*myofibrils*). Additionally, muscle tissue plays a role in the *heat economy* of the organism, since muscle contraction consumes energy, which is then liberated largely as heat.

Muscle contractions (*shivering*) are also generated to provide heat during heat loss.

In their general structure, muscle cells are similar to other cells in the body, but each muscle cell is a fiber that may reach lengths of up to 20 cm. Hence a muscle cell is also known as a *muscle fiber*. A unique feature of muscle cells (or fibers) is their high content of proteins called myofibrils, which contract on stimulaton of the muscle fiber. The *myofibrils* are composed of short protein threads, the *myofilaments*. These can be divided into *thin actin filaments* and *thick myosin filaments* (see Fig. 3.**12**). A contraction is triggered by nerve stimulation, which is transmitted from the motor end plate to the muscle by a neurotransmitter, acetylcholine. The color of muscle is due to myoglobin, a colored substance dissolved in the cytoplasm and a close relative of hemoglobin both in structure and function.

Muscle tissue is divided according to structure and function into **smooth** and **striated muscle tissue** (Fig. 3.**11a–c**).

Smooth Muscle Tissue

Smooth muscle tissue is chiefly the muscle tissue of the intestines. It forms the greater part of the *walls of the hollow viscera* (gastrointestinal tract, gallbladder, urinary tract, sex organs, blood vessels, etc.) and is found in the distal respiratory tract, the eye, the hair, and the glands. Smooth muscle is controlled by the autonomic (vegetative) nervous system, but in many organs it can be stimulated by passive distension (myogenic stimulation).

A smooth muscle cell is spindle-shaped, about 25 µm long, and has a centrally located elongated nucleus (Fig. 3.**11a**). Toward the end of pregnancy, the muscle cells in the uterus can enlarge considerably, and reach a length of some 0.5 mm (1 mm = 1000 µm). The myofibrils are located in the cytoplasm, and they generate the contraction; they are not, however, as rigidly organized as striated muscle. Smooth muscle contracts slowly, and can, for instance in the intestine, transport intestinal contents in regular contractile waves (peristalsis). It may also remain in a certain state of contraction (tone) for a long time (e. g., the pylorus muscle at the point of transition from the stomach to the duodenum). The muscle cells are connected to each other and to related structures by connective tissue

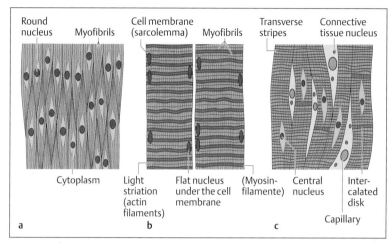

Round nucleus   Myofibrils   Cell membrane (sarcolemma)   Myofibrils   Transverse stripes   Connective tissue nucleus

Cytoplasm   Light striation (actin filaments)   Flat nucleus under the cell membrane   (Myosin-filamente)   Central nucleus   Inter-calated disk

Capillary

a   b   c

Fig. 3.**11 a–c**   **Muscle tissue in longitudinal section**
a   Smooth muscle tissue
b   Striated (skeletal) muscle (see also Fig. 3.**12**)
c   Cardiac muscle

fibers (reticular fibers). Specific chemical transmitters such as acetylcholine and epinephrine (parasympathetic and sympathetic systems, Chapter 14), trigger the contraction.

Striated Muscle Tissue

Striated muscle tissue is divided into *skeletal muscle tissue* and *cardiac muscle tissue*. The very regular arrangement of the myofibrils and their subunits (actin and myosin filaments) in the individual muscle cells can be seen in the optical microscope as *regular light and dark bands*, which have given skeletal and cardiac muscle the name striated (striped) muscle (Fig. 3.**11b**, **c**). This regular, striped arrangement of actin and myosin filaments distinguishes striated muscle under the optic microscope from the smooth variety, in which the actin and myosin filaments are distributed irregularly.

Skeletal Muscle Tissue

The skeletal musculature forms 40–50% of the total body weight, which makes it by far the most strongly developed organ of the human body. The greater part of it forms the *musculature of the active motor system*, and it is found in similar form in the face (muscles of expression), tongue, throat, larynx, eye, middle ear, pelvic floor, etc. It is supplied by the nerves of the somatic (voluntary) nervous system.

Structure of Skeletal Muscle

In a skeletal muscle, muscular fibers and connective tissue are closely interlinked (Fig. 3.**12a-e**). A strong connective tissue sheath consisting of dense collagen connective tissue (*muscle fascia*) surrounds the muscle, contains it, and allows it to slide through its related structures. Each muscle is composed of individual bundles of fibers (*fascicles*) that can be distinguished with the naked eye and are connected by areolar tissue (*epimysium*). Muscles and nerves are contained in the epimysium and by this route reach the internal part of the muscle.

The individual fiber bundles in their turn are composed of hundreds of *muscle fibers* (*muscle cells*) that are enveloped in a delicate connective tissue sheath (*endomysium*) and are also connected with each other by areolar tissue (*perimysium*). Each muscle cell is a long tube of cytoplasm surrounded by a cell membrane (sarcolemma), is without internal cell boundaries, and possesses several hundred nuclei along its margins (Figs. 3.**11** and 3.**12**). Thus, muscle cells are threadlike cells, often several centimeters long, with a diameter of 10–100 μm. They usually run the whole length of a muscle and merge at both ends into connective tissue tendons that connect the muscle to bone (Fig. 3.**12**).

■ **Muscle Spindle.** Within each muscle can be found between 40 and 500 receptor organs, the so-called muscle spindles, which contain specific stretch receptors. The receptors detect changes in length in the muscle and send this information by way of specific nerve fibers to the spinal cord (cf. Chapter 13: Spinal Reflexes). The muscle spindles are specialized muscle fibers that are contrasted as intrafusal muscle to the extrafusal muscle of the active motor apparatus. In addition to the muscle spindles, muscles contain certain tendon receptors, located at

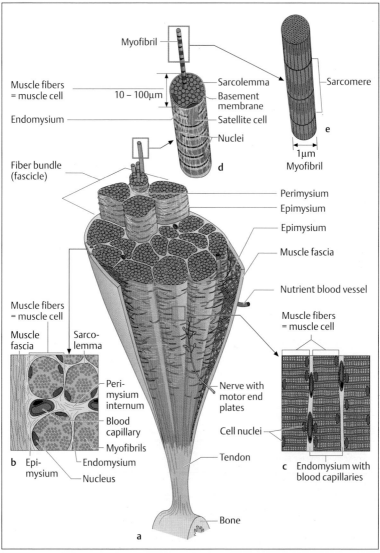

Fig. 3.**12 a–e Structure of a skeletal muscle**

a Cross-section of a skeletal muscle
b Magnified section from **a** (cross-section)
c Magnified section from **a** (longitudinal section)

d Structure of a muscle fiber
     (= muscle cell)
e Structure of a myofibril

the musculotendinous junction (Golgi tendon organ), that protect the muscle from excessive tension.

■ **T and L Systems.** The cell membranes of the muscle fibers project deep into the interior of the cell at regular intervals, in this way forming the so-called transverse tubules. They envelop the myofibrils in the form of tubules and the whole system is called the *T system* (*transverse system, transverse component of the sarcoplasmic reticulum*) (Fig. 3.**13**). This spreads the extracellular space over the whole of the muscle's cross-section and allows a rapid spread of the action potential deep into the muscle fiber. Another feature of muscle cells are tubules arranged longitudinally along the myofibrils between the transverse tubules (*longitudinal* or *L system*), a system of tubules in the endoplasmic reticulum, which in the muscle cell is called the *sarcoplasmic reticulum*. In its totality this system provides a reservoir for calcium ions, which can thus be liberated in a fraction of a second to initiate a muscle contraction on arrival of an action potential (see mechanical transformation of electrochemical excitation, Fig. 3.**15a**, **b**).

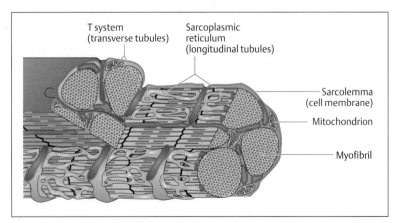

Fig. 3.**13** **Transverse and longitudinal tubules of a muscle cell (T and L system).** (After Silbernagel)

The Structural and Molecular Basis of Skeletal Muscle Contraction

■ **Actin and Myosin Filaments.** The components of skeletal muscle cells that shorten (contract)—the myofibrils—are arranged parallel to the longitudinal axis of a muscle cell. They are divided into numerous units (*sarcomeres*) about 2.5 µm long by transverse partitions called *Z disks* (Fig. 3.**14a–c**). Within the sarcomere there is another regular arrangement of myofilaments, the thin actin and the thick myosin filaments. Each actin filament is anchored to the Z disk of a sarcomere, while the myosin filaments in the middle of the sarcomere protrude on

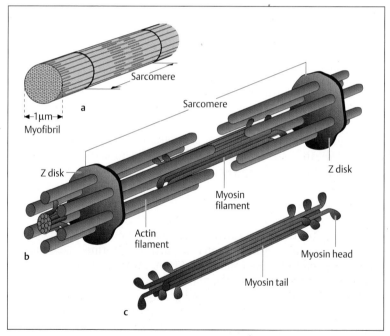

Fig. 3.**14 a–c   Schematic representation of the structure of a sarcomere.** (After Silbernagel)
a Myofibril
b Arrangement of actin and myosin filaments in the sarcomere
c Structure of a myosin filament

both sides into the actin filaments. The myosin filaments have a head (*myosin head*) and a *tail*. When a muscle shortens (contraction), the thin and the thick filaments glide past each other, so that each individual sarcomere is shortened, while the individual filaments preserve their original length. When a muscle relaxes or stretches, this process is reversed.

During a muscle contraction, the myosin heads bond to the actin filaments (formation of cross-bridges), after which they pull them toward the middle of the sarcomere by a kind of *swinging* or *rowing motion* (Fig. 3.**15a,b**). However, a single swing by all 500 or so myosin heads of a thick filament can only shorten a sarcomere by about 1 % of its original length. To achieve a stronger contraction, the cross-bridges from the myosin heads to the actin filaments must constantly be released, so that the actin and myosin filaments can continue to glide past each other as they bond and swing step by step. For maximal muscle contraction, these bonding and swinging processes must take place about 50 times in rapid succession.

■ **Muscle Metabolism and the Mechanical Transformation of Electrochemical Excitation.** The only source of energy for muscle contraction is ATP (*adenosine triphosphate*), formed in the numerous mitochondria. ATP is synthesized from a number of different fuels (e. g., carbohydrates, fatty acids), that are completely broken down to carbon dioxide and water with the help of oxygen (*aerobic metabolism, oxidation*) with little energy consumption. During intense strain, ATP metabolism briefly becomes anaerobic (independent of oxygen). However, such metabolism results in the production of *lactate*, which accumulates in the muscle, with the result that the muscle tires rapidly. Only after the blood has transported lactate to the liver can it be partly transformed back into glucose. Because of the low content of ATP in muscle, fresh ATP must be created rapidly on demand. The most important energy reserve to accomplish this is provided by *glycogen*, a form of glucose storage, and especially by *creatine phosphate*. The breakdown of creatine phosphate into creatine and phosphate liberates large amounts of energy for the generation of ATP.

Calcium ions (Ca^{2+}) are also required for muscle contraction. These are contained in high concentration in the sarcoplasmic reticulum of the muscle cell (L system) in the relaxed state (Fig. 3.**15a**). When a muscle

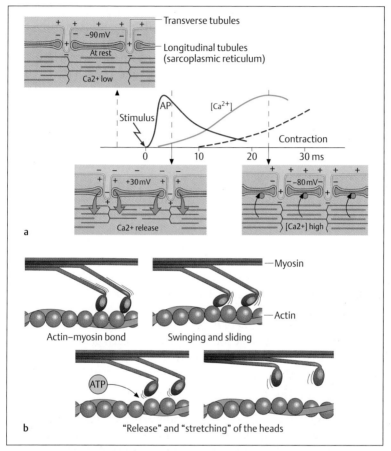

Fig. 3.**15 a, b   Mechanical transformation of electrochemical excitation**
a The role of the Ca^{2+} ion as an intermediary between electrical stimulation and muscle contraction; AP = action potential
b Gliding of the filaments

fiber is stimulated (depolarized) by a nerve impulse (action potential), calcium ions are liberated from the *sarcoplasmic reticulum* in a fraction of a second. The presence of calcium ions is necessary for the bonding of the myosin heads to the actin filaments (*electromechanical coupling*), as well as their swinging and the resulting muscle twitch.[1] Eventually ATP dissolves the bond between myosin and actin and regenerates the tension in the myosin head for the next swing, as in a spring. The energy for this process is generated by an enzyme (ATPase) in the myosin head that splits ATP into ADP (adenosine diphosphate) and phosphate. Without ATP, actin and myosin remain bonded to each other and the muscle becomes rigid (rigor mortis, see p. 96). If no further action potential reaches the cell, the calcium ions are promptly pumped back into the sarcoplasmic reticulum.

Slow and Fast (Phasic and Tonic) Muscle Fibers

The course and duration of muscle twitches in striated skeletal muscle vary considerably. Muscle fibers with a twitch duration of about 30–40 ms are called *fast* (*phasic*)*muscle fibers*, to distinguish them from *slow* (*tonic*) *fibers* with a twitch duration of about 100 ms. Because of differences in their myoglobin content—myoglobin being an oxygen-storing protein related to hemoglobin—phasic muscles are also sometimes called "*pale muscles*" (less myoglobin) and tonic muscles "*red muscles*" (more hemoglobin). While red muscles are more capable of prolonged activity (e. g., postural activity during standing) and take longer to tire, pale muscles are remarkable for their ability to reach peak performance for brief periods, although they tire more rapidly.

Isometric and Isotonic Contraction

Muscles can only develop their maximum strength when they do not shorten or shorten very little. During such an *isometric contraction* the muscle is tensed without changing in length (example: holding the barbell during weight lifting). On the other hand, during *isotonic contraction*

---

[1] A single action potential evokes a brief contraction that lasts a few milliseconds (twitch). This single twitch of skeletal muscle follows the all-or-none law: i.e., a single stimulus of sufficient strength will always evoke the greatest possible contraction of the muscle fiber. In order to obtain a longer-lasting contraction, the muscle fiber must be stimulated several times in short succession (tonic contraction).

the muscle shortens without changing its tension (example: lifting the barbell during weight lifting). Hence, very rapid movements can only be accompanied by the development of relatively little strength. The mode of operation of a single sarcomere explains this dependence of muscular strength on the speed of the muscle contraction. With rapid shortening of the muscle, the myofilaments glide past each other very rapidly. This requires that in each unit of time a portion of the myosin–actin bonds must continually be dissolved, so that the cross-bridges can always get a new hold. Consequently, only a relatively weak force can be generated. In contrast, during isometric contraction almost all the bonds between the myosin heads and the actin filaments can be completed simultaneously, since no new holds need be sought when the muscle is not shortening. Hence a large force can be developed.

Muscle Blood Flow

The blood flow in a muscle, and consequently its oxygen supply, depends on muscular work. During physical exertion the oxygen supply that must be brought to the muscle is 500 times that required at rest. Hence, during muscular work blood flow in the muscle is greatly increased (300–500 capillaries/mm^3 of muscle) and may reach 20 times that at rest. This regulation of muscle blood flow is achieved by several factors (see Chapter 5: Regulation of Organ Perfusion).

Muscle Tone

In the waking state, muscles are in a constant state of *active* (*involuntary*) *tension* (*tone*), maintained in skeletal muscle by a weak but steady stream of impulses (*reflex tone*). No individual twitches are perceptible, as the motor units are stimulated in turn. This muscle tone itself is controlled by muscle and tendon spindles. When muscle tone is absent, the condition is called flaccid paralysis; if paralysis is accompanied by increased tension it is called spastic paralysis (see Chapter 13: Lesions of the Lower Motoneuron [Flaccid Paralysis], and Lesions of the Upper Motoneuron [Spastic Paralysis]).

Special Muscular Conditions

■ **Muscle Wasting (Atrophy) and Overdevelopment 0f Muscles (Hypertrophy).** When muscles are underused or after injury to the nerve supplying a muscle, the muscle atrophies. On the other hand, with strong muscular activity, e. g., during athletic activities, the individual muscle fibers become thicker and the muscle hypertrophies. Severe damage to muscle tissue due to injury leads to a connective tissue scar, as the regenerative power of muscle is scant.

■ **Muscle Soreness.** The muscular pain that occurs after strenuous or unaccustomed physical work is known as muscle soreness. It apparently is not due, as believed for a long time, to local accumulation of lactate or other metabolic products, but is the result of very small injuries (microlesions) in the muscle. Such pains therefore occur not only in the untrained but also, for instance, after operations or muscle cramps.

■ **Muscle Cramps and Contractures.** A muscle cramp (sometimes called a "charley horse") is a mostly reversible ongoing contraction of a muscle due to increased spontaneous tension in skeletal muscle, i.e., increased muscle tone not triggered by a nerve impulse. It may, for instance, be caused by an ongoing localized depolarization resulting from a rise in extracellular K^+ concentration or liberation of intracellular Ca^{2+}. The cramps occurring with fatigue are often accompanied by a reduction or loss of energy-containing phosphates (ATP) resulting from lack of oxygen or glucose. Irreversible muscle contractions are called *contractures*.

■ **Postmortem Rigidity.** In the case of postmortem rigidity (rigor mortis), which usually supervenes about 4–10 hours after death, intramuscular metabolism stops and consequently ATP (adenosine triphosphate), which normally dissolves the bond between actin and myosin after a contraction, is absent from the muscle cell. As a rule postmortem rigidity begins with the mandibular musculature; it disappears after 1–3 days, when the structure of all tissues begins to disintegrate (autolysis).

Cardiac Muscle Tissue

Cardiac muscle tissue is a special form of striated muscle tissue. It differs from skeletal striated muscle mainly in three ways:

1. In contrast to the marginal nuclei of skeletal muscle, the nuclei of heart muscle mostly are located centrally (Fig. 3.**12c**). Heart muscle cells also have a smaller cross-section than skeletal muscle fibers.
2. Heart muscle cells, in contrast to the unbranched skeletal muscle fibers, are connected to each other in a net by the so-called *intercalated disks*. This allows an impulse originating in the sinus node to spread evenly fanwise over the atria. The impulse is then conducted with some delay by way of the AV node and the bundle of His to the ventricular myocardium, where it again spreads evenly and fanwise (see Chapter 5: Resting and Action Potential of the Heart).
3. A further unique feature of cardiac muscle is the ability of some of its cells to generate impulses not only in response to an external stimulus, but spontaneously. Additionally, the activity of cardiac muscle cells can be influenced by the autonomic nervous system; for example, the sympathetic accelerates heart rate, while the parasympathetic slows it down (see Chapter 14: The Autonomic Nervous System).

■ Nerve Tissue

Like all other tissues in the body, the structural element of the nervous system, nerve tissue, is made up of individual cells, the **nerve cells** or **neurons** and the **glia cells**. While the nerve cells are responsible for the reception of stimuli, the conduction of impulses and the transformation of stimuli, glia cells are regarded as a sort of *nervous connective tissue* (*neuroglia*). They are at the same time nutrient and supporting tissue for the nerve cells and additionally serve as a defensive system and as insulation of nerve fibers. By the latter function they take part—albeit indirectly—in the conduction of impulses. Glia cells retain the ability to divide throughout their life, as opposed to neurons, which cannot divide after birth. Hence, glia cells replace nerve cells lost through disease, lack of oxygen, or injury.

The Neuron

Within the nervous system the nerve cells (neurons) form structurally and functionally independent units, of which there are 20–50 billion in the human brain alone. The neurons connect to each other by so-called synapses and form *neuronal chains* or *loops*. The size and shape of these neurons vary within wide limits, but the basic structure is always the same. According to the direction of the impulse, a nerve cell is divided into three segments (Fig. 3.**16**):

- Dendrites (receptor structures)
- Axis cylinder or axon (effector structures)
- Perikaryon or soma (cell body, metabolic center)

■ **Dendrites.** The dendrites (up to 1000 per cell) are branching multiform processes with *special contact points* (*synapses*), that receive stimuli originating in other neurons and transmit them to the perikaryon. From there, the axis cylinder generally conducts the impulse to a receptor organ (e.g., skeletal muscle) or another neuron (Fig. 3.**16**). Stimuli from the axon of one nerve cell to the dendrites of the next are not transmitted directly but with the aid of chemical substances, the *neurotransmitters* at the synapses (see below). The junction between an axon and a muscle fiber is called a *motor end plate* (*neuromuscular junction*) (Fig. 3.**16**).

■ **Axon Cylinder.** The axon cylinder (axon, nerve fiber) originates in a narrow base from the *axon hillock*. Within its course, which varies in length from a few millimeters to almost 100 cm, it can divide into numerous side-branches (collaterals). Axons are surrounded by a myelin envelope of varying thickness (*myelin sheath*, *Schwann cell sheath*) con-

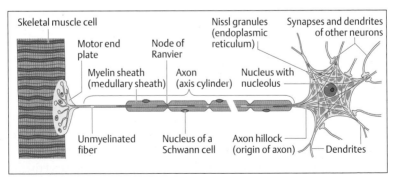

Fig. 3.**16** **Simplified representation of a motoneuron**

sisting of a phospholipid membrane with constrictions at defined intervals (nodes of Ranvier) (Fig. 3.**16**). The significance of the myelin sheath as a stimulus conductor lies in the ability of impulses to leap from node of Ranvier to node of Ranvier (*saltatory conduction*), leading to much faster conduction speeds (up to 120 m/s). The myelin sheaths are formed by certain glia cells (Fig. 3.**17a–c**), namely, Schwann cells (in the peripheral nervous system) and oligodendrocytes (in the central nervous system).

■ **Perikaryon.** The perikaryon varies in size and shape and has few cell organelles beyond the nucleus. The most prominent are the so-called *Nissl granules* (Fig. 3.**16**), granular endoplasmic reticulum arranged in clumps. Between these, ribosomes, mitochondria, and numerous neurotubules and neurofilaments enter the axon at the axon hillock. The neurotubules, for instance, route insoluble proteins (transmitters, enzymes) to the synapses. Nerve cells are classified according to the number and type of branching of their dendrites and axon processes (Fig. 3.**18a–d**):

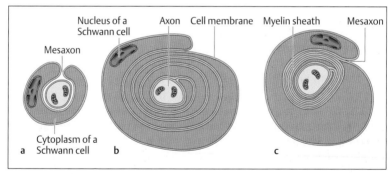

Fig. 3.**17 a–c** **Development of the myelin sheath (medullary sheath) around a nerve fiber**
a The axon is surrounded by a Schwann cell; the mesaxon is the point where the Schwann cell processes meet
b A thin cytoplasmic layer of a Schwann cell wraps itself around the axon
c The cytoplasm between the coiled cell membranes of the Schwann cell is squeezed out; what is left are several layers of membrane forming a myelin sheath around the axon

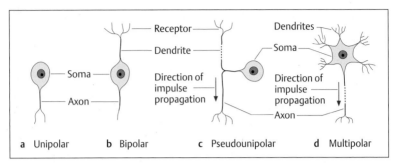

Fig. 3.**18a–d   Types of neuron**
a Unipolar neurons have a single axon
b In bipolar neurons, axon and dendrite arise from opposite ends of the cell body (soma)
c Pseudounipolar neurons originate from bipolar neurons by merging of axon and dendrite near the soma
d In multipolar neurons, numerous dendrites arise from the cell body together with one axon

▪ Unipolar
▪ Bipolar
▪ Pseudounipolar
▪ Multipolar

The Nerve Impulse (Action Potential)

The ability to be excited by a stimulus is a basic property of every cell. The rapid transmission of an impulse by specialized cell processes (axons) is confined to nerve cells. Nerve impulses or action potentials represent the *universal means of communication* within the nervous system of animals and humans. The significant parameter for such communication is not the intensity of a single action potential but the *number of action potentials per unit time* (*frequency*) received, processed, and transmitted by a nerve fiber. Hence the language or code of the neuron in the nervous system is the impulse frequency (up to 500 per second).

The generation of an action potential in a nerve cell depends on the negative resting potential (see Fig. 1.**13**) that is present in almost all cells and characterized by an *electrical potential difference* between the outer surface of the cell and the cell interior. When the nerve cell is stimulated electrically, chemically, or in any other way, the cell membrane briefly loses its external positive charge and becomes temporarily slightly negative; the membrane potential changes from –60 mV (resting potential) to +20 mV (Fig. 3.**19**). The potential regains its initial value in less than 1 ms. Since the cell loses its initial resting potential or polarization, this process is called *depolarization*; the return to resting potential is called *repolarization*. As with muscle, here too the all-or-none law applies; that is, a stimulus above a defined threshold always elicits an action potential of equal form, intensity, and duration.

■ **Mechanism.** The mechanism of the action potential is as follows. When a stimulus reaches a nerve cell, membrane pores (channels) that are permeable only to sodium ions (Na^+) are opened briefly. This allows sodium ions to move along their concentration gradient (there are few Na^+ ions inside the cell) into the cell, where they lead to an excess of positive ions. In this way, the membrane is depolarized. However, the Na^+ channels close again after less than 1 ms, and next the K^+ channels open more than usual. More potassium ions move out of the cell and re-polarize the cell membrane back to its resting potential. After the K^+ channels have also closed again, sodium ions must be removed from the cell (ion pump), with expenditure of energy (via ATP) so that the cell is ready for renewed stimulation.

The propagation of the action potential along the surface of the nerve cell or along its axon occurs because localized increases in the membrane potential open neighboring ion channels. In this way, the excitation of the membrane spreads over the whole cell and along the axon. The rate at which such an impulse travels is between a few meters per second (autonomic nerves) to 120 meters per second (motor nerves of voluntary muscles).

The Synapse

In general two processes lead to *depolarization of a nerve cell*:

1. Stimuli acting on the nervous system from outside (e. g., light stimuli, mechanical stimuli, pain stimuli or thermal stimuli)
2. Impulses transmitted through synapses from an axon to another nerve cell or a muscle or glandular cell. Such synaptic transmission

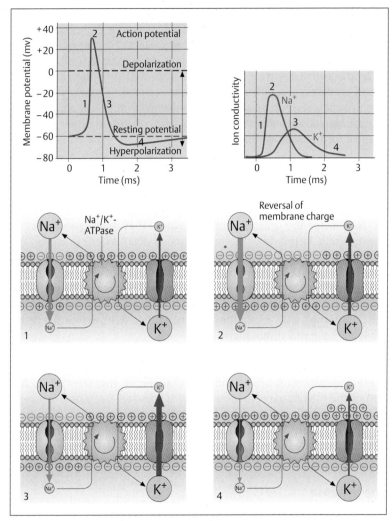

Fig. 3.**19** **Time course of an action potential**

mostly occurs by means of certain chemical agents, the *neu-rotransmitters*.

At the synapses, the cells are in intimate contact. Three components are described corresponding to their structure (see Fig. 3.**20**):

- The presynaptic membrane
- A narrow intercellular gap (synaptic cleft)
- The postsynaptic membrane

■ **Mechanism of Synaptic Transmission.** At the presynaptic membrane, the axon frequently shows a club-shaped thickening, the *synaptic terminal*, which contains numerous small vesicles, the *synaptic vesicles*. When an action potential reaches the synaptic terminal, the transmitter molecules stored in the synaptic vesicles are released into the synaptic cleft by exocytosis. They diffuse across the 10–50 nm wide synaptic cleft to the postsynaptic membrane and bind to the corresponding receptors. This binding induces either depolarization of the postsynaptic membrane, which promotes further conduction of the impulse (*excitatory synapse*), or hyperpolarization, which inhibits further conduction of the impulse (*inhibitory synapse*).

The most important excitatory neurotransmitters are acetylcholine and glutamate, while the most important inhibitory neurotransmitters are glycine and γ-aminobutyric acid (GABA). A number of neurotransmitter substances have a more complex pattern of activity and therefore cannot be classified as uniquely excitatory or inhibitory. These

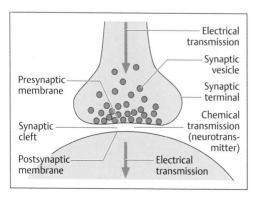

Fig. 3.**20 Schematic representation of a synapse.** (After Silbernagl and Despopoulos)

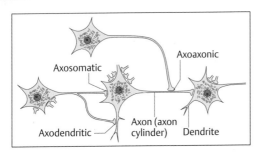

Fig. 3.**21** **Various types of synapse.** (After Duus)

include norepinephrine, dopamine, serotonin, and the endogenous opioids (endorphins, enkephalins, dynorphins).

There are several different chemical classes of neurotransmitters. Norepinephrine, serotonin, and dopamine are among the *biogenic amines*; glutamate and glycine are *amino acids*; and the endogenous opioids are *peptides* (*neuropeptides*).

So-called exogenous opioids, such as morphine, mimic the function of the endogenous opioids by binding to the same membrane receptors, thus blocking the conduction of nociceptive impulses.

Serotonin is an example of a neurotransmitter that modulates many different functions of the brain. It plays a role in the regulation of body temperature and in sensory perception, and it influences the individual's mood, drive, and state of consciousness. Many psychoactive drugs exert their effects through an alteration of serotonin metabolism.

■ **Synaptic Function.** Since the impulse always runs in one direction, e. g., from the axon terminal to the next nerve cell, the synapse can be regarded as a valve. Some synapses may facilitate conduction of an impulse or inhibit it. Finally, synapses have an important role in the functions of *memory* and *learning*. The more frequently they are used, the more easily they conduct an impulse. Synapses may also disappear or be newly formed throughout life.

■ **Types of Synapses.** From many tens of synapses up to several thousand may terminate on a single nerve cell. According to the termination of an axon, that is, whether it ends on a dendrite, the soma, or the axon of another nerve cell, the synapse may be *axondendritic*, *axonsomatic*, or *axonaxonic*, respectively (Fig. 3.**21**).

The Glia Cells (Neuroglia)

Within the peripheral and central nervous system, the following types of cell can be distinguished in the nervous connective tissue, the neuroglia (see Chapter 13: The Central and Peripheral Nervous Systems):

- Peripheral nervous system
  - *Schwann cells* (form the myelin sheath)
  - *Amphicytes* (*capsule cells*) envelop the nerve cells of the spinalganglia and the autonomic ganglia)
- Central nervous system
  - *Oligodendrocytes* (form the myelin sheath)
  - *Astrocytes* (exercise a kind of supporting function)
  - *Microglia* (phagocytic immune cells)
  - *Ependymal cells* (line the cavities of the brain and spinal cord)
  - *Choroid plexus cells* (generate the fluid surrounding the brain and spinal cord, the cerebrospinal fluid (CSF)

Blood–Brain Barrier of the Central Nervous System (CNS)

Astrocytes not only take part in the structure of the neuroglia but are also part of the structure of the so-called *blood–brain barrier*. The astrocytes envelop the outer walls of the capillaries with their pseudopodia-like processes, sealing them very effectively (Fig. 3.22); also, in contrast to capillaries elsewhere, the endothelium of the capillaries in the CNS forms so-called "tight junctions" between individual cells. The blood–

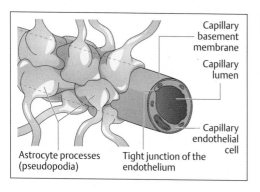

Capillary basement membrane

Capillary lumen

Capillary endothelial cell

Astrocyte processes (pseudopodia)

Tight junction of the endothelium

Fig. 3.**22** **Structure of the blood–brain barrier**

brain barrier serves as a barrier surrounding the whole brain, functioning as a regulator that allows carbohydrates, such as glucose, and proteins to pass only with the aid of special transport mechanisms, while fat-soluble substances pass almost unimpeded. Hence many substances, among them most medications, cannot cross the blood–brain barrier unless they are fat-soluble. This applies, for instance, to medications that act on the brain (e. g., levodopa in Parkinson disease).

The Nerves

Only the peripheral pathways are called nerves; the pathways in the brain and spinal cord are not commonly called nerves, but rather tracts (central pathways). One nerve contains several bundles of *nerve fibers* (fasciculi) (Fig. 3.**23a**, **b**). A mixed nerve is one in which *sensory* (*afferent*)

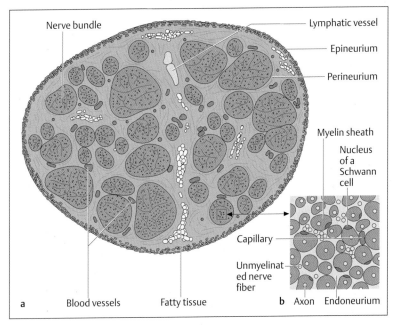

Fig. 3.**23 a, b Cross-section of a peripheral nerve**
a Overview; **b** greatly magnified section of **a**

and *motor* (*efferent*) nerves run together (see Chapter 13: Peripheral Nerves). Such a nerve therefore contains hundreds of individual axons, which are enveloped by their myelin sheath and an additional connective tissue layer, the *endoneurium* (*neurilemma*). The individual bundles of fibers in their turn are each enveloped by another connective tissue layer, the *perineurium*. The fasciculi are then bundled together as a peripheral nerve by an areolar collagen connective tissue sheath, the *epineurium* (Fig. 3.**23a**, **b**). The various sheaths not only provide *mechanical protection* for the nerves but are important for the *nutrition* of the nerve fibers by the blood vessels contained in them. Additionally, they represent an important *barrier to diffusion* and especially the perineurium.

Regeneration of Peripheral Nerves

Unlike the axons of the CNS, peripheral nerves can regenerate after injury or even complete transection. This can only occur after the two ends are joined surgically. Following a lesion, the part of the axon separated from the soma at first degenerates, while the Schwann cells remain intact. The latter serve as a *conduit* for the regenerating axons. In this way, the regenerating axons grow about 1–2 mm per day in the direction of the organ to be innervated (e. g., muscle). Complete *reinnervation* may take several months. After amputation, the axons grow in all directions, since their conduit of Schwann cells has been removed. They form a proliferative mass called an amputation neuroma.

Summary **Tissues**

Cells are connected to each other by cell junctions, which vary greatly in form according to their function in specific tissues. They can be classified into tight junctions, gap junctions, and desmosomes.

■ **Epithelial Tissues**
The cells of all epithelia rest on a thin basement membrane. They are classified as:

- Surface epithelia
- Glandular epithelia
- Sensory epithelia

Surface Epithelia

These cover the outer and inner surfaces of the body. According to their shape they are divided onto squamous, cuboid, and columnar, which can be simple, stratified, or pseudostratified. According to their function, their surface may be differentiated into microvilli, cilia, or stereocilia.

Glandular Epithelia

These produce secretions that reach their destination by secretory ducts (exocrine glands) or are secreted directly into the bloodstream (endocrine glands). Individual glandular cells may also be part of a surface epithelial group of cells.

Sensory Epithelia

These transmit sensations and are part of the structure of sensory organs.

■ Connective and Supporting Tissues

Connective and supporting tissues are made up of cells and an extracellular matrix, while other tissues are made up mainly of cells. Connective tissue ensheathes organs, vessels, and nerves, and fulfills an important metabolic function by serving as a pathway for exchange of substances between individual components. The harder tissues, namely, cartilage and bone (and also chordate and dental tissue), are designated supporting tissues, because in them the supportive function dominates, and the metabolic function takes a minor role.

Connective Tissue

Connective tissue contains tissue-specific fibroblasts that produce the extracellular matrix, and various forms of leukocyte. The extracellular matrix consists of ground substance (interstitial fluid, protein polysaccharides, glycoproteins) and connective tissue fibers (collagen fibers, elastic fibers, reticulum fibers). There are seven different types of connective tissue:

- Loose areolar (interstitial) connective tissue (e. g., the stroma of organs)
- Dense white fibrous connective tissue: dense irregular (e. g., organ capsules) and dense regular white fibrous connective tissue (e. g., tendons and aponeuroses)

- Reticular connective tissue (e. g., the connective tissue framework of lymphatic organs)
- Fatty (adipose) tissue
- Gelatinous connective tissue (umbilical cord)
- Fibroareolar tissue (e. g., ovary)
- Elastic bands (ligamenta flava, the ligaments between the laminae of the spinal column)

Supporting Tissue

Representative supporting tissues are cartilage and bone.

Cartilaginous Tissue

The cartilage cells (chondrocytes) are found in small clusters (chondrones) in the extracellular matrix, which consists of ground substance (see Connective Tissue) and connective tissue fibers. Cells form only 1–10% of cartilage (30–50% in connective tissue). Cartilage is divided into three types according to type and quantity of fibers:

- Hyaline cartilage (e. g., joint surfaces): smallest proportion of fibers (only collagen fibers), largest proportion of water (70%)
- Elastic cartilage (e. g., in the auricle): additionally contains elastic fibers
- Fibrocartilage (e. g., intervertebral disks): highest proportion of fibers (only collagen fibers)

Bone Tissue

The cells of bone (osteocytes) are connected to each other in a network. The extracellular matrix is rich in collagen fibers, while the ground substance is poor in water and consists of 50% inorganic salts (calcium salts) that are responsible for the hardness of bone. in contrast to cartilage, bone has a good blood supply. A fully differentiated bone is called cancellous bone; it consists of an outer dense compact layer and a trabeculated spongy inner layer (spongiosa). The compact layer is made up of tubular lamellar systems (osteons, haversian systems). The spongiosa consists of lamellae arranged in layers; especially at the epiphyses of long bones, they form the characteristic spongy trabeculae that develop according to their load as compression or tension trabeculae.

Precursor to the lamellar bone is a primitive bone, which can develop by direct ossification as membrane bone or by indirect endochondral ossification.

■ **Muscle Tissue**

In general, muscle cells are structurally similar to other cells in the body, but they have certain unique features:

- Muscle cells are fibers of up to 20 cm in length. Hence muscle cell = muscle fiber.
- They can be stimulated chemically and electrically.
- Certain proteins (myofibrils) allow the muscle to shorten. There are two types of muscle tissue.

Smooth Muscle Tissue

This occurs predominantly in the inner organs. The myofibrils are not organized in the cytoplasm; the contractions are slow and involuntary (autonomic nervous system).

Striated Muscle Tissue

The regular arrangement of the myofibrils gives the impression of transverse striations under an optic microscope. There are two types:

- Cardiac muscle tissue
- Skeletal muscle tissue

The skeletal musculature is the musculature of the active motor system. Skeletal muscle is composed of individual bundles of muscle fibers, each comprising many hundreds of muscle fibers (muscle cells). The whole muscle, the fiber bundles, and the fibers are each surrounded by connective tissue sheaths. Each muscle contains specialized muscle fibers (muscle spindles = intrafusal musculature) that register changes in muscle length and correct this by spinal reflexes. Processes of the sarcolemma in the form of transverse tubules (T system) and longitudinal tubules, a system of tubules of the endoplasmic reticulum (L system, serves as Ca^{2+} reservoir) enable the rapid conduction of impulses and immediate muscle contractions.

The protein structures adapted for contraction (myofibrils) are arranged in the longitudinal axis of the muscle fibers and are organized in sarcomeres. The sarcomeres consist of the myofilaments actin and myosin. These glide into each other (hence the shortening of the sarcomere, but not the filaments!) and in the process bond to each other. Bonding depends on Ca^{2+}; release depends on ATP. In the absence of metabolism, ATP production does not take place and all muscles remain contracted (postmortem rigidity). A maximal muscle contraction is made up of about 50 individual contractions that succeed each other smoothly, and during which the actin and myosin fibers continue to glide into each other.

■ Nerve Tissue

Nerve tissue consists of nerve cells (neurons) and connective tissue cells, the glia cells (neuroglia).

The Neuron

A neuron possesses the properties of stimulus reception, conduction, and processing and can be divided into dendrites, axon, and soma (perikaryon). The dendrites receive nerve impulses from other nerve cells by means of neurotransmitters at synapses, and transmit them to the soma. The axon leaving the soma in its turn transmits the impulse either by synapses to the dendrites of other neurons, or directly by the motor end plate to a muscle fiber. A myelin sheath interrupted by constrictions surrounds the axon and accelerates impulse conduction.

The Nerve Impulse (Action Potential)

The generation and conduction of action potentials depends on brief depolarization of the membrane or reversal of its charge that spreads in turn over the whole neuron including the axon. Cell membrane depolarization is generated by a stimulus acting on the nerve cell.

The Synapse

The transmission of an impulse from an axon to another neuron is effected across a synapse by neurotransmitters. These are released from synaptic vesicles close to the presynaptic membrane. The transmitters diffuse across the synaptic cleft and at the postsynaptic membrane lead to depolarization and so to transmission of the impulse.

The Glia Cells

In the peripheral nervous system, specialized glia cells (Schwann cells) form the myelin sheath of the axon. In the central nervous system, oligodendrocytes form the myelin sheath.

The Nerves

A nerve consists of several axon bundles (fascicles) and blood and lymph vessels. The axon, the fascicle, and the whole nerve are each enveloped in connective tissue sheaths.

4

The Locomotor System (Musculoskeletal System)

Contents

■ Axes, Planes, and Orientation

Axes and Planes of the Body

Any number of axes and planes may be drawn through the human body. It is customary, however, to define three main axes running perpendicular to each other in three spatial coordinates (Fig. 4.**1**):

■ A **longitudinal axis** (*vertical axis, cephalocaudal axis*) of the body, which in the upright posture runs perpendicular to the base

■ A **horizontal axis** (*transverse axis*) running from left to right and perpendicular to the longitudinal axis

■ A **sagittal** axis running from front to back and perpendicular to both the other axes

Hence it is possible to define three principal planes:

■ A **sagittal plane**, defined as any plane that is oriented along the sagittal axis (the vertical plane that divides the body into two equal halves is called the **median plane**)

■ A **transverse plane**, defined as any plane running transversely across the body

■ A **frontal plane** (**coronal plane**) that includes all planes oriented parallel to the forehead

Nomenclature of Positions and Directions

The following designations of positions and directions serve to describe accurately the positions of parts of the human body:

■ **For the trunk**

Cranial, cephalad, or superior:	Toward the head
Caudad or inferior:	Toward the coccyx (tailbone)
Ventral or anterior:	Toward the front (abdomen)
Dorsal or posterior:	Toward the rear (back)
Medial:	Toward the median plane
Lateral:	Away from the median plane
Internal:	Inside the body
External:	Outside the body
Peripheral:	Away from the trunk

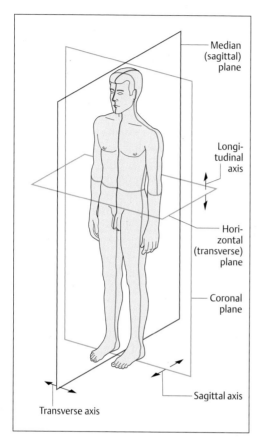

Fig. 4.**1 Major axes and planes of the human body.**
Left anterior view

- Median (sagittal) plane
- Longitudinal axis
- Horizontal (transverse) plane
- Coronal plane
- Sagittal axis
- Transverse axis

■ For the extremities

Proximal:	Toward the trunk
Distal:	Toward the extremities of the limbs
Radial	Toward the radius (thumb side)
Ulnar:	Toward the ulna (side of the little finger)
Tibial:	Toward the shin (side of the big toe)
Fibular:	Toward the fibula (side of the little toe)
Palmar (volar):	Toward the palm of the hand
Plantar:	Toward the sole of the foot
Dorsal (of hand and foot):	Toward the back of the hand or foot (upper side of foot)

■ General Anatomy of the Locomotor System

The skeleton, the supporting framework of the body, is formed by bony and cartilaginous elements, connected by connective tissue structures. Its parts are moved or held in defined positions or postures by the skeletal musculature. The overarching term *locomotor system* includes the *skeleton and the musculature*. The passive locomotor system consists of the skeleton and its joints (articulations), while the active motor system includes the striated muscles, the tendons, and their auxiliary structures (muscle fasciae, bursae, tendon sheaths, and sesamoid bones). Beside their supporting function, the skeletal elements and their joints serve to provide levers for the muscles during locomotion. The skeletal elements, joints, and skeletal musculature together form the organs of locomotion. In addition, the skeletal elements function to *protect* other organ systems (bones of the skull, vertebral canal, chest cage).

The Bones

The bony skeleton consists of bones of various structures and shapes. In the adult human, the skeleton is composed of about 200 individual bones, which are connected by cartilaginous, fibrous, and synovial joints. Each bone, with the exception of the cartilaginous joint surfaces and areas where flat tendons are attached, is enclosed in a connective tissue sheath, the *periosteum*, like a stocking.

The shape of each bone is determined genetically, but its structure depends largely on the type and extent of the mechanical demands placed on it. According to their external shape, bones are divided into *long, short, flat*, and *irregular bones*. Examples of long bones (pipe bones) are the bones of the free extremities, with the exception of the wrist and ankle bones. Long bones are composed of a *shaft* (*diaphysis*) and an *epiphysis* at each end. During growth, each diaphysis and the corresponding epiphysis are separated by the so-called *epiphyseal cartilage* (*epiphyseal plate*) (see Fig. 3.**10**, p. 85). The short bones include the cube-shaped bones of the wrist and ankle.

Among the *flat bones* are the ribs, the breast bone, the shoulder blade, and the bones of the skull. The *irregular bones* include the vertebrae and the bones at the base of the skull. Some of the bones in the skull (frontal, cribriform plate, upper jaw) contain air-filled cavities. *Sesamoid bones* are bones embedded in tendons (e. g., the kneecap). Finally, certain extra bones, occurring especially in the hand and foot, are called *accessory bones*. Their presence in a radiographic image can lead to diagnostic errors (as displaced fragment due to a fracture).

The Joints

Joints are connections between cartilaginous and/or bony parts of the skeleton. They enable movement between the individual segments of the trunk and the extremities, and transmit force. They are divided, according to the type of connection, into immovable and movable.

Immovable Joints (Synarthroses)

So-called immovable joints, or synarthroses, are those joints in which parts of the skeleton are separated by a different tissue such as cartilage or connective tissue. According to the intervening tissue these are divided into (Fig. 4.**2**):

- Syndesmoses (fibrous joints)
- Synchondroses (cartilaginous joints)
- Synostoses (bony joints), which are not true joints but bony fusions

■ **Syndesmoses.** In syndesmoses, two bones are connected by connective tissue (Fig. 4.**2**). Examples are the interosseous membrane between the ulna and radius of the lower arm; the membranous fontanelles of the newborn skull, and the sutures between the bones of the skull. The connective tissue anchoring of the roots of teeth in the upper and lower jaw, known as a peg and socket joint (gomphosis), is also a syndesmosis.

■ **Synchondroses.** The connecting tissue in synchondroses is cartilage (Fig. 4.**2**). Examples are the fibrocartilaginous intervertebral disks between vertebrae or the symphysis pubis at the junction of the two pubic bones. The connection of the bony diaphysis of a juvenile long

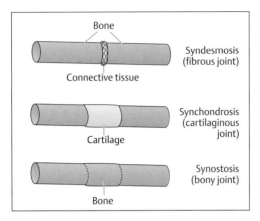

Fig. 4.**2**   **Simplified representation of the different immovable joints (synarthroses)**

bone to the epiphysis by its cartilaginous epiphyseal plate is also a synchondrosis.

■ **Synostoses.** In a synostosis individual bones are fused secondarily by bone tissue (Fig. 4.**2**). A typical example is the sacrum, which originally consists of five separate vertebrae that fuse to each other when growth is complete. Another example is the hip bone, which, until growth is completed, consists of three separate bones: the pubis, the ilium, and the ischium.

Movable Joints (Synovial Joints, Diarthroses)

In synovial joints the bones are separated by a *joint space* (Fig. 4.**3**). They are also distinguished by *hyaline cartilage* covering the *joint surfaces* and by a *joint capsule* that encloses a *joint cavity*. Some joints feature *interarticular disks* (menisci), *articular lips*, or *intra-articular ligaments*. For instance, the menisci of the knee are made of fibrocartilage, are semilunar in shape, and incompletely partition the knee joint. Disks are also a feature of the mandibular joint and the sternoclavicular joint among others. The function of disks in joints is to increase the contact between two opposing surfaces.

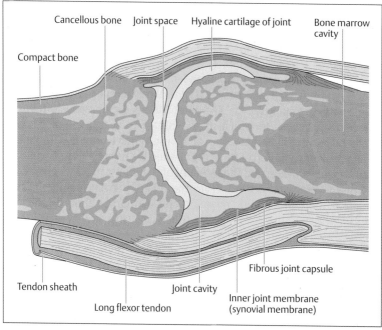

Fig. 4.**3**   **Structure of a movable joint as exemplified in the metatarsophalangeal joint of the big toe**

■ **Joint Cartilage.** The smooth surface of joint cartilage consists mostly of hyaline cartilage (Fig. 4.**3**), the mechanical and "shock absorbing" properties of which are essentially due to its extracellular matrix. Important constituents of extracellular matrix are collagen fibers, macromolecules (protein saccharides), and water. The thickness of joint cartilage varies considerably. It averages 2–3 mm, but in some places (joint surface of the patella) joint cartilage can reach 8 mm. Since this cartilage does not contain blood vessels, it must receive nutrients by diffusion from the *synovial fluid*. Optimal nutrition requires regular movement (loading and unloading) of the cartilage, so that the synovia is pressed into the cartilage. Lack of movement and unphysiologically high tensions lead to *degenerative changes* (*osteoarthritis*) in joint cartilage, especially in older people. Because there is no *perichondrium*, the regenerative power of joint cartilage is insignificant (see p. 79).

■ **Joint Capsule and Synovial Fluid.** The joint capsule (Fig. 4.**3**) is a continuation of the periosteum. It is made up of an outer dense white fibrous layer (*fibrous membrane*) and an inner loosely structured membrane rich in vessels and nerves (*synovial membrane*), which may contain a varying amount of fat. The outer fibrous membrane is often reinforced with *ligaments*, which may reinforce the capsule, guide movement, or prevent hyperextension of a joint. When a joint is immobilized over a prolonged period of time, the connective tissue fibers shorten, the joint capsule shrinks, and the mobility of the joint can be severely compromised (*joint contracture*). From the inner synovial membrane *folds and protrusions* project into the joint. This membrane abuts on the joint cavity with specialized connective tissue cells that are responsible for the secretion (production) and reabsorption (resorption) of the synovial fluid. The glairy, thick (viscous) synovial fluid not only nourishes the joint cartilage, but serves as a lubricant to reduce friction between the joint surfaces.

Slightly Movable Joints (Amphiarthroses)

Some joints are *severely limited* in their mobility by the shape of their facets and *strong ligaments*. Such joints include the tibiofibular joint and the sacroiliac joint between the sacrum and the ilium.

Types of Joint

Joints may be classified from different points of view, for example, by the number of axes of mobility, of degrees of freedom, or of components of the joint. The following is a classification by *shape and configuration* of the joint surfaces (Fig. 4.**4**):

- Ball-and-socket joints
- Condyloid joints
- Hinge joints
- Pivot joints
- Saddle joints
- Plane joints

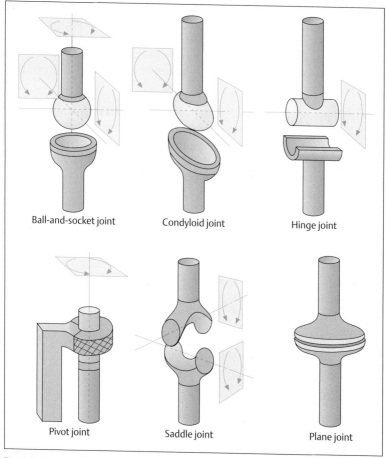

Ball-and-socket joint   Condyloid joint   Hinge joint

Pivot joint   Saddle joint   Plane joint

Fig. 4.**4** **Types of joint.** The arrows show the direction in which the skeletal parts can move around each axis.

■ **Ball-and-Socket Joints (Spheroid Joints)** consist of a *ball-shaped head* and a correspondingly *concave socket*. They have three main axes perpendicular to each other and allow *six main movements*. Typical ball-and-socket joints are the hip and shoulder joints.

■ **Condyloid Joints (Condylar Joints)** have an *elliptical head* fitted into a *convex* and a *concave socket*. They have two main axes perpendicular to each other, and they allow *four main movements*. Examples are the joint between the bones of the forearm and the wrist (proximal wrist joint) and the joint between the atlas and the occipital condyles.

■ **Hinge Joints (Ginglymus Joints) and Pivot Joints (Trochoid Joints)** are also known as trochlear joints. In hinge joints, a *cylindrical bone end* is applied to a gutterlike depression in a hollow skeletal cylinder. Because of this shape, hinge joints have only one axis of movement and *two main movements* (elbow joint). In pivot joints, a cylindrical part of the skeleton is fitted into a corresponding hollow cylinder and a ring-shaped ligament. A typical example is the superior radioulnar joint and its annular ligament. Such a joint allows rotation around one axis and two main movements.

■ **Saddle Joints** consist of two *concave curved surfaces* with two main axes of movement that are perpendicular to each other and allow *four main movements*. An example is the joint in the wrist between the first metacarpal bone and the trapezium.

■ **Plane Joints (Gliding Joints)** allow *gliding movements of plane joint surfaces*, as in the small joints of the vertebrae.

Joint Mechanics

The direction of movement in a joint is determined not only by the shape of the joint surfaces but also by the arrangement of the muscles and ligaments. Human joints cohere by force: their integrity is ensured by muscular forces, which also determine the direction and type of their movement. The shape of the joint, the muscles, ligaments, and soft tissues limit the extent of movement. Hence, limitations may be divided into *bony*, *muscular*, *ligamentous*, and *soft tissue* types.

Joints move around *movement axes*: the direction of movement is determined by the relationship of the muscles to the axes. The body can be considered to have three main axes, running perpendicular to each other (p. 115). In addition there are *axes relating specifically to the movement of each joint*, named according to its movement, e. g., the pronation/supination axis of the proximal and distal radioulnar joints around which the hand may be rotated inward and outward (pronation and supination).

Two opposite movements can occur around each axis. Examples are:

- Bending—extending (flexion—extension), e. g., the elbow joint
- Pushing out—pulling in (abduction—adduction), e. g., the hip joint
- Rolling inward—rolling outward (inner rotation—outer rotation), e. g., the shoulder joint
- Forward motion—backward motion (flexion—extension), e. g., hip joint
- Opposition—reposition, e. g., the saddle joint of the thumb

The effect of a muscle on a joint depends on the lever arm, that is, the vertical distance of its insertion to the axis of its joint (force arm). Force and load are in equilibrium when *force × force arm = load × load arm*. The product of force with force arm and of load with load arm is called the *torque* (Fig. 4.**5**).

Function and Structural Principles of Skeletal Muscle

A skeletal muscle is divided into a fleshy, variously shaped *muscle belly* and the usually markedly thinner tendons. The latter are attached to structures in the skeleton or connective tissue of the locomotor system (fasciae, interosseous membrane) and transmit the muscle pull directly or indirectly to parts of the skeleton. In the extremities, the attachment nearest the trunk (proximal) is usually considered the *origin* and that farthest from the trunk (distal) the *insertion* of the muscle. In the trunk, the origin of a muscle is always cephalad. The origin and insertion of a muscle are designated arbitrarily and should not be confused with the *fixed* and *mobile* points, the latter being where the muscle is attached to the part of the skeleton that is moved, the former to that which is fixed. Although the fixed point and the origin coincide in most movements of the extremities, this is not necessarily the case, since the fixed point could be interchanged with the mobile point in the course of a movement.

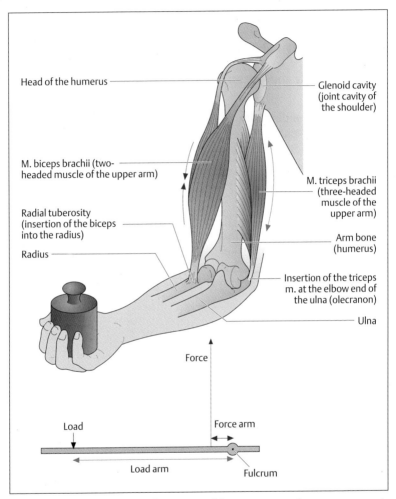

Head of the humerus

Glenoid cavity
(joint cavity of
the shoulder)

M. biceps brachii (two-
headed muscle of the upper arm)

M. triceps brachii
(three-headed
muscle of the
upper arm)

Radial tuberosity
(insertion of the biceps
into the radius)

Radius

Arm bone
(humerus)

Insertion of the triceps
m. at the elbow end of
the ulna (olecranon)

Ulna

Force

Load

Force arm

Load arm

Fulcrum

Fig. 4.**5**   **Effect of the flexors and extensors of the upper arm on forearm movement.**
Flexor at the elbow joint: *m. biceps brachii* (two-headed muscle of the upper arm). Extensor at the elbow joint: *m. triceps brachii* (three-headed muscle of the upper arm). The mechanics of muscle power are shown: load × load lever = force × force lever (the product of
force × force lever and load × load lever constitute the current torque).

At the origin of a muscle there is often a *head* (*caput*) that transitions into a *belly* (*venter*). A muscle with several origins may be two-, three-, or four-headed, all joining to form a single belly and ending in a single tendon. A muscle with a single head but one intersecting tendon is called a *digastric* muscle. A muscle may have several such intervening tendons (Fig. 4.**6**). Muscles that extend over two or more joints are called *diarthric* or *polyarthric* (*multiarticular*), respectively. Muscles that work together in one movement are *synergists*, while those with opposing actions are *antagonists*.

Muscles are also classified according to the way the muscle fibers are inserted into the tendons (e. g., *pennate muscles* from penna = feather) (Fig. 4.**6**). A muscle with *parallel fibers* can achieve considerable height of lift with relatively little force, but because of the small total cross-section of its muscle fibers (*physiological cross-section*), their lifting strength is rather small. The fibers of a *unipennate* muscle are inserted on only one side of the tendon of origin and insertion. This results in a large physiological cross-section and considerable muscular strength. Because the fibers of such a muscle are short, the height of lift is small. In a *bipennate* muscle the muscle fibers originate from a bifurcated tendon and run alongside both sides of the tendon of insertion. The physiological cross-section and so its ability to develop power is here even greater than in a unipennate muscle.

The fine structure of a muscle is determined not only by its striated muscle fibers but also by its connective tissue structures, which form the boundaries between the individual components of each skeletal muscle and are the conduit for the vessels and nerves supplying the muscle fibers (see Fig. 3.**12a–e**). Loose alveolar tissue in the form of *endomysium* forms a sheath around the individual fibers, which in their turn are grouped together by denser white connective tissue (*perimysium*). Several primary bundles are pulled together by another strong connective tissue sheath, the *epimysium*, into the secondary bundles (fleshy fibers) that are visible to the naked eye. A stout connective tissue sheath, the muscle fascia, envelops the whole muscle. Loose areolar tissue (*epimysium*) separates the muscle from the fascia. Several individual muscles can be enclosed by a *common fascia*.

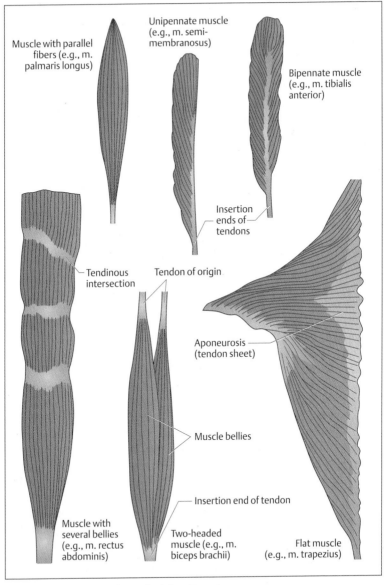

Muscle with parallel fibers (e.g., m. palmaris longus)

Unipennate muscle (e.g., m. semi-membranosus)

Bipennate muscle (e.g., m. tibialis anterior)

Insertion ends of tendons

Tendinous intersection

Tendon of origin

Aponeurosis (tendon sheet)

Muscle bellies

Insertion end of tendon

Muscle with several bellies (e.g., m. rectus abdominis)

Two-headed muscle (e.g., m. biceps brachii)

Flat muscle (e.g., m. trapezius)

Fig. 4.**6** **Various types of muscle.** (After Platzer)

The Tendons

The tendons attaching the muscles to the bones are composed of *bundles of collagen fibers of great tensile strength.* During muscle contractions they transfer force from the muscle to the skeleton. The attachments of the tendons to bone (*tendon attachments*) are of considerable functional significance, since the elasticity of the tendons at these points must be adapted to that of the bones. Tendons are classified according to their shape. When the tendons are very short and invisible to the naked eye, the muscle is said to have a *fleshy muscular attachment*, as, for example, in the case of the pectoralis major muscle. By contrast, the tendons of the muscles of the foot and hand are very long and thin. Flat tendon sheets (Fig. 4.**6**), such as those of the oblique abdominal muscles, are called aponeuroses. Tendons may run in the same direction as the muscles and act directly on the bones (sometimes called *lever tendons*), while others change their direction by running around a bone, which exerts pressure on them as they run over it. Because the bone acts as a pulley for these tendons, they are sometimes called *pulley tendons* and the bone is known as the *fulcrum*. An example of this is the tendon of insertion of the peroneus longus muscle, which runs around the side of the cuboid bone toward its insertion on the sole of the foot.

Auxiliary Structures of Muscles and Tendons

The function of **muscle fasciae**, **tendon sheaths**, **bursae**, and **sesamoid bones** is to reduce friction during muscular work, so that there is a minimum of reduction in force. *Fasciae* allow individual muscles or muscle groups to glide over each other. If tendons run next to a bone or run over a bony protrusion, they are protected by guiding channels that improve their ability to glide. The structure of the wall of such a *synovial tendon sheath* (*vagina synovialis*) is similar to that of a joint capsule and the fluid in the cavity around which the inner and outer synovial layers glide is similar to synovial fluid (Fig. 4.**7**). Where a muscle runs directly over a bone, it is protected by a *synovial bursa*, which is also filled with synovial fluid and which acts like a water cushion, distributing pressure evenly (Fig. 4.**8**). Bursae occur most often at the origins and insertions of

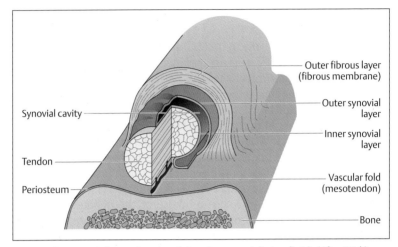

Outer fibrous layer
(fibrous membrane)

Outer synovial
layer

Inner synovial
layer

Vascular fold
(mesotendon)

Bone

Synovial cavity

Tendon

Periosteum

Fig. 4.7 **Structure of a tendon sheath (vagina synovialis tendinis).** (After Frick)
The inner layer of the synovial membrane is firmly adherent to the tendon, the outer layer
to the fibrous inner membrane of the tendon sheath. The cavity around which the two layers glide is filled with synovial fluid. The whole structure reduces friction over bone.

muscles, but they may also be found near joints. Occasionally they are
continuous with the joint capsule, and are then considered *extensions* or
recesses of the capsule. *Sesamoid bones* (*ossa sesamoidea*)are bones
embedded in tendons. Their functional significance is that they extend
the effective lever arm of a muscle and so save muscular effort. The
largest sesamoid bone in humans is the kneecap (patella). Tendon
sheaths and bursae can become inflamed by chronic irritation (tenosy-
novitis and bursitis).

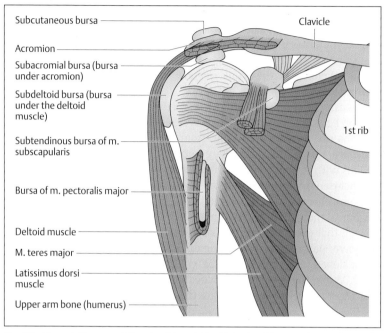

Subcutaneous bursa

Acromion

Subacromial bursa (bursa under acromion)

Subdeltoid bursa (bursa under the deltoid muscle)

Subtendinous bursa of m. subscapularis

Bursa of m. pectoralis major

Deltoid muscle

M. teres major

Latissimus dorsi muscle

Upper arm bone (humerus)

Clavicle

1st rib

Fig. 4.**8** **Synovial bursae of the shoulder girdle.** Right shoulder seen from in front. The muscles have been partially removed.

■ Special Anatomy of the Locomotor System

The fold-out at the end of the book shows the human skeleton in different views.

The Skeleton of the Trunk

With the transition to upright posture, the shape of the human body changed considerably. The *trunk*, rising vertically over the lower limbs, supports the head and the upper limbs. In this way, the lower limbs become the organs of locomotion, while the upper limbs become important "tools" for grasping and feeling. As the trunk becomes erect, the vertebral column develops the curvatures typical for the human body and the hipbones widen and combine with the sacrum to form the pelvis as a solid part of the trunk (Fig. 4.**9**).

The skeleton of the trunk includes the **spinal column** (**vertebral column**) and the **chest cage** (**thorax**), which includes the *ribs* (*costae*), the *breastbone* (*sternum*), and the *thoracic vertebrae* (Fig. 4.**9**). The spinal column contains the spinal canal (vertebral canal) with the spinal cord. The ribs run forward (ventrally) from the spinal column and form the bony structure of the *chest cavity* (thoracic cavity), which below is continuous with the *abdominal cavity* (see p. 349). The thorax and abdomen are enclosed by the bones and muscles of the trunk and abdominal wall. Anatomically, the wall of the trunk can be divided into ventral, lateral, and dorsal thoracic and abdominal walls. The back is that part of the dorsal wall that extends from the base of the skull to the tip of the coccyx. The lower part of the trunk, made up of parts of the abdominal wall and of the lower extremities, can be considered separately as the *pelvic girdle*. While the *diaphragm* divides chest and abdominal cavities, the *muscles of the pelvic floor* separate the abdomen from lower structures.

The Spinal Column

The spinal column forms the axis of the human skeleton (Fig. 4.**10**). It consists of 33–34 *vertebrae*, the *intervertebral disks*, and a number of *ligaments*. The vertebrae consist of 7 cervical vertebrae (neck), 12 thoracic vertebrae (chest), 5 lumbar vertebrae (loins), 5 sacral vertebrae (sacrum) and 4–5 coccygeal vertebrae (coccyx). The indivicual vertebrae are often designated by a shorthand notation as follows: "C5" for the fifth cervical vertebra (for example), and similarly T2, L1, S3, Co1, etc. The 24 vertebrae above the sacrum are called *true* or *presacral vertebrae*, forming the true spinal column In the adult they attain a length of 55–63 cm (ca. 35 % of the body's height). The sacral and coccygeal vertebrae are fused and form the sacrum and the coccyx (tailbone).

In the erect posture, the spinal column in the adult forms a double-S curvature in the sagittal plane, with two anteriorly oriented convexities (*cervical* and *lumbar lordoses*) and two anteriorly oriented concavities (*thoracic* and *sacral kyphoses*) (Fig. 4.**10**). This arrangement creates a flexible rod with elastic springiness that is especially fitted to cushion axial

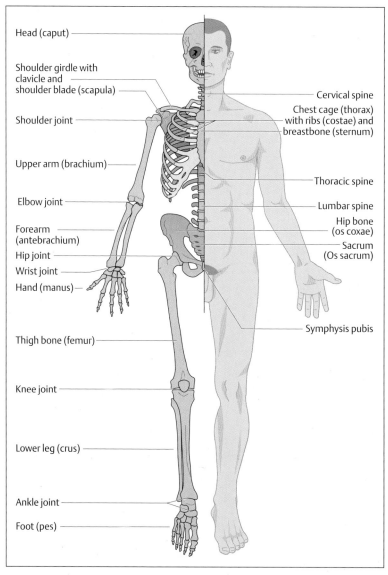

Head (caput)

Shoulder girdle with clavicle and shoulder blade (scapula)

Shoulder joint

Upper arm (brachium)

Elbow joint

Forearm (antebrachium)

Hip joint

Wrist joint

Hand (manus)

Thigh bone (femur)

Knee joint

Lower leg (crus)

Ankle joint

Foot (pes)

Cervical spine

Chest cage (thorax) with ribs (costae) and breastbone (sternum)

Thoracic spine

Lumbar spine

Hip bone (os coxae)

Sacrum (Os sacrum)

Symphysis pubis

Fig. 4.**9 Overview of the human skeleton side by side with the surface of the human body.** Cartilaginous parts are shown in light blue

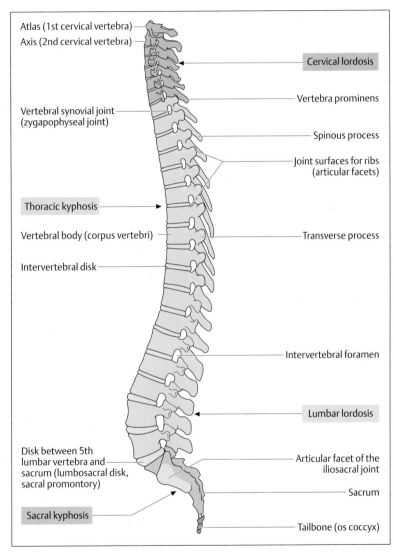

Atlas (1st cervical vertebra)
Axis (2nd cervical vertebra)

Cervical lordosis

Vertebra prominens

Vertebral synovial joint
(zygapophyseal joint)

Spinous process

Joint surfaces for ribs
(articular facets)

Thoracic kyphosis

Vertebral body (corpus vertebri)

Transverse process

Intervertebral disk

Intervertebral foramen

Lumbar lordosis

Disk between 5th
lumbar vertebra and
sacrum (lumbosacral disk,
sacral promontory)

Articular facet of the
iliosacral joint

Sacrum

Sacral kyphosis

Tailbone (os coccyx)

Fig. 4.**10** **Left lateral view of the spinal column**

(vertical) loads, e. g., during running or jumping. The degree of spinal curvature varies in each individual. Lateral curvatures are pathological and are termed *scoliosis*.

The structural principle of the spinal column recalls the structure of a *bowstring*. In the area of the trunk, the thoracic curvature represents the bow, while the abdominal muscles represent the tensed string. In the area of the cervical and lumbar lordoses, tension is achieved by the muscles and ligaments of the back. These tension systems may become unbalanced; for example, if the abdominal muscles are poorly developed, the lumbar lordosis can become exaggerated (*hyperlordosis*).

Structure of a Vertebra

Vertebrae have a common basic shape that changes in the different segments of the spinal column to adapt to their various static needs. Every vertebra—with the exception of the first cervical (atlas, C1)—has a *body* (*corpus vertebrae*), an *arch*, a *spine*, two *transverse processes*, and four *articular facets* (Fig. 4.**11a, b**). The vertebral body and arch enclose the *vertebral foramen*. All the vertebral foramina together form the *vertebral canal*, which houses the spinal cord. Corresponding to the increasing load, the size of the vertebrae increases from above down. The body and transverse processes of the thoracic vertebrae bear joint facets for the ribs. Every vertebral arch at its origin from the vertebral body is marked above and below by a *notch* (*incisura vertebralis, inferior and superior vertebral notch*). The notches of two adjoining vertebrae form the *intervertebral foramen* (Fig. 4.**10**), which transmits the spinal nerves.

Atlas and Axis: Atlanto-Occipital and Atlanto-Axial Joints

The first and second cervical vertebrae have special functions (Fig. 4.**12**). The atlas, which supports the head, has no vertebral body and is shaped like a ring. The two upper joint facets form the atlanto-occipital joint with the joint facets (condyles) of the occiput. This is a condylar joint and allows lateral inclination as well as forward and backward movement. The body of the axis carries on its upper surface a *process shaped like a tooth* (*dens axis*) that has a joint surface anteriorly. This joint connects

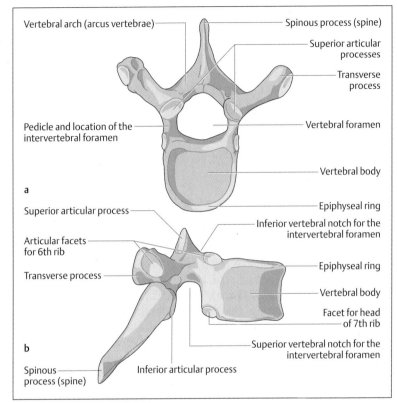

Vertebral arch (arcus vertebrae)

Spinous process (spine)

Superior articular processes

Transverse process

Pedicle and location of the intervertebral foramen

Vertebral foramen

Vertebral body

a

Epiphyseal ring

Superior articular process

Inferior vertebral notch for the intervertebral foramen

Articular facets for 6th rib

Epiphyseal ring

Transverse process

Vertebral body

Facet for head of 7th rib

b

Superior vertebral notch for the intervertebral foramen

Spinous process (spine)

Inferior articular process

Fig. 4.**11** **Sixth thoracic vertebra as an example of the basic shape of a vertebra**
a Viewed from above; **b** viewed from the right. (After Frick)
Cartilaginous articular facets are shown in light blue

the axis with the atlas. Together the atlas and axis form the *atlanto-axial joint*, which allows the head to *rotate* in both directions (total extent of rotation about 50°). The transverse processes of the cervical vertebrae each enclose a hole (*foramen transversarium*) through which the vertebral artery runs toward the head on both sides. The 7th cervical vertebra has a particularly large *spinous process* (*vertebra prominens*), which is the first one from above palpable and visible through the skin.

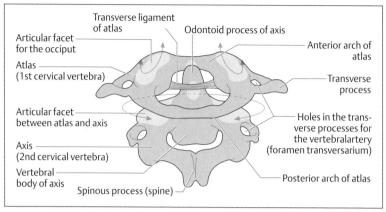

Fig. 4.**12** **Posterior view of the 1st and 2nd cervical vertebrae (atlas and axis).** The two vertebrae have been slightly separated to provide a better view. The arrows show the major directions of motion

Joints and Ligaments of the Vertebral Column

The spinal column is composed of *independently mobile segments* that are connected with each other by mobile and immobile joints. An independently mobile segment is a functional unit. It consists of the bones of two neighboring vertebrae with their connecting disk, the synovial vertebral joints of the vertebral arch (zygapophyseal joints, juncturae zygapophysiales), the ligaments, and the corresponding muscles (Fig. 4.**13a**). The *intervertebral disk* is of pivotal importance in the independently mobile segment. It is composed of an outer dense fibrous tissue ring (annulus fibrosus) and a central gelatinous core (nucleus pulposus) (Fig. 4.**13b**). The disks are attached to the neighboring vertebral bodies by synchondroses, and their position is further secured by the anterior and posterior longitudinal ligaments. Additionally, the spines, the transverse processes, and the vertebral arches are connected to each other by a strong ligamentous system. The *articular facets of the articular processes* (see Figs. 4.**10** and 4.**13a, b**) are flat and are classified as synovial joints. The variations in the directions of their facets determine the mobility of each vertebral segment.

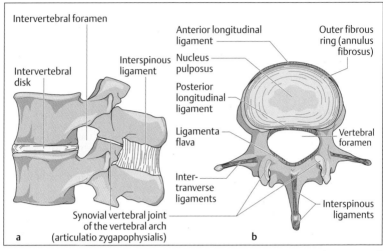

Fig. 4.13 a, b Independently mobile segments and ligaments of the vertebral column

a Lateral view of an independently mobile segment of the lumbar region. The parts of the mobile segment are highlighted in color (muscles and ligaments are shown in part only)

b Lumbar vertebra with disk seen from above. The course of the individual ligaments is shown in red

■ **Function of the Intervertebral Disk.** The function of intervertebral disks can be compared to the function of automobile shock absorbers. When a load is imposed on the disks (when erect), they are pressed down; during prolonged relief from load (when recumbent), they again assume their original shape. They resemble a "water pillow", distributing a central load evenly from the nucleus pulposus to the adjoining annulus fibrosus. In a ruptured disk the annulus fibrosus ruptures, and parts of the nucleus pulposus protrude. Compression of an emerging spinal nerve by the protruded tissue can lead to pain or weakness, e. g., of the lower extremity.

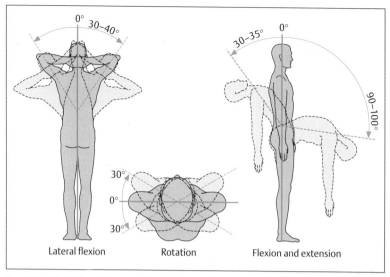

Fig. 4.**14** **Mobility of the vertebral column**. The extent of mobility from zero position (0°) is given in degrees

Movements of the Vertebral Column

The free mobility of the vertebral column results from *the sum of individual movements* in several independent regions. The degree of mobility differs in the various segments. The following main movements are observed:

- Forward and backward bending (flexion and extension) in the sagittal plane
- Lateral bending (lateral flexion) in the coronal plane
- Rotation (torsion) around a vertical axis

The cervical spine is the most mobile. The thoracic segment of the spinal column allows primarily rotation, while in the lumbar region the main possible movements are flexion and extension (Fig. 4.**14**). The degree of movement depends largely on the extensibility of the muscles, the ligaments and also body build.

The Rib Cage (Thorax)

The bones of the thorax enclose the *thoracic cavity*, which has an *inlet* and an *outlet* (*apertura superior thoracis, apertura inferior thoracis*). The thorax protects the organs of the thoracic cavity and is formed by the *breastbone* (*sternum*), the *ribs* (*costae*), and the *thoracic spine* (Fig. 4.**15**). The sternum is a flat bone and consists of the *manubrium* (*handle*), *body* (*corpus*) and a variously shaped *xiphoid process* (Fig. 4.**16**). Normally the thoracic cage is composed of 12 pairs of ribs, of which the first seven pairs, also called *true ribs*, reach the sternum. Of the remaining five pairs of ribs, the 8th, 9th, and 10th are a part of the structure of the costal margin. The remaining two pairs of ribs (*floating ribs*) usually end free in the

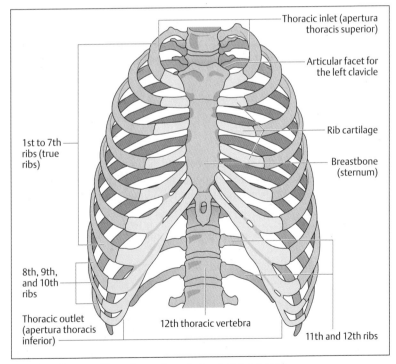

Fig. 4.**15** **Rip cage (thorax) seen from in front.** (After Feneis)

lateral abdominal muscles. The bony parts of the ribs are joined to the sternum by their cartilaginous parts, the rib cartilages, in a synchondrosis. The cartilages of the 1st to 7th ribs generally articulate with the body of the sternum by synovial joints (Fig. 4.**16**).

Each rib is divided into a *head* (*caput costae*), a *neck* (*collum costae*), and a *body* (*corpus costae*). Between the body and the neck of a rib there is a small process, the *tubercle of the rib* (*tuberculum costae*), where the rib is angled sharply forward (Fig. 4.**17**). The ribs form the costo-vertebral joints with the vertebrae. With the exception of the 11th and 12th ribs all ribs have two articular facets, one on the tubercle, the other on the head of the rib. These facets join the ribs with the transverse processes and the vertebral body (Fig. 4.**17**). The movements of both joints must work in tandem.

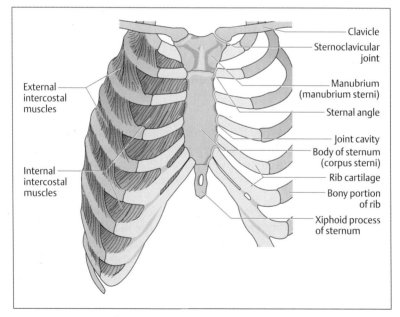

Fig. 4.**16**   **Sternum with 1st to 7th ribs and left sternoclavicular joint seen from in front.** The 1st to 7th ribs are connected to the sternum by synovial joints (double blue line). The intercostal muscles are illustrated on the right side

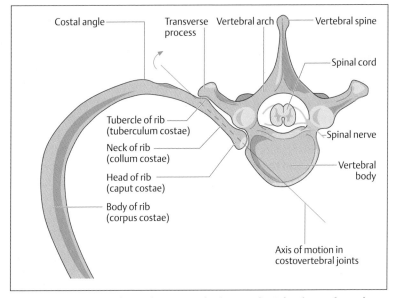

Fig. 4.**17** **Thoracic vertebra and costovertebral joints of a right rib seen from above.**
Joint facets are shown as blue double lines

The ribs are moved by the internal and external intercostal muscles located in the intercostal spaces between the ribs (Fig. 4.**16**). They serve respiration by expanding and contracting the thorax. Additional muscles, the auxiliary respiratory muscles, take part in the movements of the thorax.

The cartilaginous portion of the ribs can lose its elasticity even early in life through calcification, thus restricting the mobility of the thorax. The sternum is situated directly under the skin and, being a flat bone, contains red marrow, which is thus accessible to *sternal puncture* for diagnostic purposes.

The Muscles of the Trunk

The movements of the trunk are effected by large muscle groups that act primarily on the vertebral column. The chest and back especially are also covered by muscles of the shoulder girdle and the upper extremity in addition to the true muscles of the trunk (Figs. 4.**18a**, **b** and 4.**19**). These gradually extended their origins to the trunk in the course of phylogenetic development. The muscles of the trunk are arranged in individual segments like the skeleton. With the exception of a few muscles (e. g., the intercostal muscles), the segments are often not maintained but rather fuse with neighboring segments into larger muscles. The musculature of the trunk is divided into the muscles of the back, the chest, and the abdomen together with the diaphragm and the pelvic muscles (Figs. 4.**18a**, **b** and **4.19**).

The Back

The muscles of the back proper are applied directly to the skeleton and run in two great muscular columns on each side of the vertebral column from the neck to the pelvis. This group of muscles has the collective name *erector spinae* (see Fig. 4.**21**). It is the actual segmental musculature of the back and it may be contrasted with the muscles covering it, which encroach on the back from the upper limb and are usually classified with the muscles of the upper extremity. These encroaching muscles are the muscles of the shoulder girdle, including the *trapezius*, the *greater and lesser rhomboid muscles* (*rhomboideus major and minor*), the *levator scapulae* (elevator of the shoulder), and one of the muscles of the free upper extremity, the *latissimus dorsi* (broad muscle of the back) (Figs. 4.**18a**, **b** and 4.**19**). The trapezius muscle originates from the occipital bone and the spines of the vertebrae. It is inserted into the clavicle, the acromion, and the spine of the scapula, and is one of the most important muscles in the movements of the shoulder blade. The latissimus dorsi muscle takes its origin chiefly from the spinous processes and the iliac crest, and is inserted below the lesser tubercle of the humerus. Its chief action is on the shoulder joint, in that it pulls the arm into the body (adduction), pulls it backward (extension), and rotates it inward (medial rotation).

The Chest Wall

The muscles of the chest wall are arranged in three layers. According to the course and position of the muscles, they are divided into *external, in-*

ternal, and *innermost* (*mm. intercostales externi, interni, and intimi*) (see Fig. 4.**16**). They are the actual *muscles of respiration* and are responsible for the movement of the chest wall in inspiration and expiration. They, too, are covered by the superficial muscles. The *scalene muscles* continue the intercostal muscles cephalad. They originate from the cervical vertebrae and are inserted into the first three ribs. They are the most important muscles in quiet respiration, as they lift the thorax. They are completely covered by other muscles, e. g., the pectoralis major and the serratus anterior (Fig. 4.**18b**).

Another muscle encroaching from the upper limb is the serratus anterior (Fig. 4.**18b**), the serrations of which originate from the 1st to the 9th ribs, and which is inserted into the *medial border of the scapula*. It pulls the scapula forward, and its inferior portion (*pars inferior*) can rotate the inferior angle of the scapula forward (Fig. 4.**20**). This movement allows the arm to be elevated above the horizontal (elevation). When the shoulder girdle is fixed, the serratus anterior can lift the ribs, and so become an auxiliary muscle of respiration.

The *pectoralis major* is another muscle encroaching on the trunk from the upper limb. It is a muscle of the shoulder and originates chiefly from the clavicle, the sternum, and the ribs. It is inserted into the greater tubercle of the humerus (Figs. 4.**18b** and 4.**19**). It is a strong muscle, used to adduct the arm and to rotate it medially. It, too, can function as an auxiliary muscle in respiration by lifting the thorax when the shoulder girdle is fixed.

Another muscle that can lift the thorax is the sternomastoid (*sternocleidomastoid*). Like the trapezius, it is a muscle encroaching on the trunk. It originates from two heads attached to the clavicle and the sternum, and is inserted into the mastoid process of the occipital bone. The sternomastoid muscle acts principally on the joints of the head and the cervical vertebrae. When both sternomastoids contract, the head is thrown back toward the back of the neck; with unilateral contraction, the muscle inclines the head toward the same side and turns it to the opposite side. When the head is fixed, the sternomastoid is also a very important auxiliary respiratory muscle.

Fig. 4.**18a, b**   **View of the superficial musculature from the back and side (a) and** ▷
from the front and side (b). From a "Somso" cast

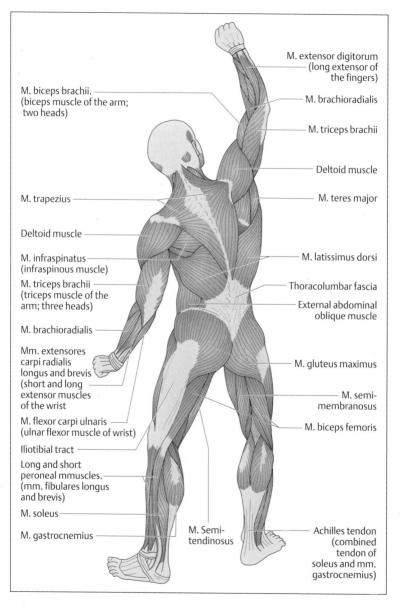

M. extensor digitorum
(long extensor of
the fingers)

M. brachioradialis

M. triceps brachii

Deltoid muscle

M. teres major

M. latissimus dorsi

Thoracolumbar fascia

External abdominal
oblique muscle

M. gluteus maximus

M. semi-
membranosus

M. biceps femoris

Achilles tendon
(combined
tendon of
soleus and mm.
gastrocnemius)

M. biceps brachii.
(biceps muscle of the arm;
two heads)

M. trapezius

Deltoid muscle

M. infraspinatus
(infraspinous muscle)

M. triceps brachii
(triceps muscle of the
arm; three heads)

M. brachioradialis

Mm. extensores
carpi radialis
longus and brevis
(short and long
extensor muscles
of the wrist

M. flexor carpi ulnaris
(ulnar flexor muscle of wrist)

Iliotibial tract

Long and short
peroneal mmuscles.
(mm. fibulares longus
and brevis)

M. soleus

M. gastrocnemius

M. Semi-
tendinosus

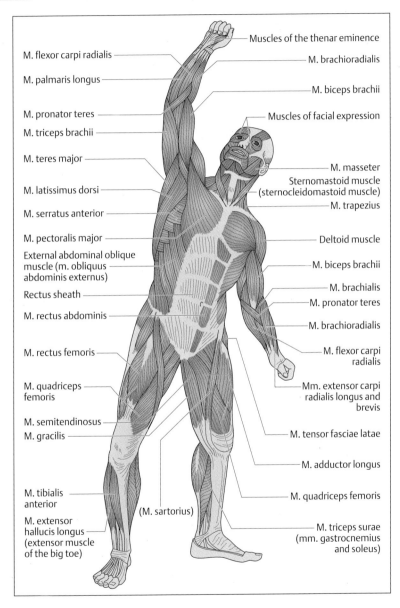

M. flexor carpi radialis

M. palmaris longus

M. pronator teres

M. triceps brachii

M. teres major

M. latissimus dorsi

M. serratus anterior

M. pectoralis major

External abdominal oblique muscle (m. obliquus abdominis externus)

Rectus sheath

M. rectus abdominis

M. rectus femoris

M. quadriceps femoris

M. semitendinosus

M. gracilis

M. tibialis anterior

M. extensor hallucis longus (extensor muscle of the big toe)

(M. sartorius)

Muscles of the thenar eminence

M. brachioradialis

M. biceps brachii

Muscles of facial expression

M. masseter

Sternomastoid muscle (sternocleidomastoid muscle)

M. trapezius

Deltoid muscle

M. biceps brachii

M. brachialis

M. pronator teres

M. brachioradialis

M. flexor carpi radialis

Mm. extensor carpi radialis longus and brevis

M. tensor fasciae latae

M. adductor longus

M. quadriceps femoris

M. triceps surae (mm. gastrocnemius and soleus)

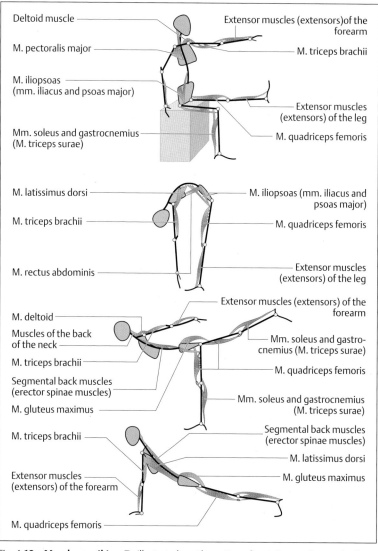

Fig. 4.**19   Muscle manikins.** To illustrate how the action of certain muscles results from their origin, insertion, and course

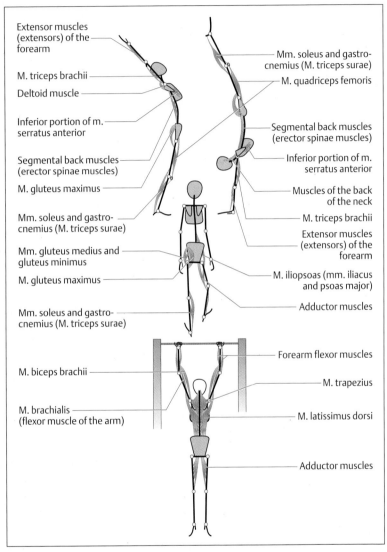

Extensor muscles (extensors) of the forearm

M. triceps brachii

Deltoid muscle

Inferior portion of m. serratus anterior

Segmental back muscles (erector spinae muscles)

M. gluteus maximus

Mm. soleus and gastrocnemius (M. triceps surae)

Mm. gluteus medius and gluteus minimus

M. gluteus maximus

Mm. soleus and gastrocnemius (M. triceps surae)

M. biceps brachii

M. brachialis (flexor muscle of the arm)

Mm. soleus and gastrocnemius (M. triceps surae)

M. quadriceps femoris

Segmental back muscles (erector spinae muscles)

Inferior portion of m. serratus anterior

Muscles of the back of the neck

M. triceps brachii

Extensor muscles (extensors) of the forearm

M. iliopsoas (mm. iliacus and psoas major)

Adductor muscles

Forearm flexor muscles

M. trapezius

M. latissimus dorsi

Adductor muscles

Fig. 4.**19** (continued)

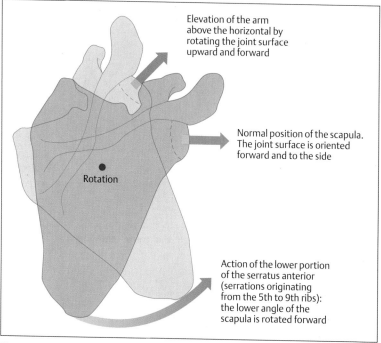

Elevation of the arm above the horizontal by rotating the joint surface upward and forward

Normal position of the scapula. The joint surface is oriented forward and to the side

Rotation

Action of the lower portion of the serratus anterior (serrations originating from the 5th to 9th ribs): the lower angle of the scapula is rotated forward

Fig. 4.**20**   **Action of the inferior part of the serratus anterior in lifting the upper arm above 90° (elevation).** The normal position of the scapula and its joint cavity is edged in green; the rotated scapula during elevation is edged in red. (After Faller)

The Abdominal Wall

The muscles of the abdominal wall are divided according to their location into *straight* (*anterior*), *oblique* (*lateral*) and *deep abdominal muscles*. The oblique muscles are arranged in three layers and their *aponeuroses* (*flat tendons*) anteriorly form a sheath (*rectus sheath*) that encloses the *rectus abdominis* (*straight muscle*) and serves it as a guiding channel (Figs. 4.**18b**, 4.**21**). The rectus abdominis has several tendons separating multiple bellies and runs from the superior border of the pubis, lateral to the symphysis, upward to the insertion of the ribs into the sternum. Of the oblique muscles, the *external oblique* runs superficially from the

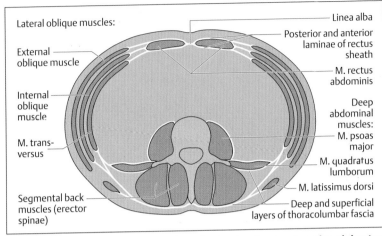

Fig. 4.**21 Schematic cross-section through the trunk, showing the abdominal muscles.** (After Faller)

lateral portions of the lower ribs obliquely forward to the iliac crest and to the rectus sheath. The *internal oblique* runs in the layer deep to this, its fibers running almost at right angles to the external oblique. Its aponeurosis also fuses with the rectus sheath. The innermost layer is formed by the *transversus abdominis*. The *psoas major* and the *quadratus lumborum* muscles, together with the lumbar spine, form the posterior abdominal wall (Fig. 4.21).

The muscles of the abdominal wall, together with their aponeuroses, form a *functional entity*, in that they exert their pull in different directions, forming an *oblique support*. The arrangement of the abdominal musculature allows rotation, flexion, and lateral inclination of the trunk. At the same time, the abdominal muscles act to exert pressure on the abdominal contents, and so assist the emptying of the urinary bladder and the rectum. They also take part in expiration by raising the diaphragm.

The Diaphragm

The dome-shaped diaphragm is the *most important muscle of respiration* and separates the abdominal from the thoracic cavity in the form of a musculotendinous partition. The muscle arises in a ring from the inferior thoracic outlet (Fig. 4.**22**). Its muscle fibers arch upward and radiate into a *central tendon* (*centrum tendineum, trefoil tendon*). According to its various origins, the diaphragm is divided into a *costal part* (*pars costalis*), a *lumbar* (*vertebral*) *part* (*pars lumbalis*), and a *sternal part* (*pars sternalis*). The inferior vena cava runs through an opening in the central tendon; the aorta and the esophagus enter the abdominal cavity from the thorax through two slitlike openings (e. g., aortic hiatus) in the lumbar part.

In life, the shape and position of the diaphragm change with breathing (Fig. 4.**23**), posture, and body position and the degree of fullness of the inner organs. When the diaphragm contracts, the thoracic cavity enlarges and thereby supports inspiration. In the relaxed state, with simultaneous contraction of the abdominal muscles, the diaphragm rises, which leads to expiration. Each displacement of the diaphragm has an effect on the abdominal organs. For instance, the inferior border of the liver descends with inspiration and rises again on expiration. In the erect posture, the left dome of the diaphragm projects to the upper border of the 5th rib during maximal expiration, while the right dome rises a little higher, to the level of the 4th intercostal space. During maximal inspiration the two domes descend by about 3–6 cm (Fig. 4.**23**).

The Pelvic Floor

The pelvic outlet, and therefore the abdominal cavity, is incompletely closed by *muscles* and *connective tissue structures*. Together they form the pelvic floor, which plays a significant role in the position of the pelvic and abdominal organs. The mechanical strength of the fibromuscular pelvic floor is limited by the emergence through it of the intestinal as well as the urinary and genital tracts (Fig. 4.**24**).

The pelvic floor consists in part of a funnel-shaped muscle, the *levator ani*, which, together with its connective tissue sheath (fascia), forms the *pelvic diaphragm*; and in part of a muscle crossed by connective tissue bands, the *deep transverse perineal muscle*, which, together with

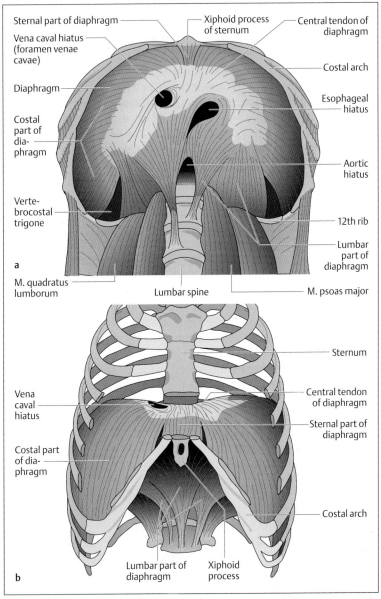

Sternal part of diaphragm

Xiphoid process of sternum

Central tendon of diaphragm

Vena caval hiatus (foramen venae cavae)

Costal arch

Diaphragm

Esophageal hiatus

Costal part of dia-phragm

Aortic hiatus

Verte-brocostal trigone

12th rib

Lumbar part of diaphragm

a

M. quadratus lumborum

Lumbar spine

M. psoas major

Sternum

Vena caval hiatus

Central tendon of diaphragm

Sternal part of diaphragm

Costal part of dia-phragm

Costal arch

b

Lumbar part of diaphragm

Xiphoid process

Fig. 4.**22 a, b** **Diaphragm, viewed from below (a) and from in front (b).** Parts of the thoracic cage have been removed. (After Benninghoff)

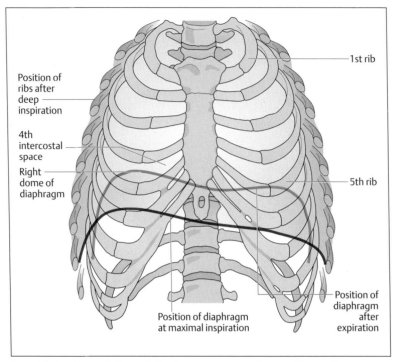

Position of
ribs after
deep
inspiration

4th
intercostal
space

Right
dome of
diaphragm

1st rib

5th rib

Position of
diaphragm
after
expiration

Position of diaphragm
at maximal inspiration

Fig. 4.**23** **Position of ribs and diaphragm at maximal inspiration and expiration.**
With maximal inspiration the thoracic cage widens and the diaphragm flattens. At maximal expiration the diaphragm arches back into the thorax and the thorax narrows. (After Frick et al)

its fascia, forms the *urogenital diaphragm* (Fig. 4.**24**). The levator ani muscle is attached to the internal surface of the true pelvis in a semicircular fashion and has an anteriorly directed opening, the tendinous arch of the levator ani. It transmits the urethra, the rectum, and in the female also the vagina. The tendinous arch of the levator ani is closed by the urogenital diaphragm, which extends in the shap of a trapezium between the pubic rami (Fig. 4.**24**).

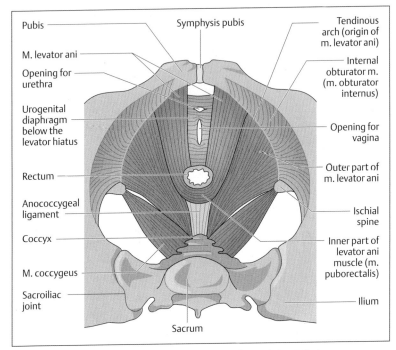

Fig. 4.**24**   **Muscles of the female perineum from above.** (After Faller)

The inner part of the levator ani (*puborectalis m.*), together with the external anal sphincter (*sphincter ani externus m.*), forms a very effective (voluntary) closing mechanism (sphincter) of the rectum (Fig. 4. **25**). The *sphincter urethrae* muscle allows the urethra to be closed voluntarily, damming urinary flow.

If the muscles of the pelvic floor are overdistended, e. g., during parturition, the internal genital organs of a woman can prolapse. Similarly, tears in the course of parturition (*perineal tears*) may damage the levator ani or the sphincter ani externus to the point of impairing control of rectal content (*rectal incontinence*).

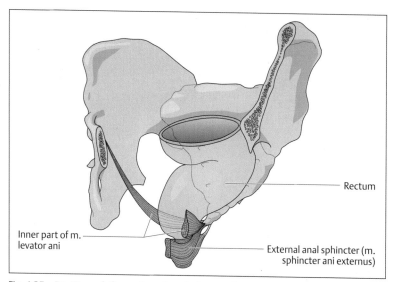

Rectum

Inner part of m. levator ani

External anal sphincter (m. sphincter ani externus)

Fig. 4.**25** **Position of the rectum in relation to the pelvic floor.** Left anterior view. Parts of the pelvic skeleton have been removed. (After Leonhardt)

The Upper Extremity

One of the essential tasks of the two upper extremities in man is to support grasping and touching. The basis for these activities is an extensive mobility of the upper limb, giving the hand as much room to move as possible. The upper extremity includes the shoulder girdle and the free upper limb. (A complete illustration of all bones and comprehensive labeling of all structures is provided in the pull-out illustration at the end of the book.)

The Shoulder Girdle—Bones, Joints, Muscles

The shoulder girdle includes the *clavicle* and the *shoulder blade* (*scapula*). It forms the base for the upper extremity and, contrary to the pelvic girdle, is not firmly anchored to the trunk (Fig. 4.**26**). It is linked to the

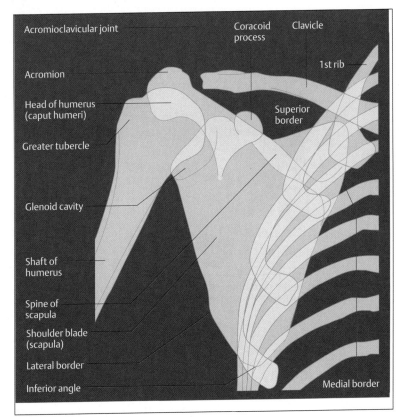

Acromioclavicular joint

Coracoid process

Clavicle

1st rib

Acromion

Head of humerus (caput humeri)

Superior border

Greater tubercle

Glenoid cavity

Shaft of humerus

Spine of scapula

Shoulder blade (scapula)

Lateral border

Inferior angle

Medial border

Fig. 4.**26** **Simplified tracing of a radiographic image of the right shoulder seen from in front.** In the radiographic image the joint cavity appears to be wider because the joint cartilage is not seen.

trunk by a joint, the *sternoclavicular joint* (Fig. 4.**27**), which, by virtue of its range of motion, functionally represents a ball-and-socket joint. The scapula is guided along the thorax by a muscular sling.

The clavicle is an S-shaped bone connecting the sternum with the scapula. It is attached to the trunk by strong ligaments to the 1st rib, the sternum and the *coracoid process*. The clavicle is joined to the scapula by the *acromioclavicular joint*. The scapula is a triangular flat

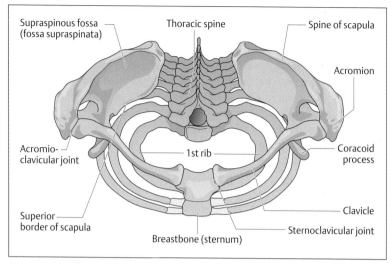

Fig. 4.**27**   **Shoulder girdle seen from above**

bone with a shallow facet (*glenoid cavity*) for the shoulder joint at its upper lateral end. The posterior surface features the *spine*, which runs obliquely upward, and the outer end bears the *acromion process*, which can easily be palpated externally (Fig. 4.**26** and 4.**27**). The acromion, the coracoid process, and the strong ligament connecting them (*coracoacromial ligament*) form a roof over the shoulder joint (*fornix humeri*) (see Fig. 4.**30b**).

The axillary and vertebral borders (*margo lateralis* and *margo medialis*) of the scapula meet at the *inferior angle* of the scapula (Fig. 4.**26**). The scapula is moved on the trunk by a muscular sling. The muscles of the shoulder girdle include the *trapezius*, the *serratus anterior*, the *levator scapulae*, and the *major* and *minor rhomboid muscles* (Figs. 4.**18a, b** and 4.**19**). (The three last-named muscles lie deep and are therefore not illustrated.)

The Free Upper Limb—Bones, Joints, Muscles

The free upper limb begins at the shoulder joint and includes the *humerus*, the two *bones of the forearm, radius and ulna*, and the *hand* (*manus*), composed of *wrist* (*carpus*), *metacarpus*, and *fingers* (*digits*). Toward the fingers, the number of bones, and therefore the possible number of joints, increases. The important joints of the free upper limb are the shoulder joint, the elbow joint, the wrist joint, the carpometacarpal joint, the saddle joint of the thumb, and the proximal, middle, and distal joints of the fingers.

The Bones of the Upper Arm, the Forearm, and the Hand

■ **Upper Arm (Brachium).** The humerus is a long bone, and it has a shaft (*corpus humeri*) as well as proximal and distal ends (*epiphyses*). The end nearest the body is formed by the *head of the humerus*, which is connected to the *glenoid cavity* (Fig. 4.**26**). At the transition to the humeral shaft there are two solid tubercles, which provide attachment to the muscles acting on the shoulder joint. In front lies the *lesser tubercle*, which distally (away from the trunk) is continued in the crest of the lesser tubercle (*crista tuberculi minoris*); laterally lies the *greater tubercle*, which is continued in the crest of the greater tubercle (*crista tuberculi majoris*). Between the two tubercles lies a groove (bicipital groove) for the tendon of the long head of the biceps (see Fig. 4.**30b**).

The distal end of the shaft of the humerus ends in the spherical *capitulum humeri*, which forms the joint with the radius, and in a markedly larger bobbin-shaped roll, the *trochlea humeri*, which forms the joint with the ulna (Fig. 4.**28a, b**). The medial and lateral sides of the distal end are marked by large bony protrusions, the medial and lateral epicondyles. Behind the larger medial epicondyle runs the ulnar nerve to the forearm and hand. Pressing this nerve against the bone elicits a brief painful sensation that radiates into the fingers ("funny bone").

■ **Forearm (Antebrachium).** The skeleton of the forearm consists of the *radius* and the *ulna*. A membrane, the *interosseus membrane* (see Fig. 4.**32**), connects the shafts of both bones and ensures their cohesion. It also distributes any pull and pressure exerted by one bone to the other and serves as origin for the forearm muscles. The ulna features at its proximal end a hook-shaped process, the *olecranon* (Fig. 4.**28a, b**). With this process the ulna grasps the trochlea of the humerus and so forms the hinge joint between the humerus and the ulna. Distally the ulna narrows and contributes only a small surface to the wrist joint. By contrast, the radius is thinner proximally and broader and more strongly developed distally. At its proximal end it bears a small flat head (*caput radii*), the cartilaginous facet of which forms joints with the humerus (*elbow joint, humeroradial joint*) and the ulna (*superior radioulnar joint, proximal radioulnar joint*). The distal end of the radius, like the ulna, bears a small process, the *condyloid process*. Both condyloid processes are easily palpable through the skin (Fig. 4.**28a**).

■ **The Hand (Manus).** The wrist consists of eight bones arranged in two rows, a proximal and a distal row (Fig. 4.**29**). The proximal row consists of the radially situated *scaphoid* (*navicular*) bone, the middle *lunate* bone, the ulnar *triquetrum*, and the *pisiform bone* (pea-shaped bone). The distal carpal bones include (from radial to ulnar) the *trapezium*, the *trapezoid bone*, the centrally situated *capitate bone*, and the *hamate bone*.

Of the five metacarpal bones, only the first metacarpal forms a mobile joint, the *saddle joint of the thumb*, with the trapezium. All the other metacarpals are joined to the bones of the wrist by plane joints with strong ligaments that limit their mobility. The metacarpal bones are continued in the bones of the fingers (*phalanges*), each finger consisting of a *proximal*, *middle*, and *distal phalanx*. The thumb has only two phalanges, lacking a middle phalanx (Fig. 4.**29**). The metacarpals are joined to the proximal phalanges and the proximal, middle, and distal phalanges to each other, by synovial joints. These are the metacarpophalangeal and the proximal and distal interphalangeal joints (Fig. 4.**29**).

The Shoulder Joint (Articulatio Humeri)

The shoulder joint is the most mobile ball-and-socket joint in the human skeleton. Because of the difference in the size of the head of the humerus and the glenoid cavity of the scapula, the joint provides little bony

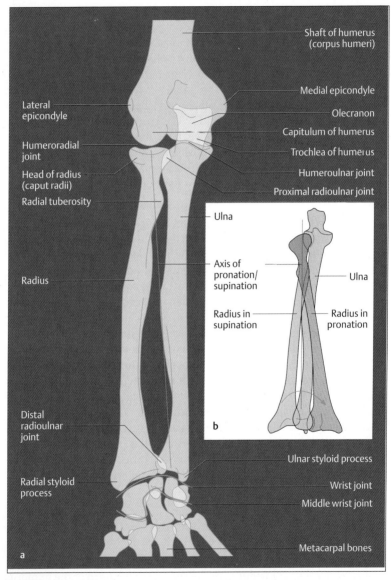

Shaft of humerus (corpus humeri)

Medial epicondyle

Lateral epicondyle

Olecranon

Capitulum of humerus

Humeroradial joint

Trochlea of humerus

Head of radius (caput radii)

Humeroulnar joint

Radial tuberosity

Proximal radioulnar joint

Ulna

Radius

Axis of pronation/ supination

Ulna

Radius in supination

Radius in pronation

Distal radioulnar joint

b

Ulnar styloid process

Radial styloid process

Wrist joint

Middle wrist joint

a

Metacarpal bones

Fig. 4.**28 a, b**

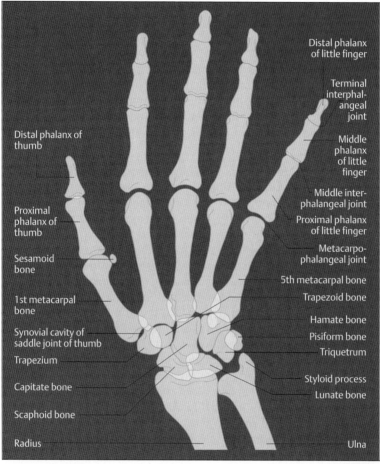

Distal phalanx of thumb

Proximal phalanx of thumb

Sesamoid bone

1st metacarpal bone

Synovial cavity of saddle joint of thumb

Trapezium

Capitate bone

Scaphoid bone

Radius

Distal phalanx of little finger

Terminal interphal- angeal joint

Middle phalanx of little finger

Middle inter- phalangeal joint

Proximal phalanx of little finger

Metacarpo- phalangeal joint

5th metacarpal bone

Trapezoid bone

Hamate bone

Pisiform bone

Triquetrum

Styloid process

Lunate bone

Ulna

Fig. 4.**29**   **Simplified tracing of a radiographic image of the right hand in dorsal view**

◁ Fig. 4.**28 a, b**   **Simplified tracing of a radiographic image of the right forearm** (the blue lines indicate the lines of the joints of the wrist)
a   In supination. Ulna and radius are parallel
b   Radius in supination and pronation

guidance. It is secured primarily by muscles and to a lesser extent by ligaments. For this reason, *dislocations* (*subluxations*) of the shoulder joint are especially common (about 45% of all dislocations affect the shoulder joint).

The glenoid cavity is bordered by a fibrocartilaginous lip (*labrum glenoidale*), about 5 mm in breadth, that increases the joint contact and so the stress-absorbing surface. The joint capsule is wide and lax, and with the arm dependent forms a recess on the medial side (Fig. 4.**30a**). This extra fold ensures that there is no resistance especially during abduction.

■ **Muscles and Movements.** The coracoid process and the acromion, together with the coracoacromial ligament (fornix humeri, Fig. 4.**30b**), limit upward mobility and at the same time secure the head of the humerus in the glenoid cavity. When the arm is lifted above the horizontal, the scapula, and so the glenoid cavity, must rotate. The movements at the shoulder joint take place in three axes, as in every ball-and-socket joint. The muscular action occurs chiefly in the *musculotendinous cuff* (*rotator cuff*, i.e., *supraspinatus*, *infraspinatus*, *subscapularis*, and *teres minor muscles*) and the *deltoid muscle*, the most important abductor of the upper arm (Figs. 4.**18a, b** and 4.**19**). In addition, the anterior part of the deltoid (pars clavicularis) flexes the arm and the posterior part (pars scapularis) extends it (Fig. 4.**31**).

The muscles of the musculotendinous cuff all have their origin on the scapula and are inserted into the greater or lesser tubercle of the humerus. While the *teres minor* and the *infraspinatus muscles* rotate the upper arm outward (external rotation), the *subscapularis muscle* is an important internal rotator. Finally, the *supraspinatus muscle* takes part in abduction, especially its initiation. The *pectoralis major*, the *latissimus dorsi*, and the *teres major muscles* adduct the arm (pull it toward the trunk) and to varying extents rotate it externally or internally (Figs. 4.**18a, b** and 4.**31**).

The Elbow Joint (Articulatio Cubiti)

The elbow joint is a hinge joint and a *compound joint* with three joint elements in the lax joint capsule. It is composed of three separate joints, the *humeroradial joint*, the *humeroulnar joint*, and the *proximal radioulnar*

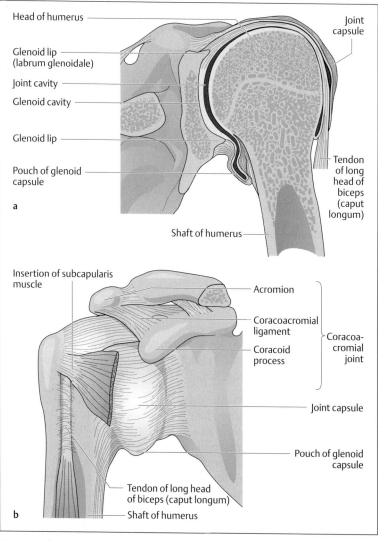

Head of humerus

Joint capsule

Glenoid lip (labrum glenoidale)

Joint cavity

Glenoid cavity

Glenoid lip

Pouch of glenoid capsule

Tendon of long head of biceps (caput longum)

a

Shaft of humerus

Insertion of subcapularis muscle

Acromion

Coracoacromial ligament

Coracoid process

Coracoacromial joint

Joint capsule

Pouch of glenoid capsule

Tendon of long head of biceps (caput longum)

b

Shaft of humerus

Fig. 4.**30 a, b** **Right shoulder joint**
a Coronal section, anterior view
b Joint capsule and acromioclavicular joint, anterior view (After Platzer)

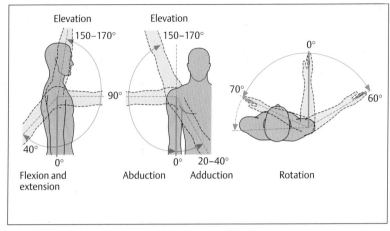

Fig. 4.**31**   **Movements of the shoulder joint**

joint. While the joint between the humerus and ulna (humeroulnar joint) acts as a typical hinge joint, allowing only flexion and extension, the head of the radius has joints with the humerus (humeroradial joint) as well as the ulna (proximal radioulnar joint) (Figs. 4.**28a**, 4.**32**).

■ **Muscles and Movements.** The proximal radioulnar joint, in combination with the distal radioulnar joint, allows the hand to be turned forward and backward (pronation and supination) (Figs. 4.**28b**, 4.**33**). As the hand turns, the radius pivots in place at the elbow joint, while pivoting around the ulna at its distal (hand) end. The position in which the forearm bones are parallel and the palm faces upward, is called *supination*. When the radius crosses the ulna, the back of the hand faces upward. This position is called *pronation*. The head of the radius is fixed by two *collateral ligaments* aided by an *annular ligament* that surrounds the radial head (Fig. 4.**32a**–c).

Muscles originating from the humerus or the shoulder girdle and inserted into the ulna include the triceps (*m. triceps brachii*), which runs along the posterior side of the upper arm and extends the elbow, and the

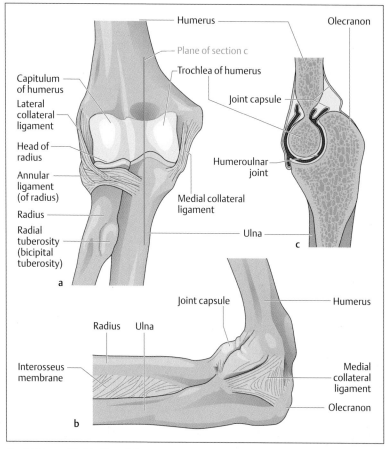

Fig. 4.**32 a–c   Right elbow joint**
a Ligaments, anterior view
b Ligaments and joint capsule, medial view
c Longitudinal section through the humeroulnar joint (After Platzer)

biceps (*m. biceps brachii*), which runs along the front of the upper arm
and flexes the elbow. Both the biceps and the triceps also act on the
shoulder joint, because one head of each originates from the scapula
(Figs. 4.**18a**, **b** and 4.**19**). Four muscles primarily take part in pronation

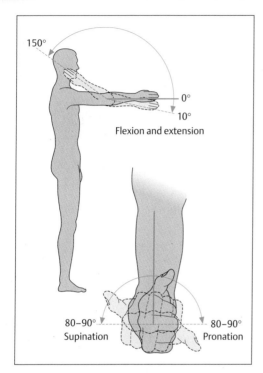

150°

0°

10°

Flexion and extension

80–90°
Supination

80–90°
Pronation

Fig. 4.**33**   **Movements at the elbow joint.** Pronation and supination additionally involve the distal radioulnar joint

and supination, two internal rotator muscles (*m. pronator teres* and *m. pronator quadratus*) and two external rotator muscles (*mm. supinator* and *biceps brachii*).

Beside its function as flexor at the elbow, the biceps, with its insertion in a roughened area of the radius (radial tuberosity) (Fig. 4.**32**), is the strongest supinator. This external rotation is especially strong when the elbow is flexed and at the same time the biceps tendon unwinds from a coiled position around the radius.

The Joints of the Hand

The proximal *wrist joint* (*radiocarpal joint*) between the radius and ulna on one side, and the wrist on the other, is a typical condyloid joint. The *middle carpal joint* is formed by the proximal and distal rows of carpal bones and forms an S-shaped joint cavity with interdigitation of the bones (Fig. 4.**28a**). The trapezium and the first metacarpal bone form an extraordinarily mobile joint, the *saddle joint of the thumb* (*carpometacarpal joint of the thumb*).

■ **Muscles and Movements.** Because of its saddle shape, the joint allows four movements: abduction, adduction, flexion, and extension of the thumb. The joint also allows a composite rotational movement—opposition—in which the thumb touches the index finger. In all nine muscles are involved in movements of the thumb. In movements of the wrist both wrist joints act in concert, though the radiocarpal joint makes the largest contribution. Flexion (palmar flexion) and extension occur around an axis running transversely to the radius and ulna. *Lateral movements* of the hand (adduction and abduction) occur around a second axis that runs vertically through a carpal bone (the capitate). Because of the interdigitation at the midcarpal joint, these movements occur exclusively at the radiocarpal joint.

With the exception of the short muscles of the hand, the muscles acting on the carpal joints and the saddle joint of the thumb originate predominantly from the forearm. Their tendons run in protective tendon sheaths to the wrist or the metacarpal bones, where they act exclusively on the wrist, or to the fingers, which they move simultaneously with the joints of the hand. Eighteen short muscles of the hand and 15 forearm muscles take part in the small movements of grasping and touching. The forearm muscles are divided by their position. The radius and ulna and the interosseus membrane between them separate the flexors anteriorly from the extensors posteriorly. A separate radial muscle group lies between these two muscle groups. Flexors and extensors are both divided into superficial and deep groups (Figs. 4.**18a**, **b** and 4.**19**).

The Lower Extremity

The lower extremities in the human are exclusively organs of *support* and *locomotion*. They can be divided into a **pelvic girdle** and a **free lower limb**. In contrast to the shoulder girdle, the pelvic girdle is solidly connected to the axial skeleton.

The Pelvic Girdle and the Pelvis—Bones, Joints, Muscles

The components of the pelvic girdle are the two *hip bones* (*innominate bones, ossa coxae*) that in combination with the *sacrum* form the *bony pelvis*. The Sacrum and innominate bones are connected to each other by the *sacroiliac joints*, synovial joints that, by virtue of their strong ligaments, are almost immobile. Anteriorly, the two innominate bones are connected by the *symphysis pubis* (Fig. 4.**34a**, **b**). The sacroiliac joints and symphysis pubis connect the bony parts of the pelvis into a stable ring and allow only very limited movement.

The bony pelvis is composed of the two innominate bones and the sacrum. The innominate bone is composed of three parts, the *ilium*, the *ischium*, and the *pubis* (Fig. 4.**35a**, **b**). The bony parts fuse at the acetabulum (articular facet of the hip joint) about the 14th to 16th years of life to form a single bone, the innominate bone. The sacrum and the innominate bone are connected on each side by two strong ligaments, which exert a strong stabilizing effect on the pelvis. The stronger band (*sacrotuberal ligament*) runs from the *ischial tuberosity* to the sacrum, while the second, weaker band (*sacrospinal ligament*) connects the *ischial spine* with the sacrum.

The pelvis is divided into the false pelvis and the true pelvis. The line between them (*linea terminalis, iliopectineal line*) is situated in the plane of the pelvic brim. It is formed by a bony line (*the arcuate line*), the upper border of the symphysis pubis, and the disk between the 5th lumbar vertebra and the sacrum (*sacral promontory*) (Figs. 4.**34a**, **b** and 4.**36**). In the erect posture the plane of the pelvic inlet forms a 60° angle to the horizontal (Fig. 4.**36**). The false pelvis is formed laterally by the iliac fossae and posteriorly by the sacrum. The upper border of the iliac fossa is termed the *iliac crest*. Anteriorly it ends in the *anterior superior iliac spine*, from which the *inguinal ligament* stretches to the *pubic tubercle* (Fig. 4.**36**).

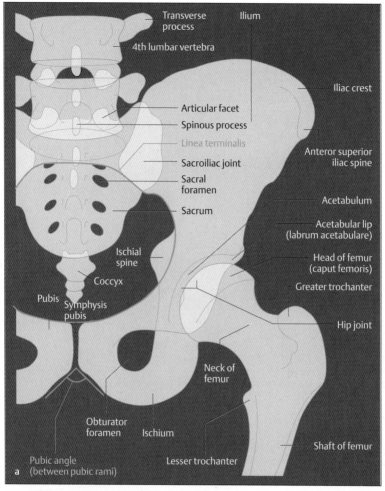

Fig. 4.**34 a** **Simplified tracing of a radiographic image of the pelvis and left hip joint (articulatio coxae) in anterior view**

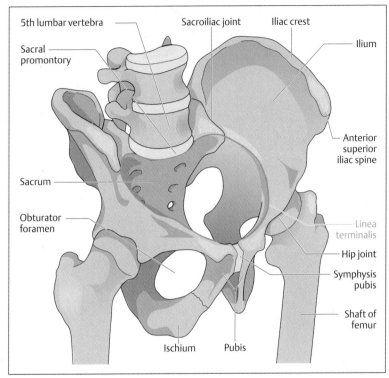

5th lumbar vertebra

Sacroiliac joint

Iliac crest

Sacral promontory

Ilium

Anterior superior iliac spine

Sacrum

Obturator foramen

Linea terminalis

Hip joint

Symphysis pubis

Shaft of femur

Ischium

Pubis

Fig. 4.**34 b**   **Bony pelvis in right anterior view** (After Schwegler)

The true pelvis is formed by the two pubic bones and the two ischial bones. Between the upper and lower branches (*superior and inferior rami*) of the pubis and the bordering ischium there is an oval opening (*obturator foramen*), closed by a connective tissue membrane (*obturator membrane*) (Fig. 4.**34a, b**). The *pelvic outlet* is bordered by the coccyx, the ischial spine, and the ischial tuberosity. Pelvic inlet, pelvic canal, and pelvic outlet of the true pelvis form the *birth canal* and as such have great practical significance.

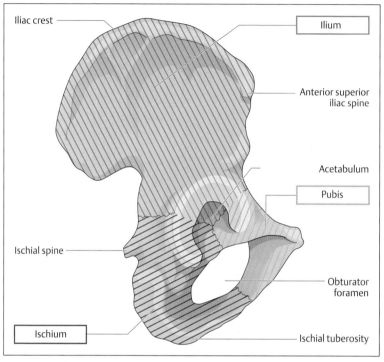

Iliac crest

Ilium

Anterior superior
iliac spine

Acetabulum

Pubis

Ischial spine

Obturator
foramen

Ischium

Ischial tuberosity

Fig. 4.**35**   **Right hip bone (innominate bone, os coxae) in lateral view**

The shape of the pelvis shows marked *sexual differences*: in the female the two iliac fossae extend more laterally. The transition from the false to the true female pelvis is oval in its transverse dimension, while in the male it is smaller and posteriorly narrowed markedly by the more prominent sacral promontory. The angle between the two inferior pubic rami is greater in the female pelvis than in the male (Fig. 4.**37**). Finally, the obturator foramen in the female pelvis is transversely oval, while that of the male is almost round. The pelvic outlet, determined by the

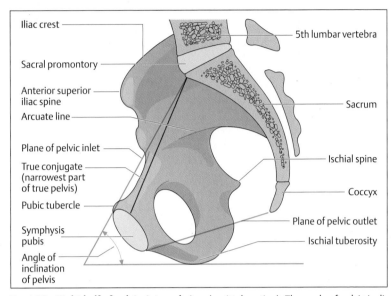

Iliac crest

5th lumbar vertebra

Sacral promontory

Anterior superior iliac spine

Sacrum

Arcuate line

Plane of pelvic inlet

True conjugate (narrowest part of true pelvis)

Ischial spine

Pubic tubercle

Coccyx

Plane of pelvic outlet

Symphysis pubis

Ischial tuberosity

Angle of inclination of pelvis

Fig. 4.**36**   **Right half of pelvis, internal view** (sagittal section). The angle of pelvic inclination between the plane of the pelvic inlet and the horizontal is about 60° in the erect posture. (After Faller)

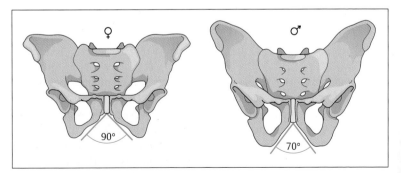

♀

♂

90°

70°

Fig. 4.**37**   **Female and male pelvis.** Female pubic angle = 90°; male pubic angle = 70°. (After Schwegler)

ischial tuberosity and the ischial spine, is also wider in the female. The musculature of the pelvis and the pelvic floor is described with that of the trunk (see above Muscles of the Trunk: The Pelvic Floor).

The Free Lower Limb—Bones, Joints, Muscles

The free lower limb is connected to the pelvic girdle by the hip joint. It consists of the *thigh bone* (*femur*), the (*lower*) *leg* (*crus*) including *tibia* and *fibula*, and the *foot* (*pes*), which includes the *ankle* (*tarsus*), *metatarsals*, and *toes* (*digits*). The movements between femur and lower leg occur at the knee joint (*genu*), which is a principal factor in the movement sequence of walking. The tibia and fibula are connected to the foot by the ankle joint. Together with the mid-tarsal (talocalcaneonavicular) joint and the other joints of the foot, this freely mobile joint enables the foot to roll during walking.

Bones of the Thigh, Lower Leg, and Foot

■ **The Thigh (Femur).** The thigh bone (femur) is the longest and strongest bone of the human skeleton. Proximally, the *shaft of the femur* (*diaphysis*) continues into the *femoral neck* (*collum femoris*), which is directed obliquely upward and which ends in the *head of the femur* (*caput femoris*). In the adult the angle of the neck to the shaft (*collodiaphyseal angle*) is about 125–126°. In the newborn the angle is markedly greater (ca. 150°), while in the elderly it may be smaller than 126° (Fig. 4.**38a–c**). At the junction between the shaft and neck there are two processes, the robust externally directed greater trochanter, and the somewhat smaller internally directed lesser trochanter (Fig. **4.34a**, **b**). Both trochanters are the site of muscle insertions. Anteriorly and laterally, the femoral shaft is smooth, while along its posterior aspect runs a rough line (*linea aspera*) with an inner and an outer lip for muscle insertions.

Distally, the femur expands to form the two *femoral condyles*, extensively covered by hyaline cartilage. Anteriorly, they are extended into a cartilaginous groove, the *patellar surface*, in which the *kneecap* (*patella*) glides downward during flexion of the knee (Figs. 4.**39** and 4.**40a**, **b**). Posteriorly, the two condyles are separated by a broad groove, the *intercondylar notch* (*intercondylar fossa*).

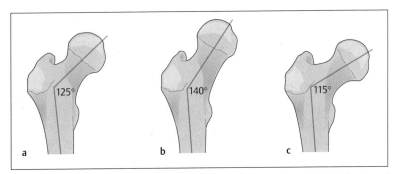

Fig. 4.**38 a–c** **Angle of the neck of the femur (collodiaphyseal angle).** Collodiaphyseal angle in the adult (**a**), in a 3-year old child (**b**), and in the elderly (**c**). (After Frick)

■ **Lower Leg.** The skeleton of the lower leg is formed by the *tibia* and the *fibula*. The tibia is the stronger bone and the true supporting pillar and connection between the femur and the foot. Proximally, the two bones are connected by the strong ligamentous tibiofibular joint (Fig. 4.**40**). Distally, the two bones are connected by a fibrous joint (syndesmosis). The *mortise* formed by the *medial* and *lateral malleoli* of these bones, together with the *trochlea of the talus*, makes up the ankle joint (Fig. 4.**41**).

Proximally, the tibia expands and features on its anterior surface the *tibial tuberosity*, into which the *quadriceps femoris* is inserted. The *superior articular surface* (Fig. 4.**40**), formed by the medial and lateral condyles, forms the knee joint with the femur. Like the radius and ulna, the tibia and fibula are connected by an *interosseus membrane*, which gives origin to some muscles in the leg.

■ **Foot (Pes).** The foot, like the hand, is divided into three groups arranged end to end (Fig. 4.**41**): the *ankle* (*tarsus*), the *intermediate group* (*metatarsus*), and the *toes* (*digits*). There are seven tarsal bones, of which the *talus*, the *navicular*, and the *three cuneiform bones* lie on the medial side, while the *calcaneum* (*calcaneus, os calcis*), and the *cuboid bone* are lateral. The calcaneum is the largest bone of the foot, its posteriorly directed *calcaneal tubercle* (*tuberculum calcanei*) forming the bony base

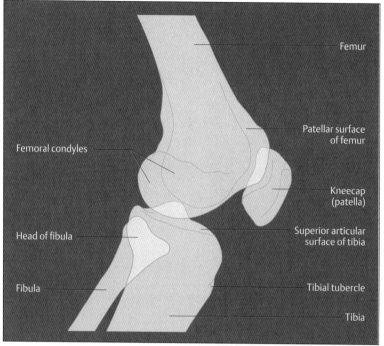

Fig. 4.**39** Simplified tracing of a lateral radiograph of the knee joint

of the heel. The five *metatarsal bones* are long bones, like the metacarpal bones of the hand. Each is divided into a base, a shaft, and a head. The first (*medial*) metatarsal bone is the thickest and strongest metatarsal bone. The 2nd to 5th toes consist of *proximal, middle and distal phalanges*, while the *1st toe* (*big toe, hallux*), only has a proximal and a distal phalanx (Fig. 4.**41**).

Inspection of the skeleton of the foot reveals that, while the talus lies above the calcaneum behind, the two bones lie side by side in the middle and in front. This arrangement creates medially a marked *longitudinal arch*, and at the level of the cuneiform bones and the metatarsal bones a

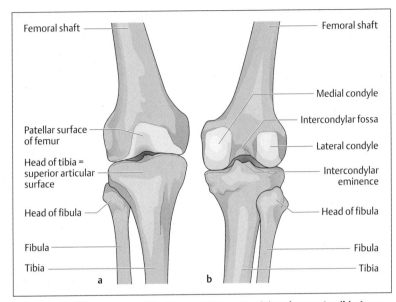

Femoral shaft

Femoral shaft

Medial condyle

Intercondylar fossa

Patellar surface
of femur

Lateral condyle

Head of tibia =
superior articular
surface

Intercondylar
eminence

Head of fibula

Head of fibula

Fibula

Fibula

Tibia

Tibia

a

b

Fig. 4.40 a, b   **Components of the knee joint, anterior (a) and posterior (b) views**

transverse arch running from medial to lateral (Fig. 4.**42a**, **b**). Muscles
and tendons serve to keep these arches intact. The calcaneal tubercle and
the heads of the 1st to 5th metatarsals may be regarded as the bases on
which all of the body weight rests on level ground.

The Hip Joint (Articulatio Coxae)

The hip joint is a ball-and-socket joint in which the *head of the femur*
moves in the *acetabulum* (Figs. 4.**34a**, **b** and 4.**43a**). The acetabulum is
formed by all three components of the hip bone, (ilium, ischium and
pubic bone, see Fig. 4.**35**). It grasps almost half the ball of the femur,
giving the hip joint a solid bony channel. The joint contact is augmented
by a fibrocartilaginous lip, (acetabular labrum), which extends the joint
beyond its equator by forming a ring around the acetabulum. In this way
the joint maintains solidity and stability in every position. The capsule of

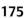

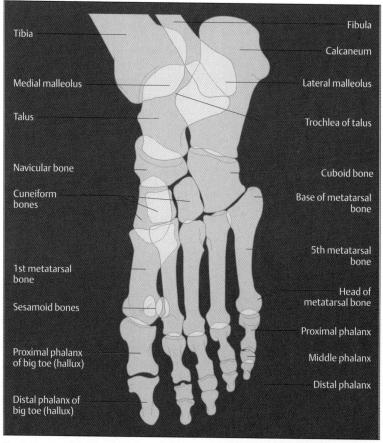

Fig. 4.**41** **Simplified tracing of a radiographic image of a plantarflexed foot in lateral view**

the joint is reinforced by three strong ligaments running from the three parts of the hip bone: the *iliofemoral*, the *pubofemoral*, and the *ischiofemoral* ligaments (Fig. 4.**43b**, **c**). The iliofemoral ligament is the strongest ligament of the body, with a tensile strength of 350 kg.

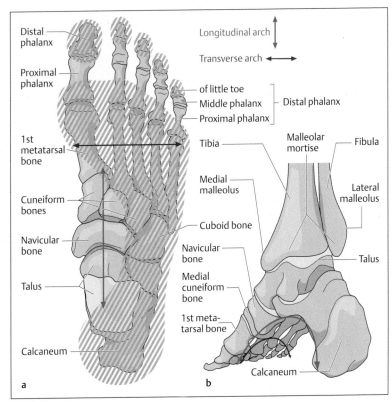

Fig. 4.42 a, b   **Longitudinal and transverse arches of the right foot**
a Skeleton of foot from above, with superimposed footprint
b Skeleton of foot with bones of the lower leg, medioposterior view

   The ligaments run a characteristic spiral course around the neck of the femur. In the erect posture they are tense, while they relax during flexion of the hip joint, allowing considerable mobility during flexion.

■ **Muscles and Movements.** Because a ball-and-socket joint has three main axes of movement, the leg can be moved around a transverse axis anteriorly and posteriorly (*flexion and extension*), a sagittal axis away from and toward the trunk (*abduction and adduction*), and a ver-

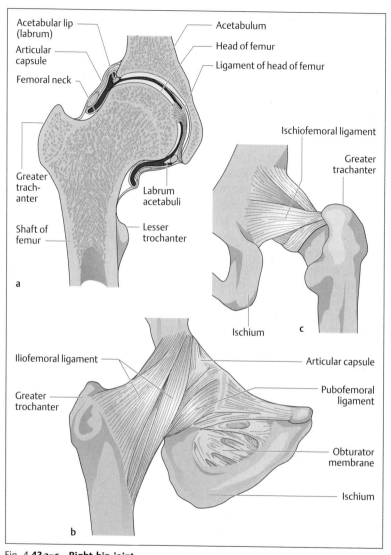

Fig. 4.**43 a–c   Right hip joint**
a coronal section; **b, c** ligaments: anterior (**b**) and posterior (**c**) views

tical axis around which it is rotated (*internal and external rotation*) (Fig. 4.**44**).

The most important hip flexors muscles include the deep *iliopsoas*, the *sartorius*, and the *rectus femoris muscles*. The extensors at the hip are the *gluteus maximus muscle* and the muscles running from the ischial tuberosity to the lower leg (*ischiocrural muscles*) (Figs. 4.**18a**, **b** and 4.**19**): the *biceps femoris*, the *semitendinosus*, and *semimembranosus muscles*). The *gluteus medius* and the *gluteus minimus muscles* function both as abductors and as internal and external rotators.

On the medial side of the thigh, between the *extensors* and the *flexors* runs a group of five muscles that adduct the thigh toward the trunk (*adductors*, e. g., *m. adductor magnus*). They take their origin from the pelvis and are inserted into the medial lip of the linea aspera of the femur. The external rotators arise from the posterior aspect of the pelvis and run to the femur, e. g., the gluteus maximus. Internal rotators are the anterior parts of the gluteus medius and gluteus minimus. During movement of the hip, the leg may be moved freely on the hip or the leg may be fixed (standing) and the hip moved against it. In walking these functions alternate.

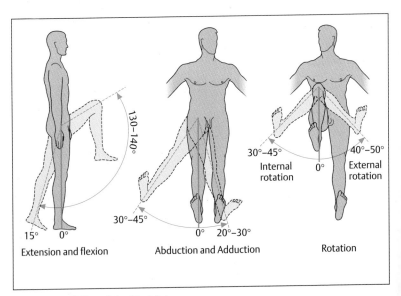

Fig. 4.**44** **Mobility of the hip joint**

The Knee Joint (Articulatio Genus)

The knee joint is the largest joint of the human body. It is a *compound joint*, formed by the combined action of the *femur, tibia, patella* and two *fibrocartilaginous disks, (menisci)* (Figs. 4.**45** and 4.**46c**). The joint consists of the joint between *the condyles of the femur and the tibia* and the joint between the *femur and the patella*. The two menisci adapt the joint surfaces of the femur and the tibia to each other and increase the *surface for the transmission of force*. When the knee joint is flexed, the femur executes a combined gliding and rolling motion over the tibial articular surface, during which the menisci are shifted more posteriorly the further the knee is flexed. The movements of the knee joint are guided by two sets of ligaments, the *medial and lateral collateral ligaments* and the *anterior and posterior cruciate ligaments* (Fig. 4.**46**).

While the collateral ligaments primarily stabilize the extended leg, the cruciate ligaments take over that function in the flexed knee joint. Because of the uneven curvature of the femoral condyles, the collateral ligaments are fully tensed only during extension of the knee joint; they are relaxed during flexion. With the knee flexed, the cruciate ligaments limit internal and external rotation of the lower leg, internal rotation being more severely limited than external rotation by the coiling of the cruciate ligaments.

■ **Muscles and Movements.** Muscles inserted into the medial surface of the tibia (e. g., *mm. semitendinosus* and *semimembranosus*) are internal rotators. The biceps femoris is inserted into the head of the fibula, and is the only external rotator of the lower leg (Figs. 4.**18a**, **b** and 4.**19**). All three muscles are flexors of the knee joint, as is the sartorius. The most important extensor of the knee joint is the quadriceps femoris, inserted by the patellar ligament into the tibial tuberosity. The patella, the largest sesamoid bone in the human body, is embedded in the patellar ligament (Fig. 4.**45**). It is triangular in shape and articulates with the anterior surface of the distal femur (patellar surface). As the knee flexes, the patella moves downward. Because there is considerable transfer of force in the joint between femur and patella, especially during flexion, this is the most highly stressed joint in the body, and is the earliest to show degenerative changes in its cartilage.

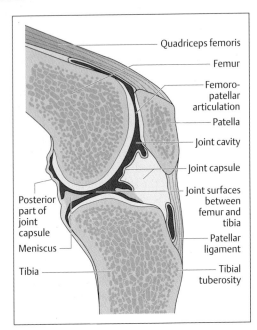

Fig. 4.**45**   **Sagittal section of knee joint**

- Quadriceps femoris
- Femur
- Femoro-patellar articulation
- Patella
- Joint cavity
- Joint capsule
- Joint surfaces between femur and tibia
- Patellar ligament
- Tibial tuberosity

Posterior part of joint capsule

Meniscus

Tibia

The Ankle Joint (Articulatio Talocruralis) and the Intertarsal Joint (Articulationes Subtalaris and Talocalcaneonavicularis)

The movements of the foot against the lower leg occur in two joints: the ankle joint and the talocalcaneonavicular joint.

■ **Ankle Joint.** The ankle joint is formed by the tibia, fibula, and talus. The distal ends of the tibia and fibula form a *mortise* made up of the medial and lateral malleoli, which grasp the *trochlea of the talus* (Fig. 4.**47a–c**). The joint is a hinge joint, the axis of which runs through the trochlea of

Fig. 4.**46 a–c**   **Ligaments of the right knee joint**
a Anterior view (patella and patellar ligament are reflected downward)
b Posterior view
c Superior articular surface of the tibia seen from above (the femur has been removed and the ligaments transsected)

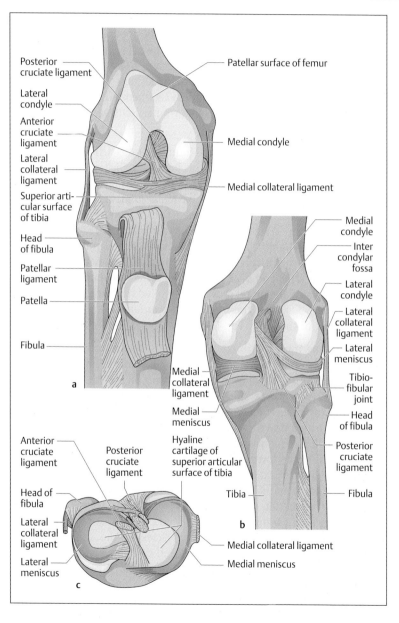

Posterior cruciate ligament

Lateral condyle

Anterior cruciate ligament

Lateral collateral ligament

Superior articular surface of tibia

Head of fibula

Patellar ligament

Patella

Fibula

Patellar surface of femur

Medial condyle

Medial collateral ligament

a

Medial condyle

Inter condylar fossa

Lateral condyle

Lateral collateral ligament

Lateral meniscus

Tibiofibular joint

Head of fibula

Posterior cruciate ligament

Medial collateral ligament

Medial meniscus

Tibia

Fibula

b

Anterior cruciate ligament

Posterior cruciate ligament

Hyaline cartilage of superior articular surface of tibia

Head of fibula

Lateral collateral ligament

Lateral meniscus

Medial collateral ligament

Medial meniscus

c

the talus and connects both malleoli. The movements at this joint are called *dorsiflexion* (lifting of the point of the foot) and *plantarflexion* (lowering the point of the foot toward the sole = plantar side of the foot). When the foot is fixed, the lower leg moves backward and forward. A strong set of ligaments stabilizes the ankle joint. It consists of three lateral ligaments and the medial deltoid ligament. The tibia and fibula are tightly joined together by a syndesmotic joint at the level of the malleoli.

■ **Intertarsal Joint.** In the intertarsal joint, the talus articulates with the calcaneus and the navicular bone. This joint is, in fact, composed of two joints that are anatomically entirely separate: posteriorly the subtalar joint, and anteriorly the talocalcaneonavicular joint. In the subtalar joint, the talus articulates with the calcaneus; in the talocalcaneonavicular joint, the ball-shaped head of the talus articulates with the calcaneus and the navicular bone. (Fig. 4.**47a–c**) The axis of movement in the talocalcaneonavicular joint runs from the center of the navicular obliquely downward, laterally, and backward through the calcaneum. The movements in this joint are lateral movements called *supination* (lifting of the inner = medial border of the foot) and *pronation* (lifting of the outer = lateral border of the foot) (Fig. 4.**48c**).

■ **Muscles.** The muscles running from the lower leg to the foot act on the ankle joint and the talocalcaneonavicular joint. They are divided onto three groups according to their position on the leg: the posterior calf muscles (*mm.triceps surae, tibialis posterior, flexor digitorum longus*, and *flexor hallucis longus*) act as supinators, plantar flexors (point of the foot turned down), and flexors of the toes (*mm. flexor digitorum longus* and *flexor hallucis longus* only). The muscles of the anterior compartment of the lower leg (*mm. tibialis anterior, extensor digitorum longus*, and *extensor hallucis longus*) act as dorsiflexors (lifting of the point of the foot) and supinators of the foot (*m. tibialis anterior* only). The muscles of the lateral compartment of the calf (*mm. peronei longus* and *brevis*) are primarily pronators and assist plantar flexion. The strongest group are the superficial muscles of the calf (*m. triceps surae*), usually considered to be composed of two muscles, the *soleus* and the *gastrocnemius muscles* (Fig. 4.**18a, b** and 4.**19**). They join to form the *Achilles tendon*, which is inserted into the calcaneal tubercle. If the Achilles tendon is torn, the triceps surae cannot act and it be-

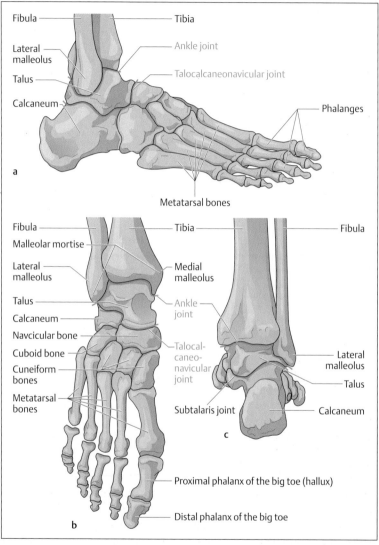

Fibula

Lateral malleolus

Talus

Calcaneum

Tibia

Ankle joint

Talocalcaneonavicular joint

Phalanges

Metatarsal bones

a

Fibula

Malleolar mortise

Lateral malleolus

Talus

Calcaneum

Navcicular bone

Cuboid bone

Cuneiform bones

Metatarsal bones

Tibia

Medial malleolus

Ankle joint

Talocal-caneo-navicular joint

Subtalaris joint

Fibula

Lateral malleolus

Talus

Calcaneum

Proximal phalanx of the big toe (hallux)

Distal phalanx of the big toe

b

c

Fig. 4.**47 a–c   Ankle joint and talocalcaneonavicular joint** (the joints are shown as blue lines)
a Lateral view
b Anterior view
c Posterior view

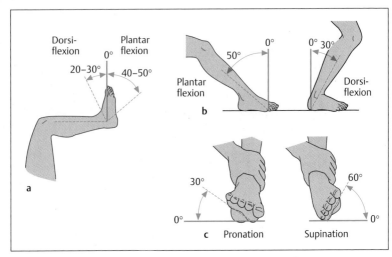

Fig. 4.**48 a–c**   **Movements of the ankle and talocalcaneonavicular joints**
a   Ankle joint (free leg)
b   Ankle joint (fixed leg)
c   Talocalcaneonavicular joint

comes impossible to stand on tip-toe; supination is also severely impaired.

Head and Neck

The Neck (Collum)

The neck joins the head to the trunk and contains the vascular and nervous pathways (blood and lymph vessels as well as nerve fibers) that run from the head to the trunk and the upper extremity. The boundary between the trunk and the neck lies at the clavicles in front and at the spine of the 7th cervical vertebra in the back. Cephalad, the neck extends to a line joining the lower border of the mandible, the two mastoid processes, and the external occipital protuberance. The neck may be divided into the posterior cervical refion (*back of the neck*, *nucha*) and the neck proper (*cervix, collum*).

The organs of the neck lie in front of the vertebral column. They include the *throat* (*pharynx*), the cervical part of the *esophagus*, the *larynx*, and the cervical part of the *air passages* (*trachea*). The thyroid gland occupies the lateral portion of the compartment containing the organs. The lateral parts also contain the vascular and nervous pathways (*common carotid artery* and its branches, *internal jugular vein, lymphatics* of the neck, *vagus nerve, sympathetic trunk*).

■ **The Neck Muscles.** The space containing the organs is enclosed on all sides by connective tissue sheaths (fascias) (Figs. 4.**49**, 4.**50**). Posteriorly, the muscular covering of the neck is formed by the segmental neck muscles, which are to a large extent covered by the *trapezius muscle*, and laterally by the *sternocleidomastoid muscle*. In front of and at the side of the cervical spine lie the derivatives of the trunk muscles (*scalene muscles*), and the prevertebral muscles (e. g., *mm. longus capitis* and *longus colli*). The organs of the neck are covered in front by the *infrahyoid muscles*. The most superficial muscle is the *platysma*, which is classified as one of the muscles of facial expression.

The Head (Caput)

The bony basis of the head is the *skull* (*cranium*). It serves partly as a bony capsule for the brain and the sense organs, and partly as support for the face; it also contains the upper ends of the digestive and respiratory tracts. It consists of a *brain case* (*neurocranium*) and a *facial skeleton* (*splanchnocranium, viscerocranium*), both sharing the base of the skull, which descends obliquely backward (see Figs. 4.**54**, 4.**55**). Externally, the boundary between the two parts can be seen to run from the root of the nose, through the upper rims of the orbits, to the external canals of the ears (external auditory meati). The internal aspect of the base of the skull separates the neurocranium from the facial skeleton and so serves as floor for the neurocranium, while anteriorly it becomes the roof of the facial skeleton. The posterior half is connected to the vertebral column by the atlanto-occipital joint and provides the origin for the neck muscles.

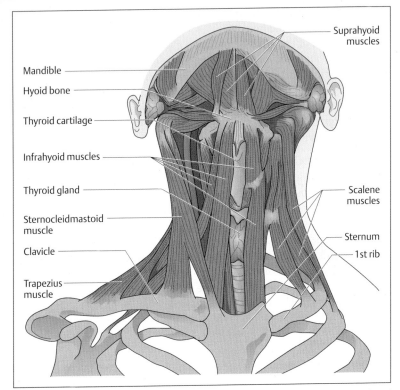

Fig. 4.**49** **Muscles of the neck, ventral view** (the platysma and fasciae of the neck and on the left side the muscles of the shoulder girdle have been removed)

General Aspects of the Skull

Both parts of the skull consist of separate bones. With the exception of the mandible, the ossicles of the ear, and the hyoid bone, they are connected by sutures or cartilaginous joints (synchndroses) or by bony joints (synostoses).

■ **The Neurocranium.** The neurocranium extends from the upper borders of the orbits (supraorbital margins) to the superior nuchal line. It includes the *frontal bone*, the two *parietal bones*, parts of the two *tem-*

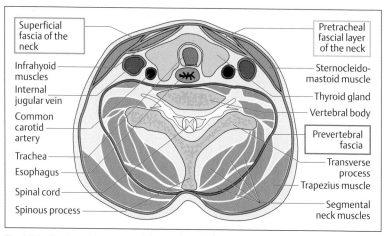

Superficial fascia of the neck

Infrahyoid muscles

Internal jugular vein

Common carotid artery

Trachea

Esophagus

Spinal cord

Spinous process

Pretracheal fascial layer of the neck

Sternocleido-mastoid muscle

Thyroid gland

Vertebral body

Prevertebral fascia

Transverse process

Trapezius muscle

Segmental neck muscles

Fig. 4.**50** **Horizontal section of the neck at the level of the thyroid gland** (the various fasciae of the neck are marked in color)

poral bones, and the uppermost part of the *occipital bone*. In front, the two parietal bones are joined to the frontal bone by the coronal suture (Fig. 4.**51**). Posteriorly, the *lambdoid suture* lies between the parietal bones and the occiput. The sagittal suture runs between the two parietal bones from the center of the coronal suture to the lambdoid suture. Laterally, the temporal bone is connected to the parietal bone posteriorly and the *greater wing of the sphenoid bone* (*ala major ossis sphenoidalis*), anteriorly by the *squamous suture*. The part of the skull visible externally is the cranial vault; the internal part, not visible from the outside, is the internal base of the skull. The latter is the internal boundary between the neurocranium and the facial skeleton.

■ **The Fontanelles.** In the newborn, broad gaps filled with connective tissue, the *fontanelles*, remain between the bones of the cranial vault (Fig. 4.**52**). The anterior, larger fontanellele is defined by the two developing halves of the frontal bone and the two developing parietal bones. It does not close completely until the 36th month of life. The posterior, triangular fontanellele lies between the two developing parietal bones and the developing occipital bone. It closes first, about the 3rd

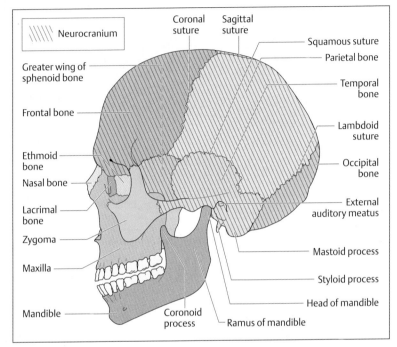

Fig. 4.**51** **Lateral view of adult skull**

month of life. The placement of the fontanelles makes it possible to determine the position of the child's head during birth.

■ **The Facial Skeleton (Splanchnocranium, Viscerocranium).** The parts of the facial skeleton are the *upper jaw* (*maxilla*), the *zygoma*, the *nasal bones*, the *lacrimal bone*, the *palatine bone*, the *vomer*, and the *lower jaw* (*mandible*) (Fig. 4.**51**). (The palatine bone is shown in Fig. 4.**54**; the vomer lies in the nasal cavity and cannot be seen in the figure.) The upper jaw takes part in the structure of the orbit, the nasal cavity, and the roof of the mouth (hard palate. In a dental process, the *alveolar arch*, it contains the roots of the upper row of teeth. It encloses the largest of the four *nasal sinuses*, the *maxillary sinus*.

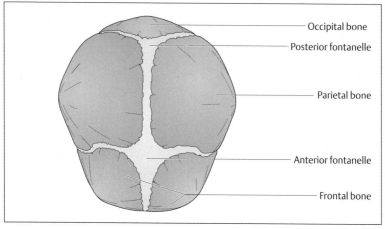

Occipital bone

Posterior fontanelle

Parietal bone

Anterior fontanelle

Frontal bone

Fig. 4.**52**   **Skull of a newborn seen from above**

The lower jaw moves on the rest of the skull at the temporomandibular joint (see Fig. 4.**58**). It consists of a body, two *condylar processes* bearing the *heads of the mandible*, and two *rami* with the muscle-bearing processes for the attachment of the temporalis muscles (*coronoid processes*) (Fig. 4.**51**) branching from them. The lower dentition is also rooted in an alveolar arch, which contains the *sockets for the teeth* (*alveoli*). A canal for the nerve and vessels to the teeth (*canalis mandibulae*) opens on the inner side of the mandibular ramus. An opening in each side allows passage of the nerves and vessels supplying the skin of the chin.

■ **Internal and External Aspects of the Base of the Skull.** The base of the skull is the floor of the cranial cavity on which the brain rests (Fig. 4.**54**). The *external surface* of the base is the part visible from the outside, looking at the skull from below. The *internal surface* (Fig. 4.**55**) is the aspect not visible from the outside.

The external surface of the base of the skull (Fig. 4.**54**) extends from the *external occipital protuberance* to the incisor teeth in the upper jaw. The lateral boundaries are formed from imaginary lines drawn between

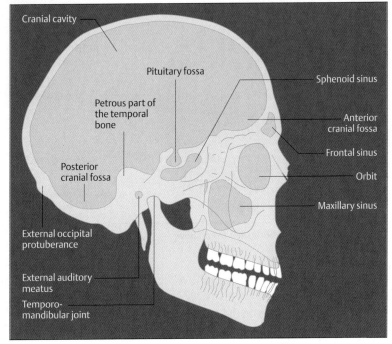

Fig. 4.**53**   **Simplified tracing of a lateral radiograph of the skull**

the alveolar arches and the mastoid processes. The anterior part forms the roof of the oral cavity and the floor of the nasal cavity. At the posterior end of the hard palate lies the entrance to the *nasal cavity (choanae)*. At the posterior end of the base of the skull lies a large opening, the *foramen magnum*, and next to it on each side sit the *occipital joint facets (occipital condyles)* that, in conjunction with the atlas, form the atlanto-occipital joint. The articular fossae for the temporomandibular joints can be found immediately in front of the mastoid processes.

Anteriorly, the internal surface of the base of the skull (Fig. 4.**55**) is formed by the frontal bone, which also forms the roof of the two orbits. In between lie parts of the *ethmoid bone*, with its *cribriform plate (lamina*

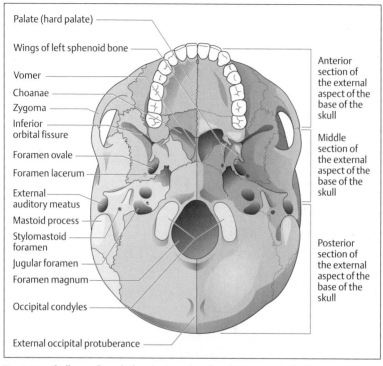

Palate (hard palate)

Wings of left sphenoid bone

Vomer

Choanae

Zygoma

Inferior
orbital fissure

Foramen ovale

Foramen lacerum

External
auditory meatus

Mastoid process

Stylomastoid
foramen

Jugular foramen

Foramen magnum

Occipital condyles

External occipital protuberance

Anterior
section of
the external
aspect of the
base of the
skull

Middle
section of
the external
aspect of the
base of the
skull

Posterior
section of
the external
aspect of the
base of the
skull

Fig. 4.**54   Skull seen from below (external surface of base of skull).** The mandible has
been removed

cribrosa), which transmits the olfactory nerves to the nasal mucosa. The
ethmoid bone takes part in the formation of the nasal cavity and the internal boundary of the orbits. In its center projects a crest like a cock's
comb (*crista galli*), which gives attachment to the *falx cerebri*. The frontal
bone and the ethmoid, combined with the lesser wing of the sphenoid,
form the two anterior cranial fossae (fossae craniis anterior).

Behind these bones lies the sphenoid bone, followed by the occipital
bone. On each side lie the temporal bones. The sphenoid bone is the
center of the base of the skull. It is composed of the body of the sphenoid
surrounding the sphenoid sinus and forming the sella turcica, the floor of
which is occupied by the *pituitary gland* (*hypophysis*). The two greater

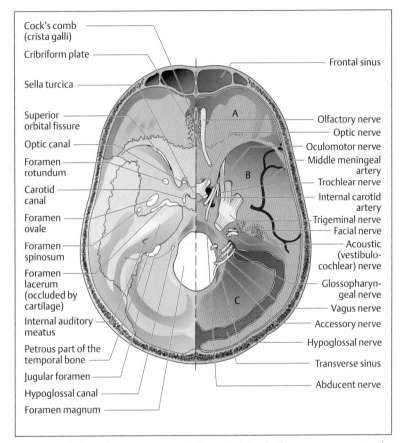

Cock's comb (crista galli)
Cribriform plate
Sella turcica
Superior orbital fissure
Optic canal
Foramen rotundum
Carotid canal
Foramen ovale
Foramen spinosum
Foramen lacerum (occluded by cartilage)
Internal auditory meatus
Petrous part of the temporal bone
Jugular foramen
Hypoglossal canal
Foramen magnum

Frontal sinus
Olfactory nerve
Optic nerve
Oculomotor nerve
Middle meningeal artery
Trochlear nerve
Internal carotid artery
Trigeminal nerve
Facial nerve
Acoustic (vestibulo-cochlear) nerve
Glossopharyngeal nerve
Vagus nerve
Accessory nerve
Hypoglossal nerve
Transverse sinus
Abducent nerve

Fig. 4.**55** **Internal surface of base of skull** (on the left side the structures covering the bone have been removed). **A** Anterior; **B** middle, and **C** posterior cranial fossa

wings of the sphenoid form a part of the middle cranial fossa (*fossa cranii media*) and below give rise to the pterygoid processes (Fig. 4.**54**). The posterior part of the middle cranial fossa is formed by the anterior superior wall of the *petrous bone* (*pyramid of the petrous bone*), which houses the middle and inner ear. The petrous bone is a part of the temporal bone. The floor of the unpaired posterior cranial fossa (*fossa cranii posterior*) is formed almost entirely by the occipital bone. Through its middle passes the foramen magnum, through which the brain is connected with the spinal cord. Anteriorly and laterally, the petrous bone takes part in the formation of the posterior cranial fossa.

Foramina (holes) and canals traverse all the cranial fossae downward, transmitting the cranial nerves and vessels (Fig. 4.**55**). Between the lesser and greater wings of the sphenoid bone lies the *superior orbital fissure*, which leads into the orbit. Nerves that run through it into the orbit include the first division of the *trigeminal nerve* (*ophthalmic nerve*) and cranial nerves III, IV, and VI (*oculomotor, trochlear,* and *abducens*) to the external muscles of the eye. The *optic nerve* and *optic artery* pass through a separate canal, the *optic foramen.* The second division of the trigeminal nerve (*maxillary nerve*) leaves the skull through the *foramen rotundum* in the greater wing of the sphenoid, while the third division (*mandibular nerve*) passes through the *foramen ovale* of the greater wing of the sphenoid. Behind it lies a small foramen, the *foramen spinosum,* which transmits the artery supplying the dura mater (*middle meningeal artery*).

Inside the petrous pyramid runs the *internal auditory meatus* (Fig. 4.**55**), through which cranial nerves VII and VIII (*facial* and *acoustic or vestibulocochlear nerves*) enter the petrous bone. On each side of the sella turcica lies a separate canal, the carotid canal, through which the *internal carotid artery* enters the skull. Between the temporal and occipital bones there is an opening (*jugular foramen*) where cranial nerves IX (*glossopharyngeal nerve*) X (*vagus nerve*), and XI (*accessory nerve*) pass through the base of the skull. Additionally, the venous blood from the brain drains through the jugular foramen into the *internal jugular vein.* Cranial nerve XII (*hypoglossal nerve*) leaves the skull through an opening (*hypoglossal canal*) immediately next to the foramen magnum.

The Muscles of the Skull

Two sets of muscles can be distinguished on the facial skeleton: the chewing muscles (muscles of mastication) and the muscles of facial expression. The muscles of mastication take their origin from the base and the lateral wall of the skull and are inserted into the mandible. The muscles of facial expression are cutaneous muscles (see below). They are of significance in facial expressions, have a protective function, and take part in the ingestion of nutrients. Both groups of muscles move and put stress on the bones of the skull and influence their shape and structure.

■ **Muscles of Mastication.** Muscles with a variety of origins and functions take part in the act of chewing (Fig. 4.**56a, b**). Muscles of mastication in the more restricted sense include the *masseter*, the *lateral* and *medial pterygoid*, and the *temporalis muscles*. They are all innervated by the third division of the trigeminal nerve. Of all these muscles, the temporalis muscle is the largest and strongest, developing almost 50% of the chewing power. The lateral pterygoid muscle occupies a special place among the chewing muscles, in that it guides the movement of opening the mandible by pulling the mandible forward. It is aided by the suprahyoid muscles, which, in addition to gravity, also take part in opening the mouth.

■ **Muscles of Facial Expression.** The muscles of expression are mostly made up of thin sheets of muscle fibers lying immediately below the subcutaneous tissue (Fig. 4.57). Unlike the skeletal muscles, they have no fascial sheaths and extend from bones to skin; hence they can move the skin. The original arrangement of the muscles of expression around the orbits, the nose, the mouth, and the pinna of the ear remains in its original state only around the eyes and the mouth. The muscles of facial expression also include the *occipitofrontalis* muscle (*m. epicranius*), which consists of a frontal and occipital belly. Both parts are connected by a strong aponeurosis, the *galea aponeurotica*, which covers almost the whole neurocranium like a bathing cap. All the muscles of facial expression are supplied by the facial nerve (cranial nerve VII).

The Jaw Joint (Temporomandibular Joint)

The temporomandibular joints are hinge joints. Their movements in the human serve not only nutritional intake but also the articulation of speech, facial expression, and singing. The temporomandibular joint connects the mandible with the temporal bone (Fig. 4.58). Between the ellipsoid joint surface of the *head of the mandible* and the *mandibular fossa* of the temporal bone lies an *articular disk*, which divides the temporomandibular joint into two completely separate chambers. The

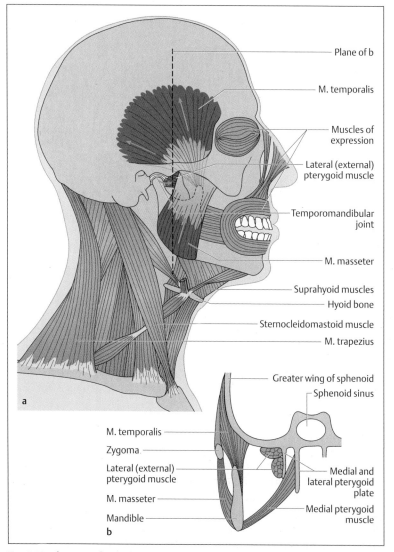

Plane of b

M. temporalis

Muscles of expression

Lateral (external) pterygoid muscle

Temporomandibular joint

M. masseter

Suprahyoid muscles

Hyoid bone

Sternocleidomastoid muscle

M. trapezius

a

Greater wing of sphenoid

Sphenoid sinus

M. temporalis

Zygoma

Lateral (external) pterygoid muscle

M. masseter

Mandible

b

Medial and lateral pterygoid plate

Medial pterygoid muscle

Fig. 4.**56 a, b**   **Lateral view (a) and coronal section (left side only) (b) of the muscles of mastication** (highlighted in red)

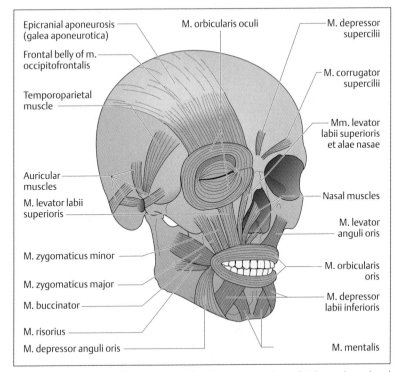

Epicranial aponeurosis (galea aponeurotica)

Frontal belly of m. occipitofrontalis

Temporoparietal muscle

Auricular muscles

M. levator labii superioris

M. zygomaticus minor

M. zygomaticus major

M. buccinator

M. risorius

M. depressor anguli oris

M. orbicularis oculi

M. depressor supercilii

M. corrugator supercilii

Mm. levator labii superioris et alae nasae

Nasal muscles

M. levator anguli oris

M. orbicularis oris

M. depressor labii inferioris

M. mentalis

Fig. 4.**57 Overview of the muscles of facial expression** (superficial muscles colored light, deep muscckes dark)

movements of the temporomandibular joint take place around one axis that runs from external and anterior to internal and posterior, and one that runs obliquely up and down. The human temporomandibular joint carries out two main functions during the act of mastication: (1) elevation (adduction) and depression (abduction) of the mandible and (2) grinding motions. Every time the mouth opens, the head of the mandible and the articular disk are pulled forward on the articular tubercle. If the forward pull occurs on only one side the result is a grinding motion.

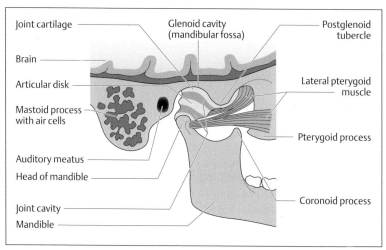

Fig. 4.**58** **Anatomy of the temporomandibular joint.** (After Faller)

Summary **The Locomotor System (Musculoskeletal System)**

■ **Locomotor System**

General Anatomy of the Locomotor System

The skeletal system and the muscles together constitute the locomotor system, in which the bones and the joints comprise the passive motor system and the striated muscles the active motor system.

The Bones

Bones may be long bones (pipe bones), flat bones (e. g., skull), short (e. g., wrist and ankle bones), irregular (e. g., vertebrae), and bones containing air-filled cavities (e. g., frontal bone), as well as sesamoid bones (e. g., kneecap).

The Joints

Joints may be movable or immovable. The immovable joints (synarthroses) include syndesmoses, synchondroses, and synostoses. In movable joints (synovial joints, diarthroses), the joint surfaces are covered with cartilage and are separated by a joint space. Inside the joint, the articular cavity is filled with synovial fluid and enveloped in a joint capsule.

Joints may be classified according to the shape of the joint surfaces as:

- Ball-and-socket joints (hip joint, shoulder joint)
- Condylar joints (wrist joint)
- Trochlear joints
  - Hinge joints (elbow joint)
  - Pivot joints (proximal radioulnar joint)
- Saddle joints (saddle joint of the thumb)
- Plane joints (articular joints of the vertebrae)
- Joints with mobility limited by strong ligaments (sacroiliac joints)

Skeletal Muscle

As a rule, a skeletal muscle consists of one or more heads, a muscle belly, and a proximal tendon of origin as well as a distal tendon of insertion connecting the muscle with a bone. A muscle may have multiple bellies if it has tendons between them, and it may be monarthric (uniarticular, monarticular) or polyarthric (multiarticular) depending on whether it runs over one or more joints.

The length and force of lift of a muscle depend on the way the muscle fibers are arranged on the tendons, that is, from the angle at which they are inserted. Because of their long fibers, muscles with parallel fibers achieve a great height of lift but relatively little force of lift, since their physiological cross-section is small. Unipennate, and especially bipennate, muscles have a large physiological cross-section and so develop considerable strength, but because of their short muscle fibers their height of lift is small.

Tendons transfer the force of a muscle contraction from the muscle to the skeleton. There are very short tendons ("fleshy" origin; e. g., pectoralis major), long, narrow tendons (muscles of the hand and foot), and flat tendons ("aponeuroses"; e. g., oblique abdominal muscles). The tendons may exert pull or pressure. In the latter case, they wind around a bone that acts as a fulcrum (e. g., tendon of insertion of the peroneus longus).

Muscle fasciae, tendon sheaths, bursae, and sesamoid bones are auxiliary structures for muscles and tendons. Their function is to reduce friction during muscular work and so reduce effort.

■ Special Anatomy of the Locomotor System
The Skeleton of the Trunk

The skeleton of the trunk includes the vertebral column and the chest cage (thorax), which includes the ribs, the breastbone (sternum), and the thoracic spine.

The Spinal Column

The spinal column consists of 33–34 vertebrae: 7 cervical, 12 thoracic, 5 lumbar, 5 sacral (fused in the sacrum), and 4–5 coccygeal (fused in the coccyx). It forms two S-shaped curves (cervical and lumbar lordoses, thoracic and sacral kyphoses); its spinal canal contains the spinal cord.

The basic vertebra consists of a vertebral body, a vertebral arch, a spinous process, two transverse processes and four articular processes. The vertebral body and the vertebral arch enclose the vertebral foramen. Together, the vertebral foramina form the spinal canal. The spinal nerves leave the spinal canal through the intervertebral foramina between two adjacent vertebrae.

Two adjoining vertebrae form one independently mobile segment, consisting of the two vertebrae, the intervertebral disk between them, the synovial joints of the vertebral arch, the ligaments, and the corresponding muscles.

The atlas supports the head and with the occipital condyles forms the atlanto-occipital joint (inclines the head laterally, forward and backward). With the axis it forms the atlanto-axial joint (rotation of the head).

The Chest Cage

The chest cage is composed of 12 pairs of ribs. The first seven of these (true ribs) are connected to the sternum directly. The 8th to 10th pairs of ribs take part in the formation of the costal margin, while the 11th and 12th ribs end unattached in the lateral abdominal wall. Each rib in the 1st to 10th pairs is connected to the vertebrae by two costovertebral joints. The movements of the ribs (expansion and contraction of the thorax) subserve respiration (muscles of respiration, including intercostal muscles).

The Muscles of the Trunk

The muscles of the trunk include back, thoracic, and abdominal muscles as well as diaphragm

The Back

- Segmental muscles of the back: m. erector spinae
- Muscles encroaching on the back: mm. trapezius, rhomboideus major and minor, together with levator scapulae (shoulder girdle muscle) and latissimus dorsi (muscle of the upper extremity)

The Thoracic Wall

- Intercostal muscles (external, internal, intimi)—inspiration, expiration; scalenus muscles—inspiration
- Muscles encroaching on the trunk: m. serratus anterior—abduction of the arm, auxiliary muscle of respiration; m. pectoralis major—adduction, internal rotation of the upper arm, auxiliary muscle of respiration; sternocleidomastoid muscle, also auxiliary muscle of respiration.

The Abdominal Wall

Muscles: m. rectus abdominis, external and internal oblique muscles, mm. transversus abdominis, psoas major, and quadratus lumborum—rotation, flexion, lateral inclination of the trunk, compression of the abdomen.

The Diaphragm

The most important muscle of respiration (contraction—inspiration, relaxation—expiration).

The Pelvic Floor

Levator ani muscle—forms the pelvic diaphragm; m. transversus perinei profundus—forms the urogenital diaphragm; medial part of the levator ani (puborectalis), m. sphincter ani externus—voluntary constriction of the anus; m. sphincter urethrae—voluntary constriction of the urethra.

The Upper Extremity

The Shoulder Girdle

- Bones: clavicle and shoulder blade (scapula)
- Joints: sternoclavicular joint, acromioclavicular joint between clavicle and shoulder blade
- Muscles: mm. trapezius, serratus anterior, levator scapulae, romboideus major and minor.

Free Upper Limb

- *Bones:* (1) Upper arm (brachium)—humerus. (2) Forearm (antebrachium)—radius and ulna. (3) Hand (manus)—wrist (carpus) with eight bones (navicular or scaphoid, lunate, triquetrum, pisiform, trapezium, trapezoid, capitate, hamate bones); metacarpus with 5 metacarpal bones; 5 fingers, each with 3 phalanges, but only two for the thumb.
- *Shoulder joint:* ball-and-socket joint between head of humerus and glenoid cavity of the shoulder blade.
  - *Muscles:* muscles of the rotator cuff (m. supraspinatus—abduction, mm. infraspinatus and teres minor—external rotation; subscapular—internal rotation of the arm), deltoid muscle (abduction, extension, and flexion of the arm), mm. pectoralis major, latissimus dorsi, and teres major (adduction, external and internal rotation).
- *Elbow joint* (*articulatio cubiti*): compound hinge joint composed of three separate joints. (1) humeroradial joint, (2) humeroulnar joint, (3) proximal radioulnar joint.
  - *Muscles:* m. triceps brachii (extension at the elbow joint); m. brachialis (flexion), biceps brachii (flexion, supination); m. supinator (supination); mm. pronator teres and pronator quadratus (pronation).
- *Joints of the hand:* (1) proximal wrist joint (radiocarpal joint—between ulna and radius as well as the proximal row of carpal bones); (2) middle carpal joint (*articulatio mediocarpea*—between the distal and proximal row of carpal bones); (3) saddle joint of the thumb (*articulatio carpometacarpea pollicis*).
  - *Muscles*: 18 short muscles of the hand, together with 15 forearm muscles (flexors, extensors, radial group). 9 muscles take part just in the movements of the thumb.

The Lower Extremity

The Pelvic Girdle

- *Bones:* the two hip bones (ossa coxae; each composed of ilium, ischium, pubic bone) and the sacrum together form the bony pelvic girdle.
- *Joints:* sacroiliac (between sacrum and ilium)
- *Muscles:* The muscles of the pelvis are part of the musculature of the trunk (see Pelvic Floor).

Free Lower Limb

- *Bones:* (1) Thigh, femur (thighbone). (2) Patella (kneecap). (3) Lower leg (crus)—tibia and fibula. (4) Foot (pes)—ankle (tarsus) composed of 7 bones (talus, navicular, 3 cuneiform bones, calcaneum, cuboid bone); metatarsus with 5 metatarsal bones; 5 toes (digits) with 3 phalanges each, except 2 phalanges for the big toe (hallux).
- *Hip joint:* ball-and-socket joint between the head of the femur (caput femoris) and the acetabulum of the hip bone (*os coxae*).
  - *Muscles:* mm. iliopsoas (flexion), sartorius (flexion), rectus femoris (flexion), gluteus maximus (extension); posterior (ischiocrural) group (mm. biceps femoris, semitendinosus, semimembranosus—extension); mm. gluteus medius and gluteus minimus (abduction, internal and external rotation); adductor group (5 muscles, e. g., m. adductor magnus—adduction).
- *Knee joint* (*articulatio genus*): compound joint. (1) Between femoral condyle and tibia, (2) between patellar surface of femur and patella.
  - Muscles: mm. semimembranosus and semitendinosus (internal rotation, flexion), biceps femoris (external rotation, flexion), sartorius (flexion), quadriceps femoris (extension).
- *Tibiofibular joint:* syndesmotic joint.
- *Ankle joint* (*articulatio talocruralis*): the distal ends of the tibia and fibula grasp the talus and trochlea of the talus in a malleolar mortise, forming a hinge joint.
  - *Muscles:* mm. gastrocnemius and soleus (triceps surae), tibialis posterior, flexor digitorum longus, flexor hallucis longus, peroneus longus and brevis (plantar flexion); flexor digitorum lon-

gus and flexor hallucis longus (plantar flexion of the toes); tibialis anterior, extensor digitorum longus, and flexor hallucis longus (dorsiflexion).

- *Talocalcaneonavicular joint:* two separate joints coupled functionally. (1) Calcaneum and talus. (2) Talus and navicular bone.
  - *Muscles:* mm. soleus and gastrocnemius (triceps surae muscle), tibialis anterior and posterior, flexor digitorum longus, flexor hallucis longus (supination); peroneus longus and brevis, extensor digitorum longus (pronation).

Head and Neck

The Neck

The neck (collum) joins the trunk to the head; the posterior region is called the nape of the neck or the back of the neck (nucha), the anterior the neck proper (cervix). The organs of the neck (throat [pharynx], cervical portion of the esophagus, larynx, cervical part of the air passages [trachea]), lie in front of the vertebral column, and are covered by the fasciae and muscles of the neck (muscles: posteriorly, segmental muscles of the neck, m. trapezius; laterally, sternocleidomastoids; anterior and lateral to the vertebral column, muscles derived from the muscles of the trunk [mm. scaleni, prevertebral muscles such as mm. longus capiti and longus colli]; anterior to the organs of the neck, infrahyoid muscles and platysma).

The Head

The bony foundation of the head is the skull, which consists of the brain case (neurocranium) and a facial skeleton (splanchnocranium) (boundary: line from the root of the nose—upper orbital rims—external auditory meati).

- *Bones of the neurocranium:* (1) Cranial vault: frontal bone, paired parietal bones, parts of both temporal bones, uppermost part of the occipital bone. (2) Internal aspect of the base of the skull: frontal bone, ethmoid bone with the cribriform plate, crista galli, sphenoid bone, occipital bone, temporal bones.
- In the newborn, gaps filled with connective tissue occupy the space between bones (fontanelles). They close between the 3rd and 36th month of life and are then replaced by bony sutures (coronal, lambdoid, sagittal, squamous sutures).

- *Bones of the facial skeleton:* upper jaw (maxilla, with a process for the teeth [alveolar arch]), zygoma, nasal bone, lacrimal bone, palatine bone, vomer, mandible (with alveolar arch).
- *Base of skull:* bony base of the cranial cavity, on which the brain rests. The foramen magnum is seen if the skull is viewed from below (inferior aspect of base of skull). This is where the vertebral column is connected to the skull by the atlanto-occipital joint. The superior aspect of the base of the skull is part of the neurocranium (see above). It forms the boundary between neurocranium and facial skeleton.
- *Muscles of the skull:* (1) Mandibular muscles (masticatory muscles): masseter, lateral and medial pterygoid, temporalis, syprahyoid muscles. (2) Muscles of facial expression: 21 muscles. They have no fascia and extend from skin to bone (cutaneous muscles).
- *Temporomandibular joint* (TMJ): hinge joint between mandible and temporal bone.

5
The Heart and Blood Vessels

Contents

In order to transport blood to the immediate neighborhood of all cells in a multicellular organism, the body needs special **circulatory organs** to move and distribute the blood. For this purpose the whole body is perfused by a special *transport system* into which the various organ systems are fitted. The circulatory organs include:

- The **heart**
- The **blood vessels**

The heart is the motor of the circulation. By its pumping action it maintains a steady blood flow. The blood circulates through a closed system of elastic pipes, the **vascular system**, which can be divided into the following segments:

- **Arteries**, which lead blood away from the heart and distribute it
- **Capillaries**, in which the exchange of substances takes place
- **Veins**, which return the blood to the heart
- **Lymph vessels**, which serve the transport of fluids and immune cells

Irrespective of their oxygen content, all blood vessels leading away from the heart are called arteries, and all blood vessels that lead toward the heart are called veins. For instance, the pulmonary artery that leads from the heart to the lungs carries oxygen-poor blood. On the other hand, the pulmonary veins, leading from the lungs to the heart, carry oxygen-rich blood. Similarly, the umbilical arteries carry oxygen-poor blood, while the blood in the umbilical veins is rich in oxygen.

The vascular system serves not only oxygen transport but also the distribution of substances absorbed from food. The blood vessels transport them to the cells (substance exchange in the capillaries), where, with the help of oxygen, they are transformed into energy (ATP) to perform the metabolic processes necessary for life, or are used to manufacture the fabric of the body.

■ The Heart (Cor)

Shape and Position

The heart is a hollow muscular organ, lying in a *connective tissue space* (*mediastinum*) between the vertebral column and the sternum. It is

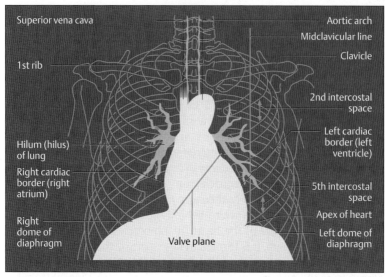

Fig. 5.**1**   **Simplified sketch of a chest radiograph with cardiac shadow.** Posteroanterior (PA) view

completely enveloped in a membrane, the *pericardium*, that extends between the pleural cavities (see p. 349), the diaphragm, and the great vessels (Figs. 5.**1** and 5.**2**). It is about one and a half times the size of a man's closed fist, but may become substantially larger through training or under pathological circumstances. It weighs about 0.5% of body weight, usually about 300–350 g. The shape of the heart resembles a truncated cone, of which the lower surface is called the *base of the heart.* The apex of the heart touches the anterior chest wall in the left intercostal space, a little inside a perpendicular dropped from the midclavicular line. The great vessels enter at the base of the heart, thereby anchoring it (Fig. 5.**1**). The apex of the heart, in contrast, is freely mobile in the *pericardial sac.*

Structure of the Heart

The **interventricular septum** completely divides the heart into a "**right heart**" for the pulmonary circulation and a "**left heart**" for the systemic circulation. Each half has an **atrium** and a **ventricle** (Fig. 5.**3c**).

Viewed from in front, the anterior wall of the heart is formed essentially by the right ventricle (Figs. 5.**3a–c**). Adjoining it on the right lies the right atrium, into which drain the *superior* and *inferior venae cavae*. A portion of the left ventricle borders on the left side of the right ventricle. In a groove between them (*anterior interventricular sulcus*) runs the anterior branch of the *left coronary artery*. The main systemic artery, the *aorta*, arises from the left ventricle, runs upward and to the right, arches over the *pulmonary artery* (*pulmonary trunk*) as it leaves the right ventricle, then continues downward behind the heart.

The *inferior surface* of the heart (diaphragmatic surface) is flat and lies on the diaphragm. It is formed in large part by the left ventricle and to a small extent by the right ventricle (Fig. 5.**3d**). Clinically, it is often referred to as the *posterior wall* (posterior wall infarcts). Viewed from behind (from the vertebral side), the left ventricular wall is separated from

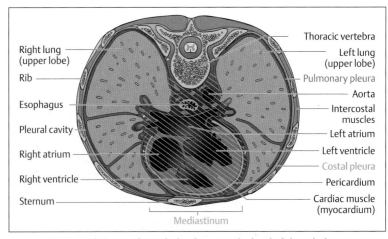

Fig. 5.**2   Horizontal section through the thorax at the level of the 8th thoracic vertebra.** (After Leonhardt)

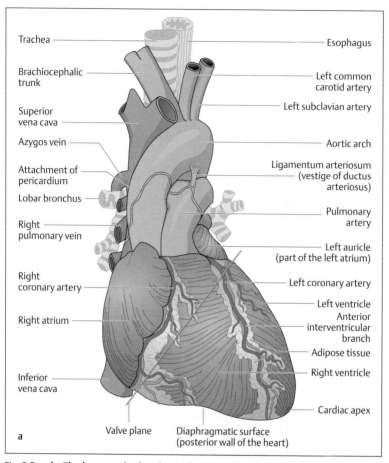

Trachea

Brachiocephalic trunk

Superior vena cava

Azygos vein

Attachment of pericardium

Lobar bronchus

Right pulmonary vein

Right coronary artery

Right atrium

Inferior vena cava

a

Valve plane

Esophagus

Left common carotid artery

Left subclavian artery

Aortic arch

Ligamentum arteriosum (vestige of ductus arteriosus)

Pulmonary artery

Left auricle (part of the left atrium)

Left coronary artery

Left ventricle

Anterior interventricular branch

Adipose tissue

Right ventricle

Cardiac apex

Diaphragmatic surface (posterior wall of the heart)

Fig. 5.**3 a–d   The heart and related vessels.** The pericardium has been removed
a Anterior view (in **b** and **c** the heart has been cut in various coronal planes)

the right ventricular wall by a groove (*posterior interventricular groove*)
(Fig. 5.**3d**). In this the terminal branch of the *right coronary artery (posterior interventricular branch)* runs toward the cardiac apex. The side of the
heart facing the spinal column contains essentially the left atrium and

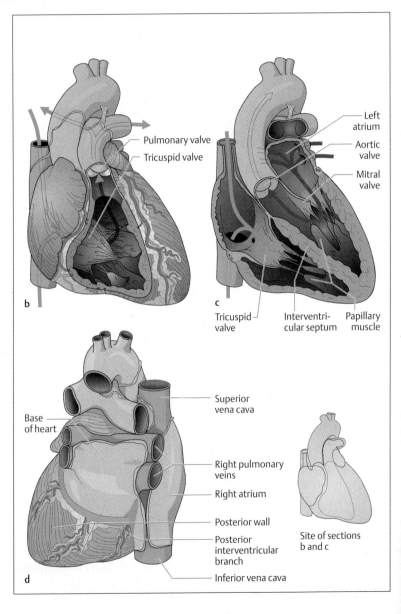

Pulmonary valve

Tricuspid valve

b

Left atrium

Aortic valve

Mitral valve

c

Tricuspid valve

Interventricular septum

Papillary muscle

Superior vena cava

Base of heart

Right pulmonary veins

Right atrium

Posterior wall

Posterior interventricular branch

Inferior vena cava

d

Site of sections b and c

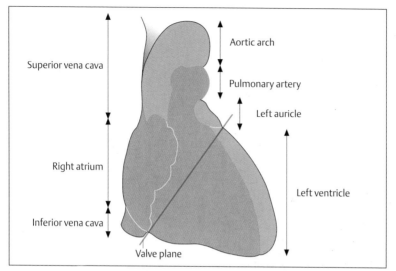

Fig. 5.**4** **Schematic representation of a radiograph of the heart and vessels related to the heart with the structures forming the contours.** Posteroanterior view. The left cardiac structures are shown in red, the right in blue; the structures forming the right cardiac border are essentially the superior vena cava and right atrium. The structures forming the left cardiac border are the aortic arch, pulmonary arteries, left auricle, and left ventricle

the *pulmonary veins* draining into it. Where the atria meet the ventricles there is a groove, *the atrioventricular groove (coronary sulcus).* It contains the large veins of the heart that drain into the right atrium by way of the **coronary sinus**.

In a posteroanterior (PA) radiographic image (the beam directed anteriorly from behind) of the chest, only the structures on the border of the *cardiac shadow* can be examined (Figs. 5.1 and 5.**4**). The right contour of the cardiac shadow is formed by the right atrium and the superior

◁ Fig. 5.**3 b–d**
   b The right ventricle has been opened (blue arrows = direction of venous blood flow)
   c In addition to the right ventricle, the right atrium and the left ventricle have also been opened (red arrows = direction of arterial blood flow)
   d Heart viewed from behind (base of heart) and below (posterior wall). (After Leonhardt)

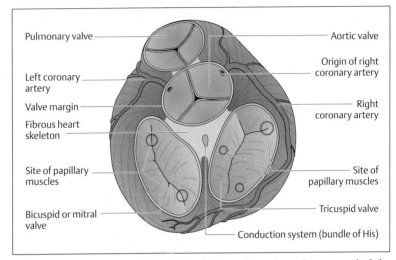

Pulmonary valve

Left coronary
artery

Valve margin

Fibrous heart
skeleton

Site of papillary
muscles

Bicuspid or mitral
valve

Aortic valve

Origin of right
coronary artery

Right
coronary artery

Site of
papillary muscles

Tricuspid valve

Conduction system (bundle of His)

Fig. 5.**5** **View from above of the plane of the cardiac valves after removal of the atria.** The site of the papillary muscles is indicated by small circles

vena cava. On the left side the following contours are visualized from above down: the aortic arch, pulmonary artery, left auricle (a part of the left atrium) and the left ventricle. Obliquely or laterally directed radiographs must be used to show the left atrium or the right ventricle.

■ **Chambers and Valves of the Heart.** Of the cardiac chambers, only the main parts of the atria have a smooth wall. In the auricles (parts of the atria) and especially in the ventricles, muscular ridges (*trabeculae carneae*) protrude into the chambers. A single layer of epithelium (*endocardium*) covers all the chambers. The four valves of the heart are anchored in dense fibrous connective tissue rings that lie nearly in a plane (Fig. 5.**3** and 5.**5**). Together with the connective tissue between them they form a unit, the so-called **cardiac skeleton**, to which the atria and ventricles are attached above and below.

The *cusps* of the valves between the atria and ventricles (*atrioventricular valves*) arise as *double layers of endocardium* from the cardiac skeleton (Fig. 5.**5**). The free ends of the valve cusps are attached by tendinous

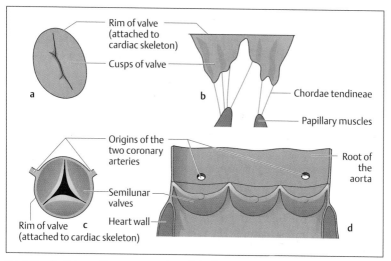

Fig. 5.**6 a–d Schematic representation of the heart valves**
a Superior view of the mitral valve (bicuspid valve)
b Open cusps of the mitral valve
c view from above of the aortic valve (valve slightly open)
d aortic valve; artery cut and valve opened

threads (*chordae tendineae*) to the *papillary muscles*. These cone-shaped processes on the inner ventricular walls, together with the chordae tendineae, prevent the cusps from flapping back during ventricular contractions (see Figs. 5.**10a, b**). A valve with three cusps (*tricuspid valve*) is situated between the right atrium and the right ventricle. A valve with two cusps (*bicuspid valve, mitral valve*) separates the left atrium and left ventricle (Fig. 5.**6**).

The *semilunar valves* are situated at the entrances to the pulmonary artery and the aorta. They prevent the blood from flowing back after a completed ventricular contraction (Fig. 5.**6**). The pulmonary and aortic valves consist of three pockets of duplicated endocardium that project into the lumen with their inferior surfaces directed toward the heart. When the margins of the semilunar valves are tightly apposed, the corresponding exit valve is closed. As the pressure in the ventricles increases, the margins of the semilunar valves draw apart, and the exit valve opens.

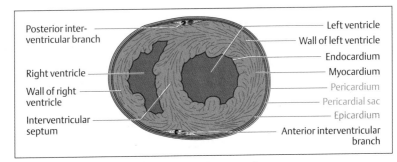

Fig. 5.**7**   **Transverse section through the two ventricles**

■ **The Wall of the Heart.** The heart wall consists of three layers of different thickness and structure (Fig. 5.**7**):

- an inner **serous coat** (**endocardium**)
- the actual **cardiac muscle** (**myocardium**)
- an **outer serous coat** (**epicardium**)

Between the epicardium and the inner side of the pericardium lies a thin *serous cavity*, scantily filled with fluid, which allows the frictionless movement of the heart in the pericardial sac. The myocardium consists of *striated cardiac muscle* and is about 0.7 cm thick in the right ventricle. The wall of the left ventricle, because of its higher pressure and the consequently increased load, averages about 1.4 cm in thickness.

The Conduction System

A comparison between the excitation of the heart, the conduction of the impulse, and contraction of the heart muscle reveals a number of differences (Fig. 5.**8**). For instance, in the presence of an adequate supply of nutrients and oxygen, a heart removed from the body can continue to beat spontaneously outside the body for a prolonged period without the need for an external nerve supply. The heart possesses an autonomous source of impulses, the sinoatrial node, that lies in the right atrium at the level of its junction with the superior vena cava. This so-called *pacemaker* has a frequency of about 60–70 beats per minute. The stimulus originates a con-

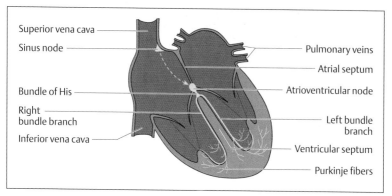

Fig. 5.**8**   **Cardiac conduction system**

traction in the atrial musculature, through which it is transmitted to the *atrioventricular node* (*A-V node*). From there, the stimulus reaches the *bundle of His*, which runs through the fibrous cardiac skeleton, and transmits it to the ventricular myocardium. There it runs first through the *bundle branches (of Tawara)* along the interventricular septum toward the apex and is distributed by the *Purkinje fibers* over the whole ventricular myocardium (Fig. 5.**8**). In this way, the cardiac musculature is stimulated along the conduction system and contracts rhythmically.

The cardiac frequency, impulse velocity, and force of contraction are influenced by the autonomic nervous system (*sympathetic* and *parasympathetic*, see p. 218). Thus cardiac activity is adjusted to the body's needs (e. g., increased cardiac minute volume during heavy physical labor).

The Coronary Vessels

The *coronary arteries* supply the heart muscle exclusively (Fig. 5.**9**). They arise from the aorta immediately above the aortic valve and send their major branches over the myocardium, their terminal branches entering the cardiac muscle from the outside.

After leaving the aorta, the *right coronary artery* (*arteria coronaria dextra*) runs in the coronary sulcus, at first under the right auricle, then around the right cardiac border toward the diaphragmatic surface of the heart. It

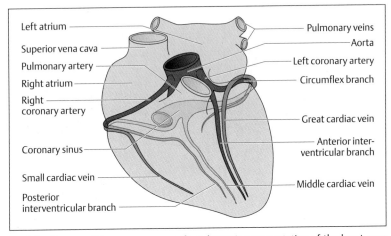

Fig. 5.**9** **Course of the coronary vessels.** Schematic representation of the heart seen from the front. (After Faller)

ends in the *posterior interventricular branch* (*ramus interventricularis posterior*), which runs to the apex of the heart (Fig. 5.**9**). The *left coronary artery* (*arteria coronaria sinistra*), after a short course, divides into the *anterior interventricular branch* (*ramus interventricularis anterior*), which runs over the anterior surface, and the *circumflex branch* (*ramus circumflexus*), which runs posteriorly. The veins collect the blood in the *small*, *middle*, and *great cardiac veins* (*venae cardiacae parva*, *media*, and *magna*), which collect in the coronary sinus and drain into the right atrium. If the coronary arteries narrow (arteriosclerosis), the affected cardiac muscle suffers from lack of oxygen and can die (cardiac infarct) if the vessel is totally occluded.

Systole and Diastole

The ventricles drive the blood in small volumes and synchronously into the pulmonary trunk and aorta. The contraction of the ventricular myocardium in this constantly repeated *biphasic cardiac cycle* is called *systole*; the relaxation is called *diastole* (Fig. 5.**10a**, **b**). Each of these phases, systole and diastole, in turn can be divided into two phases:

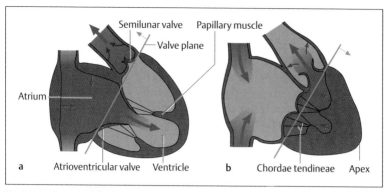

Fig. 5.**10 a, b   Simplified representation of the various actions of the heart**
a Ventricular filling phase (diastole)
b Ventricular ejection phase (systole). During the filling phase, the atrioventricular valves are open and the semilunar valves are closed; during the ejection phase, the atrioventricular valves are closed (the papillary muscles prevent prolapse of the cusps) and the semilunar valves are open. During systole the plane of the valves moves toward the apex; during diastole toward the base. (After Leonhardt)

▪ **Systole**	▪ **Diastole**
– Contraction phase	– Relaxation phase
– Ejection phase	– Filling phase

During the first part of systole, the ventricular myocardium begins to contract (*contraction phase*). Because the atrioventricular valves are closed, and the semilunar valves not yet open, the intraventricular pressure rises rapidly with no change in volume (*isovolumic contraction, isovolumetric contraction*). However, as soon as the pressure in the ventricles reaches the pressure in the aorta (about 120 mmHg) or the pulmonary artery (about 20 mmHg), the semilunar valves open, and the *ejection phase* begins. During this phase the ventricle is maximally contracted, and a volume of 70 ml of blood (*stroke volume*) is ejected into the arteries at rest. The intraventricular pressure then again falls below arterial pressure and the semilunar valves close again.

Systole is followed by diastole, during which the myocardium *relaxes* and at first the atrioventricular valves remain closed and the volume inside the ventricles (intraventricular volume) is unchanged (the so-called *end-diastolic volume* of about 70 ml). The pressure in the ventricles then falls below that in the atria, so that the atrioventricular valves open and blood flows from the atria into the ventricles (*ventricular filling*). The driving force for this movement is first of all the beginning atrial contraction, and especially the descent of the base of the heart (Fig. 5.**10a**, **b**), by which the base approaches the apex during the ejection phase, expanding the atria and thus sucking blood out of the veins. As the ventricular myocardium relaxes, the base again travels upward, and blood reaches the ventricles through the open atrioventricular valves.

Cardiac Output (CO)

Cardiac output is the volume of blood the heart pumps out in a defined time span. The *circulation volume* corresponds to the amount of blood put out by the heart per minute. The left and right heart always move equal amounts of blood, since otherwise the blood in one circulation would rapidly be dammed up, while the other would suffer from a lack of blood. If the heart at rest beats about 70 times per minute (*pulse frequency*) and each contraction ejects about 70 ml of blood into the systemic circulation (*stroke volume*), the calculated minute volume will be about 5 liters (70 × 70 ml= 4900 ml). This amounts to roughly the total blood volume of a person weighing 70 kg (see Chapter 6: The Blood).

During physical labor, the muscles, among other organs, must be perfused with more blood, and circulating blood volume and blood pressure must increase correspondingly. Heart rate and stroke volume can be raised to increase the circulating blood volume. In this way, cardiac output can increase up to 25 l/min during severe physical exertion, that is, the normal blood volume can turn over about five times. Such an increase might be achieved, for instance, if the stroke volume increases from 70 ml to 140 ml and the heart rate is briefly raised to 180 beats/min (180/min × 140 ml = 25,200 ml/min = 25.2 l/min).

Nerve Supply of the Heart

During strenuous work the heart must eject up to five times more blood. This adaptation of cardiac activity to increased demand is partly achieved by the heart itself, but is mainly guided by the *autonomic nerves* to the heart. The heart's own adaptation is achieved because greater filling stretches the cardiac muscle fibers. The stretching leads to a stronger contraction and so to a greater stroke volume.

By way of the efferent sympathetic and parasympathetic nerves (see Chapter 14: The Autonomic Nervous System), the central nervous system (CNS) (*vasomotor centers in the brainstem*) influences *heart rate* (*chronotropic effect*), *excitability* (*bathmotropic effect*), *force of myocardial contraction* (*inotropic effect*), and *impulse conductivity* (*dromotropic effect*). The effect of the *sympathetic system* is to enhance cardiac activity (e. g., acceleration of heart rate, increase in contractile force, acceleration of stimulus conduction in the A-V node), while the *parasympathetic system* inhibits or dampens cardiac activity (e. g., deceleration of heart rate, reduction in the force of contraction, decrease in the rate of spread of a stimulus from the atria to the ventricles). While activation of the sympathetic system occurs primarily through the transmitter *norepinephrine*, the parasympathetic system (vagus nerve) exerts its inhibitory action chiefly through the transmitter *acetylcholine.*

The individual effects of the autonomic cardiac nerves are expressed in different degrees, since sympathetic and parasympathetic innervation differ in the various regions of the heart. While the sympathetic innervation supplies the atria and ventricles equally, the fibers of the vagus nerve (parasympathetic) run primarily to the atria and to the sinus and A-V nodes.

Heart Sounds and Heart Murmurs

The beginning of ventricular systole and the closure of the atrioventricular valves create the *first, dull heart sound* (*lubb*). The closure of the semilunar valves can be heard as the *second, more high-pitched, brief valve sound* (*dub*). As the heart sounds are conducted along the bloodstream, the sounds are not best *auscultated* (listened to) where the valves *project to the surface* of the thorax. Rather, the best place for *auscultation* is where the bloodstream is closest to the chest wall after the closure of the respective valve (Fig. 5.**11**):

- **Tricuspid valve**, right sternal border at the level of the 5th intercostal space

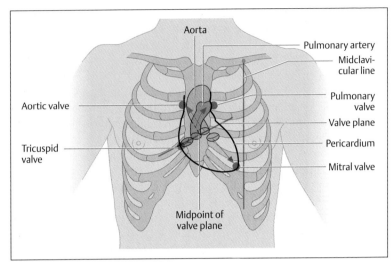

Fig. 5.**11** **Sites for cardiac auscultation.** Red circles mark the sites for auscultation. The valves lie in a plane; the arrows indicate the direction of the bloodstream (conduction of the heart sounds). (After Faller)

■ **Bicuspid** or **mitral valve**, at the apex in the left 5th intercostal space
■ **Pulmonic valve**, in the 2nd intercostal space at the left sternal border
■ **Aortic valve**, in the 2nd intercostal space at the right sternal border

When the heart valves are pathologically distorted and cannot open (*stenosis*) or close (*insufficiency*) competently, the turbulence of the bloodstream causes *heart murmurs*. The type of valve disease can be determined by the intensity and timing of the murmur in relation to the first or second heart sound at the point of auscultation.

Resting and Action Potential of the Heart

Heart muscle cells are polarized at rest similarly to skeletal muscle. Thus, there is a *potential difference* between the intracellular (negative) and extracellular (positive) spaces. This *resting or membrane potential* can be measured as an electric potential difference and is of the order of –80 to –90 mV (see Chapter 1: Membrane or Resting Potential of a Cell). When the cell is stimulated, the potential collapses (*depolarization*), followed by recovery (*repolarization*). In the course of this process, the resting potential of –80 (–90) mV reverses for a brief period up to +20 mV. This total tension or potential difference of 120 mV is defined as the *action potential*, and it is the signal for the myocardium to contract. Its mechanism is equivalent to that of the action potential in nerve cells and it results from the exchange of sodium and potassium ions (see Chapter 3: Nerve Tissue, The Nerve Impulse).

Differences between Cardiac and Skeletal Muscle

Although cardiac and skeletal muscle have much in common both structurally and functionally, they differ in important points. Under physiological conditions, skeletal muscle can only be stimulated and induced to contract by a nerve. Heart muscle, by contrast, contains *specialized muscle cells* (cells of the sinus node) that can induce impulses (action potentials) not only in response to external stimuli but spontaneously, and propagate these impulses over the cardiac conduction system. Additionally, all the cardiac muscle cells are connected with each other in a network by gap junctions at the *intercalated disks* (Fig. 3.**11c**). By this mechanism, an impulse originating in the sinus node is first propagated fanwise over the atria, and after a brief delay conducted over a narrow muscular bridge (A-V node) to the ventricular myocardium. The delay at the A-V node ensures that the ventricles are stimulated only after the atria have contracted, thus achieving adequate filling of the ventricles.

The Electrocardiogram (ECG)

The electrocardiogram is a diagnostic procedure that provides information on the development, spread, and return of the electrical impulse over the myocardium of the atria and the ventricles. It also allows conclusions to be drawn concerning the *position of the heart, heart rate*, and *cardiac rhythm*.

ECG Leads

The *potential difference* of about 120 mV between a depolarized and a resting area of heart muscle generates in the area of the heart an electric field that projects to the body surface. Consequently, potential differences of up to 1 mV (1000 mV = 1 V) arise between individual points on the surface of, for example, the right arm and the left leg during the spread and recovery of the cardiac impulse. These potential differences can be detected by electrodes and measured and amplified. They may then be recorded as a tracing on paper or on a monitor. The electrodes may be arranged as *unipolar* or *bipolar* leads, each displaying a different projection of the cardiac impulse on the surface. The height and shape of the various depolarizing waves depend on the direction of the waves toward or away from an electrode (vectors).

The electrocardiograph commonly used in medical practice consists of 12 standard surface leads: 6 limb leads (I, II, III, aV_R, aV_L, aV_F) and 6 precordial (chest) leads (V_1–V_6). The limb leads include the bipolar (Einthoven) leads I, II, III and the augmented unipolar leads aV_R, aV_L, aV_F (Fig. 5.**12**). The limb leads project cardiac electrical activity to the frontal plane of the body, while the unipolar precordial (Wilson) leads V_1–V_6

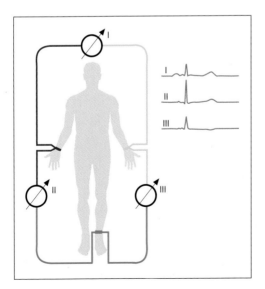

Fig. 5.**12** **Positioning of the limb leads**

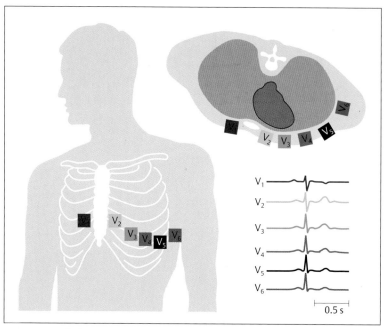

Fig. 5.**13** **Lead placements for ECG (chest leads).** The standard chest leads V_1–V_6 are unipolar leads. V_1 and V_2 are placed in the 4th intercostal space immediately to the left and right of the sternum. V_3 to V_6 are placed lower and more to the side. (After Schwegler)

represent the projection of electrical activity of the heart to the horizontal plane (Fig. 5.**13**).

ECG Tracing

The ECG tracing contains several waves, named by convention as shown in Fig. 5.**14**. The *P wave*, for instance, which lasts less than 0.1 seconds, is the result of the spread of the excitation over the atria. The *Q wave* with the *R* and *S waves*, the so-called *QRS complex*, signals the beginning of the excitation of the ventricles and also lasts less than 0.1 seconds. Next comes the *T wave*, which is the expression of the end of ventricular excitation. The interval between the beginning of the P wave and the Q wave (*PQ interval*) therefore corresponds to the conduction delay (0.1–0.2 sec-

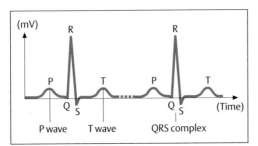

Fig. 5.**14**   **ECG tracing.**
Recording of two complexes
(see text for description)
(chest lead V$_4$)

onds), i.e., the time from the beginning of the excitation of the atrium to
the beginning of the excitation of the ventricles. The *QT interval* (Q wave
to the end of the T wave) is the time required for depolarization and repolarization of both ventricles. The duration of the QT interval is
frequency-dependent (0.32–0.39 seconds).

Heart Rate

The interval between two successive R waves corresponds to the duration of one cardiac cycle. This allows the heart rate to be calculated from
moment to moment.

■ **60 s/R-R interval (s) = beats/min (e. g., 60/0.8 = 75)**
At rest the heart beats about 70 times a minute (normal sinus rhythm). A
rise in frequency is called *tachycardia*, while a slowing is called *bradycar-
dia*. Causes of disturbances of rhythm (*arrhythmias*) may include irregular development of the excitation in the sinus node, transmission delays
in the A-V node, or the generation of spontaneous excitations (*extrasys-
toles*) in the myocardium. Atrial fibrillation is defined as an atrial
frequency in excess of 350 beats/min. Ventricular fibrillation is especially dangerous, because when it occurs the heart no longer moves any
blood.

Blood Pressure

The *arterial blood pressure* (BP) is the pressure against which the left ventricle must eject blood. The pressure wave so generated can be palpated as a pulse wave with a finger placed on a superficial artery (e. g., the radial artery = radial pulse). However, blood pressure is never constant, but alternates between a systolic level (maximal blood pressure during the ejection phase = *systolic blood pressure*) and a diastolic level (minimal blood pressure at the opening of the aortic valve = *diastolic blood pressure*). The systolic blood pressure normally is about 120 mmHg, the diastolic about 80 mmHg. The 40 mmHg difference is called the *pulse pressure*. During physical exertion the systolic pressure may briefly attain 200 mmHg. Resting diastolic pressure ≥90 mmHg or systolic pressure ≥140 is called *high blood pressure* (*hypertension*). The value of the blood pressure is the resultant of cardiac output and vascular resistance (vascular diameter and elasticity) (see Regulation of Organ Perfusion). If the elasticity of the vessels is impaired, e. g., by deposits in their walls (arteriosclerosis), the diastolic pressure rises first, followed later by the systolic, which then remains elevated even at rest.

Measurement of the Blood Pressure

Blood pressure is most commonly measured by the *indirect method*. An inflatable rubber cuff attached to a *manometer* is placed around the upper arm of the sitting patient (Fig. 5.**15**). This is inflated until the brachial artery is completely occluded (the radial pulse can no longer be felt). If now the pressure in the cuff is slowly released, and a stethoscope is applied to the elbow, a pulsating sound (the so-called *Korotkoff sound*) can be heard at the point where systolic blood pressure just overcomes the cuff pressure and blood enters the artery with every systole. At this point the systolic pressure and the cuff pressure are identical. When the cuff pressure continues to be lowered the sounds initially become louder, then increasingly softer until nothing more can be heard. At this point the blood can again flow unimpeded and the cuff pressure therefore corresponds to the diastolic pressure. The sounds are caused by *turbulence* in the blood where the artery is narrowed by the cuff.

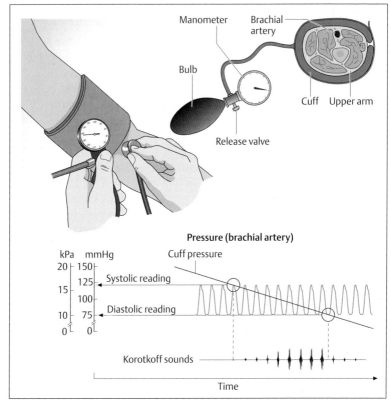

Fig. 5.**15 Blood pressure measurement by the indirect method.** (After Silbernagl and Lang)

Examination of the Heart

The following *clinical examinations* are the main ones used to evaluate the size, activity, and performance of the heart.

■ **Physical Examination (Inspection, Palpation, Percussion, Auscultation).** Inspection of the supine patient provides information about pulsations in the region of the heart. By palpation (feeling with the hand) the position of the *apical impulse* in the 5th intercostal space inside the midclavicular line (Fig. 5.**11**) can be determined. By determining cardiac dullness, percussion (striking with a short, sharp blow to detect underlying sounds) provides information about the shape and size of the heart. Cardiac rhythm (regular, irregular), heart sounds (valve closure), and heart murmurs (due to valvular disease or openings in the separating walls [septa] of the heart) can be determined using a stethoscope (auscultation, listening) (see Fig. 5.**11** for sites where sounds are best heard).

■ **Electrocardiogram (ECG).** The ECG permits the evaluation of impulse propagation and the condition of the heart muscle (see above).

■ **Radiographic Examinations.** *Radiographic examination* of the heart is best undertaken with the patient standing, using PA (posteroanterior—beam from posterior to anterior; Fig. 5.**1**) and left lateral images. In the radiographic image of the heart, the chambers filled with blood are superimposed on the great vessels and their walls. Size, shape, and contours can be evaluated especially well. Successive sections of the heart not obscured by superposition of intracardiac (atrial and ventricular) and intravascular (coronary arteries, great vessels) spaces can be displayed by *computerized tomography* (CT scanning) with contrast enhancement.

■ **Echocardiogram.** In cardiac imaging the use of ultrasound is called echocardiography. Currently this is the most important noninvasive procedure used to display the cavities and valves of the heart, and the great thoracic vessels. Echocardiography can be used not only to display the cardiac image, but also to evaluate the functioning of the chambers and valves of the heart.

■ **Cardiac Catheterization.** In *angiocardiography*, a technique used for the radiographic examination of the heart, a contrast agent is delivered through a catheter to show the chambers of the heart and the great vessels. The catheter can be advanced into the right heart through a peripheral vein (e. g., leg or arm vein) or into the left heart through a peripheral artery (e. g., leg or arm artery) (*left and right heart catheterization*). In *coronary angiography*, the coronary arteries are shown by selective injection of contrast agent.

■ **Magnetic Resonance Imaging (MRI).** MRI, like CT scanning, allows the display of sections of the heart free from superposition of intracardiac and intravascular structures; in addition to the horizontal, it can also display sagittal and coronal planes.

■ The Vascular System—Structure and Function

The Blood Vessels: Arteries, Veins, and Capillaries

The circulatory system connects the *capillary bed*, which serves the exchange of substances, with the heart through the arteries and veins. The function of the arteries and veins is strictly to channel the blood, not to exchange substances. Arteries and veins may be distinguished by the fact that pressure in the arteries is high and that in the veins is low.

The Structure of Arteries and Veins

Arteries and veins resemble each other in that *their walls contain three coats*. However, the vessels adapt to their different circulatory tasks by differing in the structure of these coats (Fig. 5.**16**). The *inner coat* (vascular endothelium, *tunica intima*) consists of a single layer of endothelial cells applied to a thin connective tissue layer, the basement membrane. The *middle coat* (*tunica media*) contains primarily smooth muscle and elastic tissue fibers. The *outer coat* (*tunica adventitia*, adventitious coat) embeds the vessel in its surroundings and consists mainly of connective tissue. In addition, the arteries have an elastic, fenestrated membrane

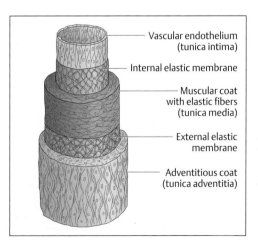

Vascular endothelium (tunica intima)

Internal elastic membrane

Muscular coat with elastic fibers (tunica media)

External elastic membrane

Adventitious coat (tunica adventitia)

Fig. 5.16 **Coats of the wall of an artery.** (After Leonhardt)

(*membrana elastica interna*) between the inner and middle coat. Usually another, thinner elastic membrane (*membrana elastica externa*) lies between the middle and the outer coat.

Arteries are distinguished by an especially well developed muscle coat, which contains a varying amount of elastic fiber according to its site (predominantly *elastic* and predominantly *muscular* arteries). This layer is the driving force of the blood vessels (Fig. 5.**17**): by dilating (*vasodilatation*) and constricting (*vasoconstriction*) the diameter of the blood vessels, it regulates blood flow and blood pressure. The arteries near the heart contain a high proportion of elastic fibers and this creates an *elastic recoil* (Fig. 5.**18a**, **b**). The blood ejected during systole is partly stored by expansion of the arterial wall, and is then moved forward during diastole by elastic recoil, thus achieving a *continuous blood flow*.

Veins in general have wider lumina and thinner walls than arteries. The three coats are less well defined and the muscular coat is less well developed. Most veins, with the exception of those close to the heart, contain *venous valves* (Fig. 5.**17**). These endothelial folds, projecting like pockets into the lumen of the vessel, act as one-way valves that guide the blood toward the heart and prevent backward flow.

Structure of the Capillaries

In the smallest blood vessels, the capillaries, the coats are reduced to one, the tunica intima (Figs. 5.**16** and 5.**17**); this facilitates the exchange of *fluids* and *gases*. The exchange of substances basically occurs in both directions: from the blood through the endothelium and basement membrane into the surrounding tissue, and in the reverse direction.

Lymph Vessels

The lymphatic system runs parallel to the venous side of the circulation (see Fig. 5.**25**). It begins near the capillaries as *"blind" lymphatic capillaries* that reabsorb fluid that has not been taken up from the tissues by the blood vessels (lymphatic fluid [lymph], ca. 10% of the fluid filtered during substance exchange—see p. 249). Small and large lymph vessels then return the lymph to the venous blood. The wall of the lymph vessels consists of an endothelium, and a thin layer of rhythmically contracting

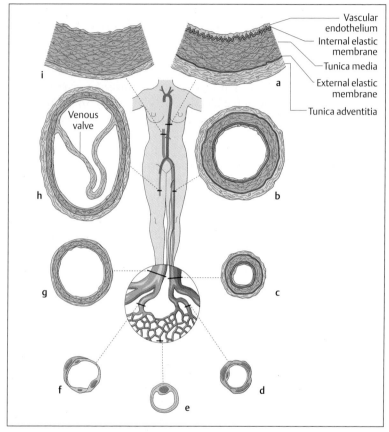

Fig. 5.17   Structure of the blood vessels in each segment of the systemic circulation. (After Leonhardt)

a–d Arteries
e   Capillary
f–i Veins

a Structure of the aortic wall (elastic artery)
b Large artery (muscular artery)
c Small artery
d Arteriole with 1 or 2 layers of smooth muscle cells

e Capillary wall consisting of only endothelium and a basement membrane
f Venule
g Small vein
h Large vein containing a valve
i Structure of the wall of a vena cava; elastic fibers confined to the muscle layer

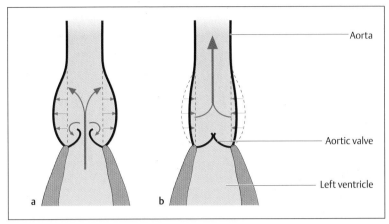

Fig. 5.**18 a, b** **Elastic recoil of the aorta.** During systole a portion of the stroke volume is stored in the elastic wall of the aorta (**a**) to be moved forward in diastole (**b**). (After Leonhardt)

smooth muscle cells. Similarly to the situation in the veins, numerous valves further the transport of the lymph. The course of the lymph vessels is interrupted by *lymph node stations*, which represent a kind of *biological filter* and fulfill important functions in *immune defense* (see Chapter 6: The Lymphoid Organs).

The lymph vessels coming from the legs and the abdomen join along the posterior wall of the upper abdomen to form the *thoracic duct*, which runs upward from there between the vertebral column and the aorta. It drains into the junction of the left subclavian and internal jugular veins (*left venous angle*), which also receives the lymphatic drainage from the chest, neck, head, and arm on the left side. The lymphatic ducts of the right side drain into the *right venous angle* (Figs. 5.**19** and 5.**24**).

Systemic and Pulmonary Circulation

Functionally the circulatory system can be divided into two parts: a *greater* (*systemic*) and a *lesser* (*pulmonary*) circulation (Fig. 5.**20**). The deoxygenated (venous) blood from the lower and upper body travels through the great venous trunks to the right atrium and then through

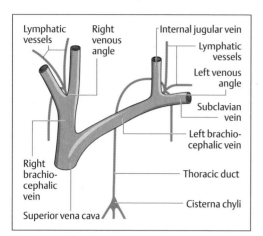

Fig. 5.**19** **Junctions of the great lymphatic trunks into the venous system**

the right ventricle and the pulmonary artery to the lung (*pulmonary circulation*). The blood is enriched with oxygen (arterialized) in the lung and flows through the pulmonary veins back into the left atrium of the heart. From there it reaches the left ventricle, which pumps the blood by way of the aorta into the greater circulation (*systemic circulation*). The blood is distributed through the whole body in the larger and smaller arteries (*distributing function*) and eventually reaches the terminal vessels, the capillaries. After exchanging substances and gases in the tissues, the blood returns to the heart through the venous part of the systemic circulation.

Of special significance in the systemic circulation is the *portal system* (see Chapter 9: The Liver). In this circulation, two capillary beds are linked serially. The blood supplying the gastrointestinal tract and the spleen is collected together with the nutrients taken up by the mucosa of the small intestine in a first capillary bed (see also Chapter 9: Mucous Membrane of the Small Bowel) and brought by the portal vein to a capillary bed in the liver. Here, among other processes, carbohydrates are stored in the form of glycogen, fats are metabolized and broken down, and detoxification (e. g., of medications) takes place. The blood then continues its path through the hepatic veins into the inferior vena cava. The nutrients remaining in the blood now pass through the lungs, where the blood is enriched with oxygen, and then reach the systemic

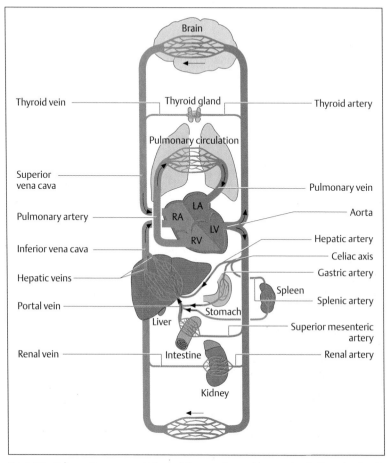

Fig. 5.**20   Schematic representation of the greater and lesser circulations (systemic and pulmonary circulation)**
LA = Left atrium   LV = Left ventricle
RA = Right atrium   RV = Right ventricle
The arrows indicate the direction of blood flow

capillaries (site of substance exchange). From there they reach the tissue cells, where, together with oxygen, they are used for metabolic processes.

The Fetal Circulation

The prenatal circulation differs in essential points from that of the new-born. Since the lungs of the unborn child are not yet aerated, and therefore there is no gas exchange, the blood must *short-circuit* the lungs (Fig. 5.**21a**, **b**). A large part of the blood passes directly from the right into the left atrium through a hole in the atrial septum (*foramen ovale*) and so by-passes the pulmonary circulation. That part of the blood that reaches the pulmonary artery through the right atrium flows through a short circuit (*ductus arteriosus*) into the aorta and so also avoids the pulmonary circulation. The necessary gas exchange of the antenatal circulation takes place in the *placenta* (*afterbirth*). *Oxygen-poor blood* flows through the two *umbilical arteries* to the placenta, and *arterialized blood* returns to the infant's body by way of the *umbilical vein.*

After birth, the lungs expand and the pulmonary circulation develops from their greatly increased perfusion. At the same time, the foramen ovale and the ductus arteriosus close as a result of the changed pressure differences. This process completes the change that aligns the two circulations in series.

The Arterial System

All systemic arteries flow from the aorta (Fig. 5.**22**). After the origin of the two coronary vessels (Fig. 5.**9**) the aorta ascends somewhat to the right (*ascending aorta*), arches to the left as the *aortic arch*, and then runs downward on the left side in front of the vertebral column (*descending aorta = thoracic aorta*). After piercing the diaphragm through the **aortic hiatus** it runs as the *abdominal aorta* to the level of the 4th lumbar vertebra, where it divides into the two common iliac arteries (*aortic bifurcation*).

The two great vascular trunks supplying the head and upper limb branch off from the aortic arch. The first branch arises on the right side and is the common trunk (*brachiocephalic trunk, innominate artery*) of the *right subclavian* and *right common carotid arteries*. The second and third branches leaving the aortic arch are the *left common carotid artery* and the *left subclavian artery*. The two common carotid arteries run cephalad and divide into the *external* and *internal carotid arteries* at the

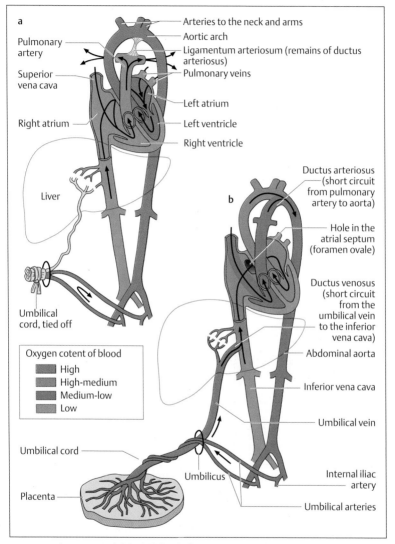

a

Arteries to the neck and arms

Aortic arch

Pulmonary artery

Ligamentum arteriosum (remains of ductus arteriosus)

Pulmonary veins

Superior vena cava

Left atrium

Right atrium

Left ventricle

Right ventricle

Liver

b

Ductus arteriosus (short circuit from pulmonary artery to aorta)

Hole in the atrial septum (foramen ovale)

Ductus venosus (short circuit from the umbilical vein to the inferior vena cava)

Abdominal aorta

Inferior vena cava

Umbilical cord, tied off

Oxygen cotent of blood
- High
- High-medium
- Medium-low
- Low

Umbilical vein

Umbilical cord

Umbilicus

Internal iliac artery

Placenta

Umbilical arteries

Fig. 5.**21 a, b   Neonatal (a) and fetal (b) circulation.** The pulmonary circulation is formed, but is essentially bypassed by short circuits. (After Leonhardt)

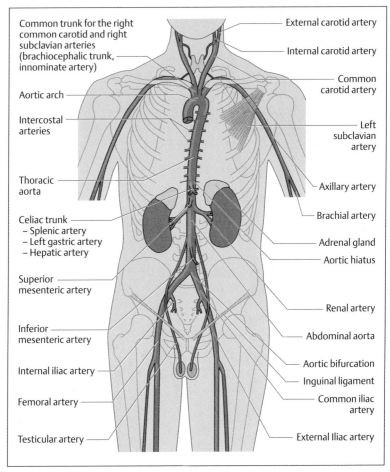

Common trunk for the right common carotid and right subclavian arteries (brachiocephalic trunk, innominate artery)	External carotid artery
	Internal carotid artery
	Common carotid artery
Aortic arch	Left subclavian artery
Intercostal arteries	
Thoracic aorta	Axillary artery
	Brachial artery
Celiac trunk – Splenic artery – Left gastric artery – Hepatic artery	Adrenal gland
	Aortic hiatus
Superior mesenteric artery	Renal artery
Inferior mesenteric artery	Abdominal aorta
Internal iliac artery	Aortic bifurcation
	Inguinal ligament
Femoral artery	Common iliac artery
Testicular artery	External Iliac artery

Fig. 5.**22**   **Overview of the great vessels arising from the aorta**

level of the 4th cervical vertebra. While the external carotid artery supplies the external regions of the face and head, the internal carotid artery runs through the base of the skull to the brain.

The subclavian artery continues in the axilla (armpit) as the *axillary artery* and in the upper arm as the *brachial artery* (Fig. 5.**23**). At the level

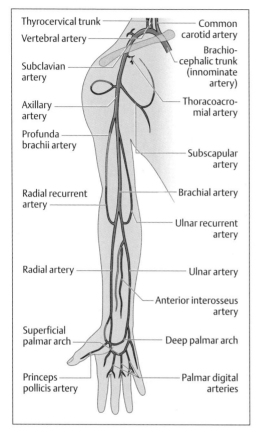

Fig. 5.**23** **Overview of the arteries of the upper extremity**

Thyrocervical trunk

Vertebral artery

Subclavian artery

Axillary artery

Profunda brachii artery

Radial recurrent artery

Radial artery

Superficial palmar arch

Princeps pollicis artery

Common carotid artery

Brachio-cephalic trunk (innominate artery)

Thoracoacro-mial artery

Subscapular artery

Brachial artery

Ulnar recurrent artery

Ulnar artery

Anterior interosseus artery

Deep palmar arch

Palmar digital arteries

of the elbow it divides into the *radial* and *ulnar* arteries, which supply the forearm and the hand. On the palm of the hand the two arteries and their branches form the *superficial* and *deep palmar arches*, from which arise the arteries to the fingers (*palmar digital arteries*).

From the thoracic aorta the paired *intercostal arteries* run to supply the intercostal muscles. Other branches supply the esophagus, the pericardium, and the mediastinum. After passing through the diaphragm (Fig. 5.**22**), the aorta gives rise to paired branches to the inferior surface of the diaphragm (*inferior phrenic arteries*), the kidneys (*renal arteries*), the adrenal glands (*suprarenal arteries*), and the gonads (*ovarian* or *testicular arteries*). The upper abdominal organs are supplied by the *hepatic artery*, the *left gastric artery*, and the s*plenic artery*, all arising from a single trunk (*celiac trunk, celiac axis*) (Fig. 5.**22**). Immediately below it an unpaired branch, the *superior mesenteric artery*, arises to supply primarily the small intestine. The unpaired *inferior mesenteric artery* arises from the abdominal aorta further down, below the origin of the arteries to the gonads, and supplies the large intestine.

The divisions of the aorta, the left and right common iliac arteries, each divide into the *internal* and *external iliac artery* (Fig. 5.**24**). While the internal iliac artery supplies the pelvic viscera (urinary bladder, sex organs, and rectum), the external iliac artery runs toward the lower extremity and continues as the *femoral artery*. It gives rise to the *profunda femoris* artery and then runs behind the knee joint to become the *popliteal artery*.

On the back of the lower leg this artery divides into the *peroneal artery*, as well as the *anterior* and *posterior tibial arteries*. After penetrating the interosseus membrane to the anterior side of the leg, the anterior tibial artery proceeds to the foot, where it continues as the *dorsalis pedis* artery, and eventually the *arcuate artery*. The arcuate artery gives off the *deep plantar artery* to anastomose with the arteries of the sole of the foot and then the *dorsal metatarsal arteries* to the metatarsal bones. The posterior tibial artery runs on the posterior side of the lower leg, also toward the foot. At the level of the medial malleolus it divides into the *medial* and *lateral plantar arteries* to the sole of the foot. These two arteries meet in the *plantar arch*, from which vessels arise to supply the metatarsals and the toes.

The Venous System

With the exception of a few large vascular trunks, arteries and veins have the same names (e. g., femoral artery and vein). The venous system in general is divided into a superficial venous net, embedded between muscle fascia and skin, and a deep system. The *superficial* and *deep venous systems* are connected with each other by so-called *perforating veins*. Large arteries are accompanied by a single venous trunk, smaller

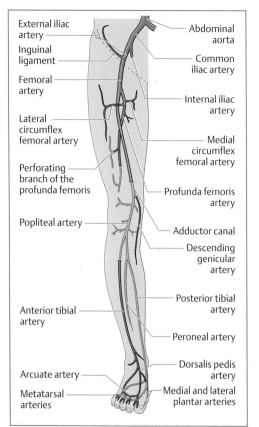

Fig. 5.**24** **Overview over the arteries of the lower extremity**

External iliac artery

Inguinal ligament

Femoral artery

Lateral circumflex femoral artery

Perforating branch of the profunda femoris

Popliteal artery

Anterior tibial artery

Arcuate artery

Metatarsal arteries

Abdominal aorta

Common iliac artery

Internal iliac artery

Medial circumflex femoral artery

Profunda femoris artery

Adductor canal

Descending genicular artery

Posterior tibial artery

Peroneal artery

Dorsalis pedis artery

Medial and lateral plantar arteries

arteries as a rule by two. In the extremities, the large vessels always run on the flexor side of joints.

At numerous sites in the systemic circulation, blood can reach certain regions by indirect routes, which detour normal flow. If these other routes can enlarge to the point where adequate circulation is maintained even when the main blood supply is interrupted, the circulatory detour is called *collateral circulation*. This is true for veins as well as arteries.

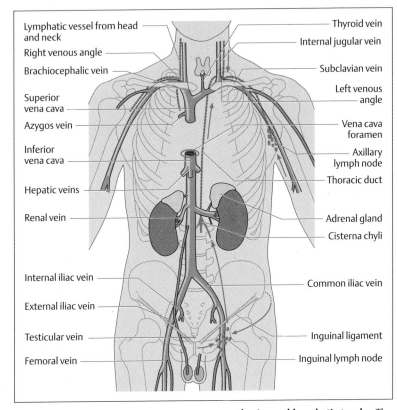

Fig. 5.**25**   **Overview of the most important central veins and lymphatic trunks.** The arrows indicate the direction of lymph flow (green)

At the level of the trunk, the whole venous system is arranged on a different principle from that of the arteries. The *superior vena cava* collects the blood from the head, neck, and arm (Fig. 5.**25**). It is formed by the confluence of two short venous trunks, the *brachiocephalic veins* (*innominate veins*), each of which is formed by the junction of the left and right *subclavian* and *internal jugular veins*. The left brachiocephalic vein also receives the thyroid vein. Additionally, the superior vena cava receives the *azygos vein*, which among other areas drains the intercostal

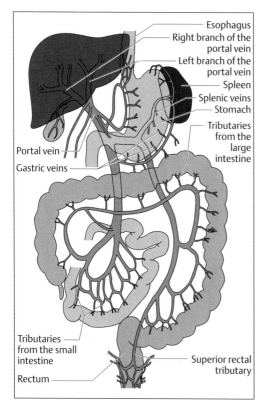

Esophagus
Right branch of the portal vein
Left branch of the portal vein
Spleen
Splenic veins
Stomach
Tributaries from the large intestine
Portal vein
Gastric veins
Tributaries from the small intestine
Rectum
Superior rectal tributary

Fig. 5.**26** **The portal system.** (After Schwegler)

spaces. The subclavian veins collect the blood from the superficial and deep veins of the upper arm (see Fig. 5.**27**).

The *inferior vena cava* is formed on the right side by the junction of the *right* and *left common iliac veins* between the 4th and 5th lumbar vertebrae. It is the largest vein in the body, with a diameter of about 3 cm (Fig. 5.**25**). In its cephalad course it receives the two *renal veins* and, just before piercing the diaphragm (*caval opening, foramen venae cavae*), the three *hepatic veins*. Immediately above the diaphragm it enters the right atrium. The blood from the unpaired abdominal organs, such as the stomach, small intestine, large intestine, spleen, and pancreas is channeled by the *portal vein* to the liver (Fig. 5.**26**).

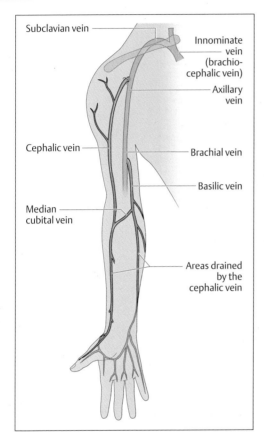

Subclavian vein

Innominate vein (brachio-cephalic vein)

Axillary vein

Cephalic vein

Brachial vein

Basilic vein

Median cubital vein

Areas drained by the cephalic vein

Fig. 5.**27** **Overview of the most important veins of the upper extremity**

The blood from the pelvis (*internal iliac veins*) and the lower extremity (*external iliac veins*) reaches the *inferior vena cava* through the *common iliac veins* (Fig. 5.**28**).

At the inguinal ligament the external iliac vein continues as the *femoral vein*, which receives among others the *great saphenous vein* (Fig. 5.**28**). The *small saphenous vein* drains into the *popliteal vein*, a deep vein of the leg, which collects blood from the muscles of the lower

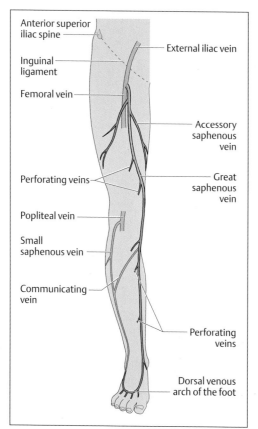

Anterior superior
iliac spine

External iliac vein

Inguinal
ligament

Femoral vein

Accessory
saphenous
vein

Perforating veins

Great
saphenous
vein

Popliteal vein

Small
saphenous vein

Communicating
vein

Perforating
veins

Dorsal venous
arch of the foot

Fig. 5.**28** **Overview of the most important veins of the lower extremity**

leg and channels it to the femoral vein. The saphenous veins communicate with the deep veins of the leg by way of the so-called *perforating veins.*

■ The Vascular System—Physiological Principles

Flow, Pressure, and Resistance in the Vascular System

If we use the universal laws of physics for blood flow through the vascular system, then Ohm's law for electrical circuits states:

■ Intensity (flow rate) $= \dfrac{\text{Pressure difference}}{\text{Vascular resistance}}$

i.e., *flow rate* increases with increasing pressure difference, and decreases with increasing *vascular resistance*. The flow resistance to be overcome is created by the internal friction of the flowing fluid. Blood flows relatively easily through the large vessels, but the smaller arteries, and especially the arterioles and capillaries, oppose flow by the high resistance created by their small diameter (*peripheral resistance*). Thus, the greater the peripheral resistance, the greater the pressure necessary to overcome it.

In principle, then, the functioning of the vascular (=circulatory) system rests on the *generation of a fall in pressure* from arteries to veins, which maintains blood flow. Since in the systemic circulation the *mean arterial pressure* declines from about 100 mmHg (the mean of systolic pressure of 120 mmHg and diastolic pressure of 80 mmHg) to about 3 mmHg, the pressure gradient is about 97 mmHg. Hence the performance of the circulation can be adapted to the body's needs by changing the flow rate (*pumping performance of the heart = cardiac output*) and the resistance to flow (peripheral resistance). For the systemic circulation therefore:

■ Cardiac output $= \dfrac{\text{Blood pressure difference}}{\text{Peripheral resistance}}$

Since the elevated pressure in the systemic circulation always places a considerable load on the vascular walls, it is maintained as constant as possible. Adaptation to altered conditions in the circulation then occurs preferentially by changing the pumping performance of the heart or the peripheral resistance. When, for example, the total need for blood rises because of increased muscular activity, cardiac output rises and peripheral resistance is lowered by dilation of the vessels in the muscles. In this way, lowering or raising the peripheral resistance in specific organs can give rise to the redistribution of the cardiac output according to need from some organs in favor of others.

Distribution of the Cardiac Output (CO)

The *distribution of blood flow* to various organs at rest and during activity varies a great deal and depends on the requirements at each site (e. g., *oxygen consumption* and *metabolic activity*) but also on the local anatomy. Thus the organs in the systemic circulation that are connected in parallel (e. g., brain, gastrointestinal tract, kidneys, muscles, skin) receive only a part of the CO, whereas the serially connected pulmonary circulation receives the whole CO. As a rule, an active muscle must be perfused better than a resting one, though certain organs such as the kidneys must be maximally perfused even at rest.

The *distribution of cardiac output* to the various organs depends on the widely varying *regional flow (vascular) resistances*. For instance, 15–20 % of resting cardiac output goes to the muscles, but during strenuous physical activity this may increase to 75 %. During digestion, a relatively large portion of the CO goes to the gastrointestinal tract. The perfusion of the skin is also increased during strenuous physical activity or with raised outside temperatures, in order to facilitate heat loss. Other organs, such as the brain, which is very sensitive to oxygen deprivation, must always receive an adequate blood supply (about 15 % of CO). To maintain their control and elimination functions, the kidneys also must receive about 20–25 % of the CO even at rest and so are well perfused in relation to their weight (0.5 % of body weight).

Regulation of Organ Perfusion

The perfusion needs of any one organ can be met in two principal ways:

- Increase in the arterial blood pressure
- Reduction in the peripheral resistance

A rise in blood pressure, however, is not the most suitable solution, since all organs would receive more blood flow, and moreover a doubling of the blood pressure (240/160 mmHg) would only result in doubling of the flow. Reduction in the peripheral resistance, however, by *localized vasodilatation* (*widening of the blood vessels*) leads to a significant change in blood flow. This is because of hemodynamic physics, by which the resistance to fluid flow in a tube (blood vessel) depends on the length of the tube, the viscosity of the fluid, and the fourth power of the radius of the tube (r^4) (*Hagen–Poiseuille law*). Thus, a reduction in arterial radius of just 16 % would double the resistance. On the other hand *doubling the radius of the vessel* would result in a *16-fold increase in blood flow*.

Since the greater part of all the peripheral resistance is located in the small arteries and the so-called "*precapillary arterioles*," these may be described as the *vascular resistance*. The regulation of peripheral blood flow therefore depends above all on the regulation of the muscle tone of small arteries and arterioles. Thus the vessels narrow (vasoconstriction) with contraction (increased tone) of their smooth muscles, while if the muscle fibers relax the vessels dilate passively. The *state of contraction of the vascular musculature* can essentially be influenced by local factors (*autoregulation*) or by hormonal or nervous signals.

Autoregulation of Vascular Tone

Among other factors, *lack of oxygen* leads to *vasodilatation*, so that blood flow and with it oxygen transport rise. Similarly, an accumulation of metabolic products (e.g., carbon dioxide, hydrogen ions) *increases local blood flow*. In this way, blood flow adjusts itself to local need.

Nervous and Hormonal Control of Vascular Tone

With few exceptions, the *state of contraction of the vessel wall* depends on the autonomic nervous system, essentially the sympathetic system (*vascular sympathetic*). The primary circulating *vasoactive hormones* that act on the muscles of the blood vessels are *epinephrine* and *norepinephrine*, which are liberated from the adrenal medulla by sympathetic stimulation (see Chapter 7: Adrenal Medulla). According to their effect on different receptors (α and β receptors), stimulation can result in *vasoconstriction* or *vasodilatation*. In contrast to these systemically (affecting all blood vessels) acting hormones, localized blood flow changes (e.g., resulting from mechanical or chemical stimuli) are triggered by so-called *local hormones* (bradykinin, prostaglandin, histamine).

Reflex Regulation of Circulation and Blood Pressure

Whenever there is an *increased demand for blood*, e. g., with increased muscle blood flow due to physical activity, cardiac output must be increased at the same time in order to maintain blood pressure or to prevent it from falling too low. The reflex adjustments to changing loads on the circulation (*short-term regulation of the blood pressure*) and the blood pressure are controlled by the autonomic nervous system (sympathetic and parasympathetic systems) and coordinated especially by the *vasomotor centers in the brain*. The *long-term regulation of the blood pressure* depends above all on maintaining the volume of the extracellular fluid, and thereby the blood volume, at a constant level. The kidney plays an important role in this task by regulating *salt and water balance* (see Chapter 10: Renal Tubules and Collecting Ducts).

Pressure and Stretch Receptors

The actual blood pressure is detected by special *pressure receptors* in the aortic arch and the carotid sinus, which is situated at the division of the common carotid artery. The information is transmitted to the vasomotor centers in the form of nerve impulses over specific *afferent nerves* (vagus and glosspharyngeal nerves). These centers also receive information by special *stretch receptors* in the venae cavae (superior and inferior) about the filling of the vessels, the two atria of the heart, and the left ventricle. In turn, *efferent nerve impulses* from the vasomotor centers in the brainstem reach the heart (cardiac nerves) and the smooth muscles of the blood vessels, especially the arterioles. By this means, the *work of the heart* (rate, stroke volume, and force of contraction) and the *diameter of the vessels* can be controlled so that a normal mean arterial pressure is maintained.

Regulation

If the blood pressure falls, e. g., because flow through the aorta increases (with increased muscle blood flow), the *sympathetic cardiac nerves* stimulate the heart to increased output. Additionally, the flow through resting organs is reduced by vasoconstriction and the venous return to the heart is increased by constriction of all veins (*emptying of the venous blood reservoir*). These measures are put in motion as it were prophylactically, even before a pending fall in blood pressure. For this, the motor centers in the cerebral cortex transmit a copy of their commands to the muscles to the vasomotor centers in the brainstem and so inform them of the impending increase in work. If renal blood flow is also decreased, the *renin–angiotensin system* (see Chapter 10: Renal Tubules and Collecting Ducts) induces vasoconstriction in the vascular arterial resistance, providing another means of raising blood pressure. Thus the kidney plays an important role in blood pressure regulation.

On the other hand, when the blood pressure is elevated, cardiac output is diminished by the vagus nerve, while inhibition of the sympathetic innervation of the blood vessels results in vasodilatation with consequent reduction of peripheral resistance.

Postural Hypotension

The circulatory reflexes just described also play an important role during *postural changes* (e. g., lying down/standing). During the transition from lying down to standing, the blood is redistributed. Gravity and dilatation of the veins of the lower body cause about 0.5 liter of blood to pool for a short period (*postural hypotension*). This reduces venous return to the heart, so that stroke volume and systolic pressure decrease briefly. If the normal circulatory responses (see above) are delayed too long, the decrease in blood pressure results in a brief reduction in cerebral blood flow and sometimes to dizziness or a brief period of unconsciousness (*syncope*).

Shock

Similarly, sudden blood loss or excessive reduction in the peripheral resistance (e. g., *heat stroke, anaphylactic shock due to allergic reactions*) can result in an excessive fall in blood pressure, with consequent circulatory collapse (*circulatory shock, hypovolemic shock*). The most important therapeutic measure in such a situation is to *increase venous return* (place the patient supine, with the legs elevated) and to provide more fluid to the heart by blood transfusions or infusions of blood substitutes, in order to restore the blood pressure.

Capillary Circulation

When a vessel (aorta) divides into many smaller vessels (capillaries), the total diameter increases while the rate of flow decreases. The greater the total cross-section, the slower is the flow rate. The *total cross section* of all capillaries of the human body is 3200 cm², which is almost *800 times greater than the cross-section of the aorta* (4 cm²). Correspondingly, the flow rate of the blood decreases from about 50 cm/s in the aorta to about 0.05 cm/s in the capillaries. From the capillary bed the flow rate slowly increases again and is about 10 cm/s in the great veins. Thus the capillaries, with their extremely thin walls (endothelium and basement membrane), and their total estimated number of about 40 billion, with a *total surface area of 600 m²*, are especially well suited for the *exchange of substances and fluids.*

Substance Exchange between Blood and Tissues

Every day about 20 liters of fluid is filtered from the capillaries into the surrounding interstitial space. This is where the exchange of substances takes place. The driving force for this filtration is the *hydrostatic blood pressure* at the arterial end of the capillaries of about 35 mmHg (Fig. 5.**29**). The *colloid osmotic pressure* (p. 31) of the plasma proteins, which opposes blood pressure, is about 25 mmHg, so that fluids and dissolved particles (e. g., nutrients) are *"pressed"* (filtered) into the tissues by the positive pressure difference (35–25 = +10 mmHg). The blood cells remain in the vessels during this substance exchange. Since blood pressure declines further to the end of the capillary (to about 15 mmHg), while the colloid osmotic pressure hardly changes, the blood pressure at the end of the capillary is below the colloid osmotic pressure (15–25 = -10 mmHg). Consequently fluid with dissolved particles (e. g., metabolic products) flows back into the vessel (*resorption*). Of the 20 liters of fluid (see above) leaving the capillaries daily only about 18 liters (90%) are resorbed. About 10% of the filtered amount (2 liters) are removed and transported as lymph by the lymphatic system (see Chapter 6: The Lymph Nodes)

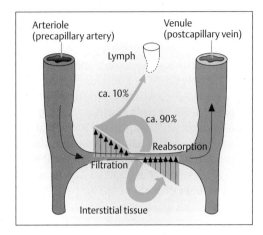

Fig. 5.**29 Schematic representation of the mechanism of fluid exchange in a capillary** (for explanation see text)

Edema Formation

Edema is a collection of fluid in the interstitial space. It may be formed in several ways:

- A rise in blood pressure caused by back pressure in the venous limb of the capillaries (e. g., *right heart failure*). In this case filtration predominates, so that fluid accumulates in the tissue.
- Change in *capillary permeability*, caused by histamine release during *allergic reactions.*
- Change in protein content (e. g., reduction in albumin) of blood plasma with consequent reduction of the *colloid osmotic pressure.*
- Reduction in lymphatic drainage, due to constriction or obliteration of lymph vessels.

Venous Return to the Heart

The following mechanisms return the blood to the heart:

- *The suction effect of the heart:* negative pressure is created as the base of the heart descends toward the apex (Fig. 5.**10**), sucking blood into the atria.

- *The influence of respiration*: inspiration creates negative pressure in the thorax (fall in thoracic pressure p. 364), which leads to distension of the intrathoracic veins, increasing the inflow of blood. This inflow is boosted by the simultaneous increase in intra-abdominal pressure during inspiration (descent of the diaphragm).
- *Venous valves:* the valves of the veins, which resemble the semilunar valves of the heart, prevent the blood from flowing backward, especially in the veins below the heart. The distance between valves in the smaller veins is a few centimeters, but in the larger veins may be up to 20 cm.
- *Companion veins:* two veins usually run in close proximity to large and small peripheral arteries. Arteries and veins are tied together into a vascular bundle by connective tissue. As the artery is distended by the regular pulse wave, it presses on the veins running close to it. Because of the valves, the blood in the veins can only flow in the opposite direction (toward the heart).
- *Muscular pump:* when skeletal muscles contract, they exert pressure on the veins and squeeze the venous walls, sending the venous blood toward the heart. Here, too, valves prevent backflow of blood.
- *Vasoconstriction of smooth muscles:* action of the CNS, which plays a role in the regulation of blood pressure.

Impedance of Venous Flow

Because of the greater hydrostatic pressure, impedance of blood flow on the venous side is primarily confined to the lower extremities. *Varicose veins* (*varices*) consist mainly of dilated veins with structural changes in the vascular coats (smooth muscle is partly replaced by connective tissue). This leads to insufficiency of the venous valves and backflow of venous blood. Moreover, there is interference with the resorption of fluids filtered from the blood at the level of the capillaries (increased pressure in the venous side of the capillary bed). With inadequate lymphatic drainage, this leads to fluid retention and edema. The raised tissue pressure increasingly also strangles the arterial blood supply, with resulting impedance to perfusion.

Summary **The Heart and Blood Vessels**

The heart and vascular system have the task of transporting the blood and its dissolved components (e. g., oxygen, nutrients) to all cells in the body in a closed circuit. The heart is the driving force. The actual transport system, the vascular system, has two parts. One part, namely, arteries (all blood vessels leading away from the heart, regardless of their oxygen content), capillaries (smallest vessels, site of substance exchange), and veins (all blood vessels leading blood toward the heart, regardless of oxygen content) transports the blood. The other part, the lymph vessels, transports lymph and immune cells.

■ **The Heart**

The heart and the pericardium in which it is enclosed lie in a connective tissue space (mediastinum) in the thorax. The dividing wall of the heart (atrial and ventricular septa) divides the heart into a right ventricle and atrium for the pulmonary circulation, and a left ventricle and atrium for the systemic circulation. The pulmonary veins enter the left atrium at the base of the heart (vertebral side = dorsal). The inferior aspect of the heart (mainly left ventricle, partly right) lies on the diaphragm and is defined as the posterior wall of the heart. The anterior wall of the heart is formed mainly by the right ventricle, partly by the left. The extreme end of the left ventricle, the apex, lies at the level of the 5th intercostal space a little inside the midclavicular line.

The wall of the heart is made up of three layers (from inside out: endocardium, myocardium = actual cardiac muscle, epicardium). Outside the epicardium lies the pericardial sac, which contains some fluid, and the actual pericardium.

The Valves of the Heart

The four cardiac valves lie in one plane (base of the heart) and are anchored by the skeleton of the heart:

- *Atrioventricular valves:* valves between the atria and the ventricles: (1) tricuspid valve (with three cusps) between the right atrium and right ventricle; (2) bicuspid or mitral valve (with two cusps) between the left atrium and the left ventricle.
- *Semilunar valves:* (1) pulmonary valve (at the entrance to the pulmonary artery); (2) aortic valves (entrance to the aorta).

The Conduction System

The sinus node is the autonomic impulse generator and pacemaker. Unlike skeletal muscle cells, which must be stimulated by a nerve, the cells of the sinus node and the conduction system are specialized muscle cells that are able to form action potentials spontaneously. The stimulus passes through the atrioventricular node (A-V node) and the bundle of His to reach the ventricular myocardium. From here it is distributed throughout the ventricular myocardium through the bundle branches and then the Purkinje fibers. The heart muscle cells form a network connected by gap junctions at the intercalated disks. This allows stimulation and the ensuing contraction to spread evenly at first through the atria, and subsequently equally evenly through the ventricles.

Through the sympathetic and parasympathetic nerves (autonomic cardiac nerves), the vasomotor centers in the brainstem of the CNS adjust cardiac work to the needs of the body (the sympathetic innervation of the heart acts primarily on the myocardium of the atria and ventricles, the vagus nerve on the sinus and A-V nodes).

The Coronary Vessels

These supply the myocardium:

- *Coronary arteries:* (1) right coronary artery (with posterior interventricular branch); (2) left coronary artery (with anterior interventricular and circumflex branches).
- *Coronary veins:* small, middle, and great cardiac veins drain into the coronary sinus and thence into the right atrium.

Systole and Diastole

(1) Contraction of the ventricular myocardium = systole: isovolumic phase, (closure of the atrioventricular valves, semilunar valves still closed); ejection phase (opening of the semilunar valves). (2) Relaxation of the ventricular myocardium = diastole: relaxation phase (closure of the semilunar valves, atrioventricular valves still closed); ventricular filling phase (atrioventricular valves open). Driving force: descent of the base.

- Stroke volume = the volume of blood ejected into the arteries during systole (about 70 ml at rest)

- Cardiac output (CO) = the volume of blood pumped by the heart in a defined time
- Circulation volume = the volume of blood pumped by the heart in one minute (about 5 liters at rest)
- Heart rate = number of heart beats per minute (at rest about 70 beats/min)

Heart Sounds

First, dull heart sound: closure of the atrioventricular valves. Second, high-pitched heart sound: closure of the semilunar valves. The sounds are best heard where the bloodstream from the closed valve approaches the chest wall most closely.

The ECG

The ECG provides information about the heart rate and the conduction of the impulse over the heart. Leads are either bipolar limb leads or unipolar chest leads. The waves of the ECG tracing are always designated by the same letters and each represents a specific phase of the spread of the impulse.

Blood Pressure (Arterial)

This is the pressure against which the left ventricle must eject blood: systolic value (normal 120 mmHg) = maximal blood pressure during the ejection phase; diastolic value (normal 80 mmHg) = minimal blood pressure at the opening of the aortic valve. High blood pressure (hypertension): diastolic value ≥ 90 mmHg. Most blood pressure measurementss are taken by the indirect method.

Clinical Examination

Inspection, palpation (feeling with the hand), percussion (striking with a short sharp blow to examine underlying sounds), auscultation (listening), ECG (echocardiography), radiography (PA or lateral), computerized tomography (horizontal sections), fluoroscopy (live radiographic examination), cardiac catheterization (angiocardiography, coronary angiography), MRI (magnetic resonance imaging—horizontal, sagittal and frontal sections).

■ **The Vascular System**
The Blood Vessels

Arteries and veins have similar structures, with three layers. Arteries, however, have a well-developed muscular layer and elastic membranes between the layers. Arteries close to the heart have a high proportion of elastic fibers (elastic recoil). Veins have thinner walls and most have venous valves, folds of the vascular endothelium. The capillary walls are reduced to a vascular endothelium (inner layer).

The Lymph Vessels

The walls consist of endothelium, some with folds (valves) and a thin muscular layer.

The Circulation

The circulation consists of two parts:

1. **Lesser (pulmonary) circulation:** deoxygenated blood from the lower and upper regions of the body through the superior and inferior venae cavae into the right atrium, through the right ventricle into the pulmonary artery—enriched with oxygen in the lungs—oxygenated blood through the pulmonary veins and the left atrium into the left ventricle.

2. **Greater (systemic) circulation:** oxygenated blood from the left ventricle into the aorta—distributed by the arterial system over the whole body—substance and gas exchange in the capillaries—deoxygenated blood back to the right atrium by way of the venae cavae.

   – **Portal circulation** (insertion of a venous capillary bed into the systemic circulation): venous blood from the gastrointestinal tract and the spleen carrying nutrients reaches the liver through the portal vein. In the liver it passes through a predominantly venous capillary bed (detoxification, storage, metabolism of substances absorbed from the intestines), then through the hepatic veins to the inferior vena cava and the right atrium. By this path the *absorbed nutrients* pass through the lesser circulation with the deoxygenated blood, and then together with the oxygenated blood through the systemic circulation into the capillaries and so to the "end users," the cells of the body.

– **The fetal circulation:** by-passing of the pulmonary circulation, as the lungs are not yet functional: (1) Hole in the atrial septum (foramen ovale); blood passes directly from the left into the right atrium. (2) Short circuit between the pulmonary artery and the aorta (ductus arteriosus); gas exchange in the placenta; umbilical veins bring oxygenated blood to the inferior vena cava of the fetus through the ductus venosus.

Important Arterial Trunks

The great paired vascular trunks to the head (common carotid arteries) and arm (subclavian arteries) branch from the aortic arch. Branches from the thoracic aorta go to the intercostal muscles, the esophagus, the pericardium, and the mediastinum. Below the aortic hiatus in the diaphragm, the aorta continues as the abdominal aorta. From above downward it gives off branches to the inferior surface of the diaphragm, the kidneys (renal artery), and adrenals, a common trunk (celiac trunk, celiac axis) for the arteries to the liver, stomach and spleen, branches to the small intestine (superior mesenteric artery), the gonads (testicular and ovarian arteries), and the large intestine (inferior mesenteric artery). At the level of the 4th lumbar vertebra, the abdominal aorta divides into the two common iliac arteries that supply the pelvic organs (internal iliac artery) and the lower extremity (external iliac artery). At the level of the inguinal ligament the external iliac artery is continued as the femoral artery.

Important Venous Trunks

Two venous networks, the superficial and deep, are connected by perforating veins. The superior vena cava is formed by the junction of the two brachiocephalic veins, which collect blood from the head, neck, and arm. The inferior vena cava is formed by the junction of the two common iliac veins that collect blood from the lower extremities (external iliac veins) and the pelvic organs (internal iliac veins). On its way to the right atrium the inferior vena cava is joined by the veins from the kidneys (renal veins) and before piercing the diaphragm (foramen venae cavae) by the three hepatic veins.

The Lymphatic Channels

The lymphatic channels run parallel to the veins and begin blindly in the capillary bed. Lymph is that part of the fluid filtered in the capillaries that is not reabsorbed (10%). Through small and large lymph vessels and lymph nodes (immune defense), the lymph returns to the venous system at the left and right venous angles.

The Regulation of the Circulation and Blood Pressure: Physical and Physiological Fundamentals

Blood flows more easily through large vessels than through small arterioles and capillaries, the narrow diameter of which presents a high resistance to the blood flow. Hence, they are called the vessels of the peripheral resistance (vascular resistance = peripheral resistance, which requires increased pressure to overcome). The circulation of the blood is maintained by this pressure gradient.

Distribution of the bloodstream according to need (distribution of the cardiac output) can be achieved by regional changes in vascular resistance, e. g., by vasodilatation (relaxation of smooth muscles) or vasoconstriction (contraction of smooth muscle). Local muscle tone is regulated by localized influences (autoregulation, e. g., vasodilatation due to lack of oxygen), or nervous (vascular sympathetic) or hormonal (epinephrine, norepinephrine, tissue hormones such as histamine) messages.

In order to avoid blood pressure drops during increased blood flow requirements (e. g., to muscles during physical activity), cardiac ouput (CO) must increase. The vasomotor centers in the brain receive nerve impulses from pressure receptors in the aorta and stretch receptors in the venae cavae as they register actual blood pressure. In order to maintain median blood pressure, constriction occurs in (1) the vessels of resting organs, (2) the vessels of peripheral resistance (renin–angiotensin system, raises blood pressure), and (3) the veins (increases venous return); and (4) the work of the heart is adjusted to the increased need. Both effects are regulated reflexly by the vasomotor centers. The kidneys also play a role in the regulation of blood pressure (regulation of salt and water balance, renin–angiotensin system).

During normal circulation, other mechanisms influence **venous return**: suction mechanism of the heart, negative intrathoracic pressure during inspiration, venous valves, effect of arterial pulsation, muscular pump.

Circulation of the Blood and Substance Exchange in the Capillaries

The total surface in the capillaries is very great (600 m²), the flow rate is very low because of the high resistance, and the capillary walls are very thin: these are ideal circumstances for substance exchange. Every day an average 20 liters of fluid is filtered into the interstitial space, where substance exchange takes place. The driving force is hydrostatic pressure, which is above the colloid osmotic pressure at the arterial end of the capillaries. Consequently, fluid and dissolved particles (e. g., nutrients) are filtered into the tissues under pressure. At the venous end of the capillaries, blood pressure falls below colloid osmotic pressure. Consequently, fluid and dissolved particles (e. g., metabolic products) flow back into the vessel (resorption). Of the 20 liters of fluid about 18 liters are resorbed, while 2 liters (10 %) are transported in the lymph vessels as lymph.

6

Blood, the Immune System, and Lymphoid Organs

Contents

The cells of the blood and the immune cells are free connective tissue cells and are in part of identical origin. Developmentally they both originate from the mesenchyme. For the most part they are formed in the same site, the *bone marrow*, but they differ considerably in their location and the site of their functioning (blood vs. connective tissue).

■ The Blood

Blood may be viewed as tissue—a sort of *fluid transportation tissue*, of which the intercellular substance is the **blood plasma** (plasma). The cellular components of this tissue are the **red** (**erythrocytes**) and **white** (**leukocytes**) **blood cells** and the **platelets** (**thrombocytes** (Fig. 6.**1a**, **b**). The proportion of the total blood volume occupied by all blood cells in percent is called the *hematocrit* (see Fig. 6.**3**). It averages 45%, and is usually a little higher in men (47%) than in women (43%).

■ **Total Blood Volume.** The total circulating blood volume in humans is about 8% of body weight; i.e., the total blood volume of a person weighing 70 kg is about 5.6 liters.

Functions of the Blood

Blood has multiple functions closely connected with its components and with the vascular system. While a function of the blood vessels is to distribute the blood overall (heat regulation and distribution of substances), the formed and unformed blood components have some very specific functions.

The red blood cells, for instance, are responsible for the *transport of blood gases* from the lung to the tissues (oxygen) and from the tissues back to the lungs (carbon dioxide).

White blood cells serve to defend against pathogens and foreign bodies (*immunity*). They perform these tasks most of the time outside the blood vessels, in the connective tissues. In this case the blood serves solely as a means of transportation from the site of cell formation (bone marrow) to the site of action.

The fluid portion of the blood, the plasma, subserves several different transportation tasks. For instance, it undertakes the transport of

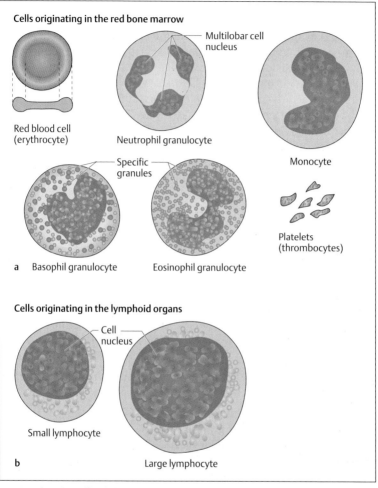

Cells originating in the red bone marrow

Multilobar cell nucleus

Red blood cell (erythrocyte)

Neutrophil granulocyte

Monocyte

Specific granules

Platelets (thrombocytes)

a Basophil granulocyte

Eosinophil granulocyte

Cells originating in the lymphoid organs

Cell nucleus

Small lymphocyte

b

Large lymphocyte

Fig 6.**1 a, b The cells of the blood.** The cells of the blood are formed in the red bone marrow from a common ancestor, the blast cell, and released into the peripheral blood-stream after a certain maturation period. Throughout life all the cells of the blood are formed in the red bone marrow, with the exception of lymphocytes, which also multiply in the lymphoid organs

nutrients from where they are absorbed (intestinal villi) to where they are utilized (organs), of metabolic products to the excretory organs (kidneys), and of substances acting inside the body to their sites of activity (hormones). Simultaneously, blood transports heat from the metabolically active organs to the surface.

Another task of blood is coagulation. When blood vessels are injured, the clotting factors carried in the blood, such as fibrinogen and platelets, are of vital importance. In addition to water, blood plasma contains a number of salts (electrolytes), proteins (albumins and globulins), lipids (fatty acids and cholesterol), and carbohydrates (blood glucose), and numerous vitamins, trace elements, and enzymes. Other noteworthy features of blood include its essentially constant composition, relatively constant osmotic pressure, and a pH value that varies only within narrow limits (7.2–7.4) (the so-called *"constant internal milieu"*).

The Cells of the Blood

The following are average values per microliter (1 µl = 1 mm³) for the formed elements of the blood:

- **Erythrocytes**   4.5–5.5 million
- **Leukocytes**   4000–8000
- **Thrombocytes**   150 000–350 000

The white blood cells (leukocytes) are further subdivided into (differential white cell count):

- **Neutrophils (neutrophil granulocytes)**   60–70 %
- **Eosinophils (eosinophil granulocytes)**   2–3 %
- **Basophils (basophil granulocytes)**   0.5–1 %
- **Lymphocytes**   20–30 %
- **Monocytes**   4–5 %

The Erythrocytes

The erythrocytes (red blood cells) are round, disk-shaped structures with an average diameter of 7.5 µm. They are concave on both sides and this gives them an optimal *surface to volume ratio* (Fig. 6.**1a**). The shape favors oxygen uptake and release (through short diffusion distances) and facilitates passive deformation during passage through narrow capillaries. The content of the cell consists almost entirely of the red iron-containing pigment *hemoglobin*, which binds oxygen reversibly. When hemoglobin is oxygen enriched (arterialized blood) it appears bright red, while it appears dark red when oxygen-poor (venous blood).

The normal red cell count in a man is about $5.3 \times 10^6/\mu l$, while in a woman it is $4.6 \times 10^6/\mu l$, the number depending on the oxygen needs of the body and the availability of oxygen in the lung. For instance, at high altitudes the number increases (polycythemia). If the formation or lifespan of the red cells is insufficient as a result of pathological processes, the result is anemia (p. 277). The commonest causes of anemia are iron deficiency, vitamin B_{12} deficiency, and folic acid deficiency.

Formation, Lifespan and Breakdown

The site of the formation and maturation of erythrocytes is the red bone marrow, where they develop from stem cells. In the course of their maturation they lose their nucleus and cell organelles and are extruded into the peripheral bloodstream. In humans, about 160 million red cells are formed every minute. In blood the least mature erythrocytes (reticulocytes; about 1%) can be recognized by a granular structure visible with a special stain. The reticulocyte count in peripheral blood is increased, for example, after loss of blood.

The lifespan of red blood cells is on an average 120 days. They are mostly broken down in the spleen and in the liver. The part of the hemoglobin molecule that does not contain iron forms bile pigments (bilirubin). The liberated iron is stored and reused for the formation of hemoglobin.

In *hypertonic solutions* red cells lose water and shrink (crenated cells), while in *hypotonic solutions* they take up water and burst (hemolysis). When this happens, hemoglobin is liberated and the cells become transparent (ghost cells, achromocytes).

The Leukocytes

In addition to the red blood cells, the blood contains cells that are relatively colorless, the white blood cells (leukocytes). These include the granulocytes (polymorphonuclear leukocytes, polymorphs), the lymphocytes, and the monocytes (Fig. 6.**1a**, **b**). Their lifespan, in contrast to that of the red cells, varies a great deal and can be from a few hours to years. Together with the lymphoid organs (the spleen, thymus, lymph nodes, tonsils, etc.), the white blood cells form the *immune system*, which is divided into a nonspecific and a specific immune system (p. 282).

The number of white blood cells varies between 4000 and 8000/µl. The number can increase considerably above 10000/µl (*leukocytosis*). If the leukocytes are diminished to below 2000/µl, the condition is called *leukopenia* (e. g., after damage to the site of their formation). The leukocytes, like the erythrocytes, are generated in the red bone marrow and after maturation and proliferation they are released into the bloodstream. The lymphocytes form an exception, in that their stem cells are located in the bone marrow but they may multiply and differentiate in other lymphoid organs (e. g., in the thymus or the lymph nodes) (see Specific Immunity [T and B lymphocytes] below).

Most of the white blood cells use the blood only as a means of transportation from their generation in the bone marrow to the site of their activity. They fulfill their immune functions almost exclusively outside the vascular system, i.e., in the connective tissue and in the lymphoid organs. There they can move autonomously by their ameboid motion after passing through the walls of the capillaries and postcapillary venules (*leukocyte diapedesis*).

Granulocytes

Granulocytes are divided into *neutrophils, eosinophils*, and *basophils* according to the granules they contain (granular cell inclusions) (Fig. 6.**1a**). They all have a multilobar nucleus (polymorphonuclear leukocytes, polymorphs). In contrast, immature stages can be distinguished by their bandlike nuclei (band cells, stab cells).

Neutrophil granulocytes are also termed *phagocytes* because they phagocytose (Greek *phagein* = to ingest) foreign material. They are a part of the nonspecific immune system, and they are the first to reach the site of an inflammation. Their granules contain a number of lysosomal enzymes that destroy pathogens and cell debris, rendering them harmless. In so doing, the polymorphs mostly perish themselves (resulting in pus formation).

Eosinophils are also capable of phagocytosis, especially of antigen–antibody complexes (see p. 286). They take part in allergic reactions by bonding to and inactivating excess histamine that has been released from mast cells or basophil granulocytes. Hence their chief task is to limit allergic reactions. Additionally, their granules contain a number of aggressive enzymes that are released when needed to damage their target cells.

Basophils form a very small part of human blood cells. Their granules contain mainly histamine and heparin. Histamine plays a part in immediate hypersensitivity (increase in vascular permeability, contraction of smooth muscle tissue), while heparin has anticoagulant properties.

The Lymphocytes

The lymphocytes present in the bloodstream (small lymphocytes) are about the size of erythrocytes, while the so-called large lymphocytes occur mainly in the lymphoid organs (Fig. 6.**1b**). Lymphocytes have a noticeably large nucleus and their cytoplasm is rich in cell organelles. They are the cells of specific immunity and they are also formed in the red bone marrow. However, they reach the various lymphoid organs by way of the bloodstream and there develop into specific immune cells (see The Immune System, p. 282).

Monocytes

The monocytes are the largest of the white blood cells (Fig. 6.**1a**). Their nucleus is oval or kidney-shaped and their cytoplasm contains numerous lysosomes. Like the other leukocytes they are generated in the red bone marrow, but after their release into the bloodstream they remain there only about 20–30 hours. After that time they leave the blood vascular system and are transformed into *macrophages* in the tissues. Monocytes and macrophages have multiple tasks in the immune system and take part especially in nonspecific immunity. Their function includes phagocytosis and intracellular destruction of bacteria, fungi, parasites, and autologous damaged cells. Beyond that they also take part in specific immunity, in that they pass information about foreign antigens to the lymphocytes (antigen presentation, see p. 283).

The Platelets

Platelets or thrombocytes play a major role in coagulation of the blood and in hemostasis. They are formed in the bone marrow by cytoplasmic extrusions from *giant cells* (*megakaryocytes*), to be released into the bloodstream in the form of irregularly shaped platelets (Fig. 6.**1a**). Their cytoplasm has no nucleus and few cell organelles. Thrombocytes have a lifespan of about 5–10 days, after which they are destroyed in the spleen. They are deposited on the vessel wall when a blood vessel is injured and break down, liberating enzymes (e. g., thrombokinase) that combine with other factors (thrombin, fibrinogen) to coagulate the blood.

Blood Groups and Blood Transfusions

The surface membrane of erythrocytes contains a large number of various saccharides (glycolipids, glycoproteins), the so-called *blood group antigens.* They are called antigens because in foreign organisms they induce the formation of antibodies (see The Immune System, p. 282). Human blood contains more than 100 such antigens, of which especially the *ABO* and *Rh* systems are of clinical importance.

Blood Groups

The ABO (O = none, from German *ohne*) system consists of four blood groups: erythrocytes with the A antigen (blood group A), the B antigen (blood group B), antigens A and B (blood group AB), or neither antigen (blood group O). Additionally, plasma contains antibodies against whichever antigen is missing, i.e., persons with blood group A have antibodies against B (anti-B). Correspondingly, the plasma of blood of group B contains antigens against A (anti-A). In the case of blood group AB, the plasma contains neither antibody; and blood group O plasma contains both anti-A and anti-B. Unlike normal antibody formation, the formation of antibodies of the ABO system does not require contact with foreign antigens. They develop in the first months of life. Because of their agglutinating effect they are also called *agglutinins*, while the erythrocyte antigens are called agglutinogens (Table 6.**1**).

Table 6.**1** **Blood group antigens (agglutinogens) and the corresponding antibodies (agglutinins)**

Erythrocyte antigen (blood group)	Antibody in the serum*
A	Anti-B
B	Anti-A
AB	None
0	Anti-A and Anti-B

* Serum = plasma without fibrinogen

Blood Transfusion

During the transfusion of *incompatible* blood, the red cells clump together (agglutinate) as a result of the interaction of the blood group antigens with their corresponding antibodies. This damages the red cells, which hemolyze. Such a *transfusion reaction* is especially severe when the plasma of the recipient contains antibodies against the red cells of the donor. In the reverse case, where the donor blood contains antibodies against the red cells of the recipient, the reaction is less marked, because the antibodies are diluted in the recipient's bloodstream.

To avoid such reactions, the precise blood group of donor and recipient must be determined before any transfusion and *matched serologically*. For this, a few drops each of donor and recipient blood or banked blood is mixed with prepared test sera containing respectively antibodies against antigen A (anti-A) and antigen B (anti-B). This method is simply a test for blood groups of the ABO system (Fig. 6.**2**). To determine antigens and antibodies that are not part of the ABO system (e. g., the Rh system), blood is also subjected to Coombs' tests. The direct Coombs' test measures the presence of antibodies on the surface of erythrocytes, while the indirect Coombs' test measures the presence of antibodies to erythrocytes in serum.

The Significance of the ABO System

In populations of middle European descent, blood group A occurs in about 44% of people, group O in about 42%, group B in about 10%, and group AB about 4%. In other ethnic populations, these percentages may

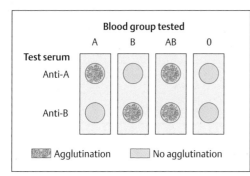

Fig. 6.**2 Determining blood groups.** Simplified representation of the agglutination reaction after addition of various test sera (anti-A and anti-B)

vary considerably. The ABO blood group system is inherited according to Mendelian laws, and therefore the possible blood groups of children can be predicted if the blood groups of the parents are known. On the other hand, if the blood groups of the mother and child are known, it is possible to determine whether a man with a certain blood group is the father of that child (*forensic paternity exclusion*). The ABO antigens used to be important for forensic medical assessment because they occur in other bodily secretions, such as saliva, sperm, sweat, and gastric secretions, in about 85 % of subjects. Meanwhile this method has been superseded by DNA analysis, which is 100 % reliable.

The Rh Factor

Beside the ABO system the *Rh (rhesus) blood group system,* consisting of 40 different groups of antigens, has important clinical applications. These antigens were discovered by accident, when guinea-pigs were repeatedly injected with red cells of the rhesus monkey. It was found that they formed antibodies that agglutinated not only the erythrocytes of the rhesus monkey, but also human erythrocytes when these were injected in later studies. This reaction was caused by the most powerful and important Rh antigen (R1, D, Rh_0). Hence people whose blood agglutinates in this way, that is, who possess the antigen, are labeled "*Rh-positive*" (Rh+), while the rest, whose erythrocytes do not carry the antigen, are "*Rh-negative*" (Rh–). In most Rh+ people, agglutination is linked to antigen D on the erythrocyte.

Unlike the ABO antibodies, Rh antibodies do not occur naturally, but are formed only when blood from Rh-positive donors is transfused into Rh-negative recipients. In such a case the recipients become sensitized to the Rh antigen, that is, they form antibodies against Rh-positive erythrocytes. Subsequently, during a second transfusion, large numbers of antibodies are formed rapidly, and these promptly agglutinate the erythrocytes of the Rh-positive donor.

Similarly, Rh antibodies may be formed automatically during pregnancy, for example, when the mother is Rh-negative and the father and child are Rh-positive. During labor, Rh-positive erythrocytes from the child can pass through leaks in the placenta into the maternal bloodstream, eliciting the formation of so-called *anti-D antibodies* (*Rh antibodies*) in the mother. These antibodies belong to the class G immunoglobulins (IgG) and are diffusible through the placenta; in case of another pregnancy, these antibodies can pass through the placental barrier from the maternal blood into the fetal circulation. If this child also possesses Rh-positive erythrocytes, the antibodies can cause the fetal cells to agglutinate and eventually destroy them (hemolysis). The unborn child develops a sometimes severe anemia, which can be fatal. This disease is known as hemolytic anemia of the newborn (erythroblastosis fetalis).

Often these children can only be saved by a timely blood transfusion. In order to prevent the formation of Rh antibodies in the mother after the first pregnancy, Rh-negative mothers are given *anti-D prophylaxis*. Immediately after delivery, previously prepared anti-D antibodies (immunoglobulins against Rh antigen developed in an animal) are injected into the mother. This renders harmless Rh-positive fetal erythrocytes that may have reached the maternal bloodstream, before the Rh-negative mother can be sensitized.

The Plasma

If the cellular blood components (e.g., erythrocytes, leukocytes, thrombocytes) are separated by centrifugation from blood that has been made incoagulable, the resulting fluid is *plasma* (Fig. 6.**3**). In contrast, the liquid phase of blood that has already clotted is called *serum* (serum = plasma without the clotting factor fibrinogen, see

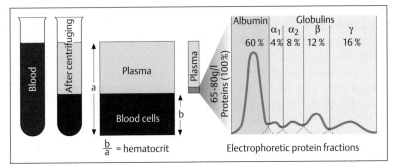

Fig. 6.**3** **Composition of blood.** (After Silbernagl and Despopoulos)

below). Plasma consists of 90% water and 10% dissolved substances. Of the dissolved substances, about 70% are proteins (plasma proteins), 20% are low-molecular-weight substances (e.g., nutrients, metabolic products, vitamins, trace elements, hormones), and 10% are electrolytes.

Plasma Proteins

The 100 or so different proteins occurring in plasma (about 70 g/l) have a role in transportation (e.g., lipids, hormones, vitamins), form important constituents of the clotting system, and constitute the antibodies of the immune system. By electrophoresis, an analytical method, they can be roughly separated into five groups by their electric charge and their molecular size and shape (Fig. 6.**3**):

- **Albumins** (3.5–5.5 g/dl plasma)
- **α_1-Globulins** (0.1–0.3 g/dl plasma
- **α_2-Globulins** (0.2–1.1 g/dl plasma)
- **β-Globulins** (0.5–1.2 g/dl plasma)
- **γ-Globulins** (0.5–1.5 g/dl plasma)

Albumins

Albumins are proportionally the most important plasma proteins and their primary function is to maintain the osmotic pressure of the blood

(p. 31). They also play a role in the transport of calcium ions, fatty acids, bilirubin (breakdown product of hemoglobin), bile acids and a few hormones and vitamins. They also serve as a protein reserve in albumin deficiency.

α_1-, α_2- and β-Globulins

The proteins in these three groups serve chiefly for the transport of lipids (lipoproteins), free hemoglobin (haptoglobin), iron (transferrin), vitamin B_{12} (transcobalamin), and adrenal cortical hormones (e. g., transcortin). Some of them also form important constituents of the clotting system (e. g., fibrinogen, prothrombin).

Of major importance in this connection are the proteins that transport lipids that are insoluble in plasma (e. g., cholesterol). *Lipoproteins* are divided into several classes according to their proportion of fat and protein. They are classified in descending order of size and increasing density:

- **Chylomicrons**
- **Chylomicron remnants**
  - very-low-density lipoproteins (VLDL)
  - low-density lipoproteins (LDL)
  - high-density-lipoproteins (HDL)

The various densities depend essentially on the proportion of fat (e. g., cholesterol, triglyceride, phospholipid) in each lipoprotein. This is very high in the VLDLs (about 90%) and significantly lower in the HDLs (about 50%). The LDL lipoproteins are rich in cholesterol and transport lipids from the liver, where they are formed, to the tissues. The HDL lipoprotein, on the other hand, transports excess cholesterol formed in the tissues back to the liver. There are a number of indications that a high plasma LDL level combined with a low HDL level is an important factor in the genesis of arteriosclerosis. In this disease, cholesterol is deposited in previously damaged cells in the walls of the blood vessel (e. g., when at the same time the blood pressure is high), and this markedly increases the risk of vascular occlusion by localized blood clots. Since the cholesterol content of blood is made up of VLDL, LDL, and HDL, the total cholesterol content has only conditional predictive value. A high HDL content is very favorable, a high LDL content, as previously noted, is very unfavorable. Hence, the HDL and LDL *ratios* in blood should always be determined.

γ-Globulins

The group of γ-globulins consists mainly of immune globulins, the immune substances in the blood plasma (antibodies). They are *glycoproteins* (proteins conjugated with carbohydrates) that are spilled into the plasma after being secreted by plasma cells, parts of the specific immune system (p. 286) derived from B lymphocytes. Human immunoglobulins can be divided according to their functions into five groups of immunoglobulins (prefixed "Ig"): IgA, IgD, IgE, IgG, and IgM.

Immunoglobulin A (IgA). These specialize in immune processes at mucosal surfaces and therefore occur chiefly in the gastrointestinal tract and in bodily secretions (saliva, sweat, tears, maternal milk, and intestinal secretions).

Immunoglobulins D (IgD). These are found only in small amounts in the plasma. Their function is still largely unknown. They may at times play a role as surface receptors during the differentiation and maturation of B lymphocytes.

Immunoglobulin E (IgE). Of all the immunoglobulins these occur in the plasma in the smallest concentration. They are increased especially in allergic reactions and parasite infections. IgE can bind e. g., to mast cells and induce the liberation of histamine from mast cells (anaphylaxis, anaphylactic shock).

Immunoglobulin G (IgG). Quantitatively these are the most important antibodies (75% of all immunoglobulin). Apart from the plasma, they also occur in the interstitial fluid. IgG is the only human immunoglobulin able to pass through membranes and by crossing the placenta can reach the circulation of an unborn child. By this means maternal IgG provides immunological protection during the first six months.

Immunoglobulin M (IgM). These are the largest antibodies and are the first immunoglobulins to be formed after contact with an antigen (e. g., infection with a microorganism) (early antibodies). Their early forms are attached to B lymphocytes.

Low-Molecular-Weight Plasma Constituents

The low-molecular-weight plasma constituents are mostly transported bound to proteins. They include the following substances:

- Nutrients, vitamins, trace elements
- Metabolic products (e. g., lactic acid, pyruvic acid)
- Nitrogenous excretory products of protein and purine metabolism (e. g., urea, uric acid, creatinine)
- Hormones and enzymes
- Fatty substances (e. g., cholesterol, phospholipids, triglycerides, free fatty acids)

Plasma Electrolytes

The electrolyte composition of the plasma differs from the intracellular electrolyte concentration in specific ways. While sodium, calcium, and chloride ions have relatively high concentrations in plasma, potassium, magnesium, and phosphate ions have a higher concentration in the cells. The most important osmotic ion is common salt (NaCl) with about 0.6–0.7 g/100 ml plasma. The total electrolyte osmotic pressure in plasma is about 290 mOsm/l (osmolarity = concentration of all osmotically active particles per unit volume). More accurate, however, is the determination of mOsm/kg H_2O (osmolality), since the volume of a solution depends on the temperature and the volume of the dissolved substances.

When, for instance, saline solutions are needed for infusions, they must have the same osmotic pressure as the plasma, i.e., they must be *isotonic*. Solutions with a higher osmotic pressure are called *hypertonic*; solutions with lower osmotic pressure are *hypotonic.* Hypertonic solutions would lead to diffusion of water from the cells and so to shrinking of the cell. Hypotonic solutions, on the other hand, would allow water to flow into the cells and cause them to rupture.

The Erythrocyte Sedimentation Rate (ESR)

In incoagulable blood the red cells slowly sediment, because of their higher specific gravity. The erythrocyte sedimentation rate is usually determined by the Westergren method after 1 or 2 hours and is 6–10 mm in women and 3–6 mm in men in the first hour. The sedimentation rate depends on a number of factors (among others the quantity and composition of plasma proteins). An elevated ESR must be considered a nonspecific sign of illness. The sedimentation rate can reach 100 mm in the first hour, especially in cases of inflammation and of increased tissue destruction due to tumors. The cause is a strong tendency for the erythrocytes to form rouleaux (clumps). This reduces their surface-to-volume ratio, resulting in a reduced resistance to flow and more rapid sedimentation.

O_2 and CO_2 Transport in the Blood

Hemoglobin Transport of O_2

The red pigment hemoglobin (Hb) consists of a protein moiety, globin, and the actual pigment, heme. The molecule is composed of four subunits, each with a heme group attached, with a bivalent iron atom arranged in its center. In the lung, each iron atom takes up one molecule of oxygen (O_2). This is transported into the tissues where it is split off (Fig. 6.**4**). The taking up of O_2 is called *oxygenation*, its splitting off *deoxygenation*.

CO_2 Transport

About 10 % of carbon dioxide (CO_2), the end product of oxidative metabolism in the tissue cells, is transported in the blood in physical solution and 90 % in chemically bound form. The greater portion of carbon dioxide first diffuses out of the tissue cells into the plasma, and from there into the red cells. There it is converted by enzymes into the much more *soluble bicarbonate* (HCO_3^-), bound chemically, and transported in the plasma. The creation of CO_2 from HCO_3^- is greatly accelerated by an enzyme, carbonic anhydrase (new name: *carbonate dehydratase*) present in the erythrocytes (Fig. 6.**4**).

$$CO_2 + H_2O \rightleftharpoons HCO_3^- + H^+$$

The larger part (about 50–60 %) of the bicarbonate formed diffuses back into the plasma out of the erythrocytes in exchange for chloride ions. It is

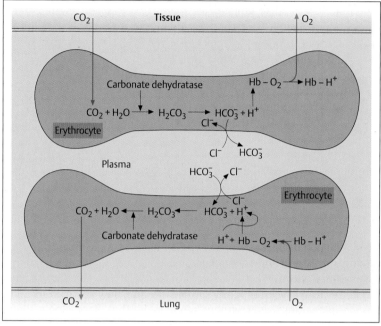

Fig. 6.**4** · Simplified representation of the reactions in erythrocytes during CO_2 and O_2 transport. Hb-O_2 = oxygenated hemoglobin; Hb-H^+ = deoxygenated hemoglobin

transported into the lungs (see respiratory organs) and exhaled after conversion into CO_2. Both processes, formation of HCO_3^- and liberation of CO_2 are linked respectively to the deoxygenation and oxygenation of hemoglobin. Deoxygenated hemoglobin is a markedly stronger base than oxygenated Hb and can take up more H^+ ions (*buffer function of hemoglobin*), and so promotes the formation of HCO_3^- in the tissue capillaries. In the capillaries of the lungs, HCO_3^- again passes from the plasma into the erythrocytes, takes up H^+ ions and is transformed back into CO_2. This process is furthered by the fact that oxygenated blood liberates more H^+ ions.

A much smaller portion of CO_2 (about 5–10%) is bound directly to hemoglobin and transported as carbaminohemoglobin.

Hemoglobin and Carbon Monoxide

Carbon monoxide (CO) is a colorless, odorless gas that is formed during incomplete combustion and, like oxygen, can combine reversibly with hemoglobin. However, the affinity of carbon monoxide for hemoglobin is markedly greater than that of oxygen. Hence, with even a 0.3% CO content in inspired air, 80% of hemoglobin is bound to carbon monoxide (HbCO). Since carbon monoxide is released from its combination with hemoglobin 200–300 times more slowly than oxygen, the toxic effect of carbon dioxide is due to the fact that hemoglobin can no longer carry oxygen. In heavy smokers, for instance, 5–10% of hemoglobin is present as HbCO, while at 20% acute toxic symptoms appear (headache, dizziness, nausea), and 65% can be fatal.

Hemoglobin Concentration (Hb)

The hemoglobin concentration in human blood is about 16 g/dl (160 g/l) in men and 14 g/dl (140 g/l) in women. Since every gram of hemoglobin can combine with 1.33 ml oxygen, about 200 ml O_2/l can be carried in the blood. Because oxygen is poorly soluble in water, only about 3 ml O_2/l of blood can be transported without hemoglobin; thus, hemoglobin allows an almost 70-fold increase in the amount moved.

Mean Corpuscular Hemoglobin (MCH)

Often, in order to assess hemopoiesis or to distinguish between different anemias, the mean corpuscular hemoglobin of a single erythrocyte is determined MCH). It is calculated by the formula:

$$\blacksquare \quad MCH = \frac{\text{Hemoglobin content (g/100 ml blood)}}{\text{Erythrocytes } (10^6/\mu l)} \times 10$$

The value of mean corpuscular hemoglobin lies between 38 and 36 picograms (pg) (1 pg = 10^{-12} g). Erythrocytes with a normal MCH are described as *normochromic* (*orthochromic*). If the MCH is low (e. g., due to chronic blood loss or iron deficiency), the erythrocytes are said to be *hypochromic*, if it is high (e. g., pernicious anemia due to vitamin B_{12} deficiency, see below), they are *hyperchromic*.

The Anemias

Anemia is defined as an erythrocyte deficiency or a diminished hemoglobin content of the blood. The diagnosis of anemia is usually made by looking at the hemoglobin concentration, the lower limit of normal being about 14 g/dl in men and 12 g/dl in women. A noticeable symptom in almost all forms of anemia is pale color of the skin and mucous membranes. Often the heart rate increases markedly (accelerated circulation) during physical exertion and oxygen reduction in the tissues results in shortness of breath. Dizziness and easy fatigability can also occur.

Besides iron deficiency anemias and chronic blood loss due, e. g., to bleeding ulcers or tumors in the gastrointestinal tract (**hypochromic anemias**), anemia may also be due to deficiencies in vitamin B_{12}, folic acid, or erythropoietin (see p. 278, The Regulation of Erythrocyte Generation). Vitamin B_{12} and folic acid are involved in the synthesis of DNA in immature bone marrow cells and hence especially influence the division and maturation of red cells (erythropoiesis). When they are deficient, fewer erythrocytes are formed, but these are markedly enlarged because of an increased hemoglobin content (macrocytes, precursors: megaloblasts), since the hemoglobin content of the blood is almost unchanged (**hyperchromic, megalobastic, macrocytic anemia,** see above).

Vitamin B_{12} deficiency is often due to a disturbance in absorption of the vitamin from the intestines, less often to insufficient nutritional intake. This so-called **pernicious anemia** is most often the result of chronic inflammation of the gastric mucosa, with reduction in the production of gastric secretions. Vitamin B_{12} can only be absorbed from the intestine when it combines with a factor found in gastric secretion (*"intrinsic factor"*) that prevents it from being destroyed by the digestive juices of the stomach. Since the liver can store large amounts of vitamin B_{12}, it may take 2–5 years before an impairment of absorption in the intestine has an effect on erythrocyte formation. Like vitamin B_{12} deficiency, a deficiency of folic acid, another B vitamin, leads to disruption of erythropoiesis in the bone marrow.

There are two other causes of anemia. One is the destruction of the bone marrow (bone marrow aplasia) by radioactive radiation (e. g., after an accident in a nuclear power plant) or due to toxic reactions to medication (e. g., by cytostatics) (**aplastic anemias**); the other is the reduction in erythrocyte lifespan due to destruction or increased breakdown (**hemolytic anemias**). With severe hemolytic anemias (e. g., following mismatched transfusions), a yellowish discoloration of the skin and mucous membranes may be observed besides anemic pallor. This jaundice (hemolytic icterus) is caused by the increased degradation of hemoglobin to bilirubin (yellow bile pigment) in the liver (see liver metabolism). This causes an increase in the plasma bilirubin level and bilirubin is deposited in the tissues.

An example of an anemia due to a genetic disorder of hemoglobin synthesis, clinically manifest as hemolytic anemia, is **sickle cell anemia**. In this disease, which occurs almost exclusively in black populations, there is a molecular defect leading to the substitution of sickle cell hemoglobin (Hb S) for normal hemoglobin. In Hb S the amino acid valine is substituted for glutamic acid. The erythrocytes containing this abnormal hemoglobin take on a sickle shape in the deoxygenated state. The sickle erythrocytes are inflexible and become wedged in the capillaries. Where the genetic defect occurs in homozygotes (proportion of Hb S in the total hemoglobin 70–99 %), it results in the occlusion of small vessels and hence permanent damage to organs. Those affected usually only reach adulthood with intensive treatment (e. g., partial exchange transfusions, analgesics, avoiding hypoxia, and at times bone marrow transplants). In some tropical African regions with a high incidence of malaria, 40 % of the population are heterozygous carriers of the gene (Hb S less than 50 %) and are asymptomatic. The defective gene gives them resistance to malarial infections (selective advantage).

The Regulation of Erythrocyte Generation

The generation of erythrocytes is regulated by the renal hormone *erythropoietin*. The body contains a simple but very effective regulatory system to keep oxygen content and with it the number of red cells relatively constant. If the oxygen content of the blood declines below a certain value, e. g., after large losses of blood or during a stay at high altitudes, formation of erythropoietin is repeatedly stimulated. The result is that the formation of erythrocytes in the bone marrow is stimulated, increasing oxygen carrying capacity. Once the oxygen deficiency has been re-

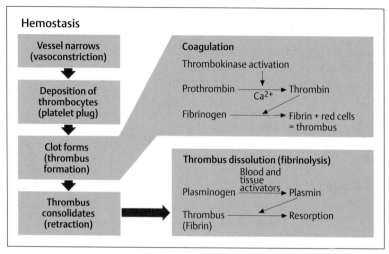

Fig. 6.**5** Schematic overview of the processes occurring during hemostasis, coagulation, and fibrinolysis

medied by the increased availability of erythrocytes, the formation of erythropoietin is again reduced. Patients requiring dialysis with disturbed renal functions (e. g., chronic renal failure) often suffer from marked deficiency in erythropoietin and therefore almost always suffer from concurrent anemia.

Hemostasis and Coagulation of the Blood

After injury to the vascular system, the body must be protected from life-threatening blood loss. Immediately after an injury, physiological mechanisms of hemostasis and coagulation are set in motion to minimize blood loss as far as possible. Besides platelets (thrombocytes), various plasma components (coagulation factors) and the vessel walls play a role in this (Fig. 6.**5**). *Bleeding time* is defined as the time between injury and the arrest of bleeding (normally 2–4 minutes). *Clotting time* (*coagulation time*) is the time to definitive hemostasis by the formation of a solid thrombus. For a small stab wound it amounts to about 8–10 minutes.

Hemostasis

Arrest of bleeding (*hemostasis*) can be divided into successive steps, ending in coagulation. Immediately after an injury, the vessels constrict (*vasoconstriction*) by contraction of the smooth muscle in the vessel wall. The second step is the formation of a platelet plug at the site of injury by deposition of thrombocytes on the injured vessel walls. At this stage the platelets are activated and change their shape, liberate substances from vesicles in which they were stored, and initiate the formation of the actual clot (thrombus) by aggregation (sticking together).

Coagulation of the Blood

At the same time, coagulation of the blood is set in motion. In the course of this process a cascade of reactions leads to enzymatic conversion of the soluble plasma protein fibrinogen into a fibrous meshwork of insoluble fibrin molecules. This process consists of numerous individual reactions, in which a total of 13 *coagulation factors* take part. According to the site of liberation of these factors, coagulation of the blood can be initiated in two different ways, namely, by tissue injury (*extrinsic mechanism*) or by processes that begin on the inside of a vessel (*intrinsic mechanism*). In both instances the enzyme thrombokinase is activated, either from thrombocytes or from the injured tissue (Fig. 6.**5**). In the presence of calcium ions this enzyme converts a protein precursor, prothrombin, that is carried in solution in the plasma, into the enzyme thrombin. Under the influence of thrombin, in turn, fibrinogen is converted to fibrin, which forms a feltlike meshwork of fibers. The deposition of more blood cells then leads to the formation of the final clot, which solidifies after coagulation and retracts.

Fibrinolysis

When the thrombus has fulfilled its task of wound closure, the fibrous clot must be dissolved in the course of wound healing (fibrinolysis). This is accomplished by the enzyme plasmin (Fig. 6.**5**), which is present in plasma as an inactive precursor (plasminogen) and is activated by a *plasminogen activator* present in blood or the surrounding tissues.

The Regulation of Blood Clotting

In order to prevent uncontrolled blood clotting from occurring in the blood vessels, a number of mechanisms maintain a constant balance between activation and inhibition of blood clotting. The smooth walls of the vessels, with their negatively charged surfaces, prevent platelet adhesion and consequent activation of thrombokinase. Additionally, the thrombin created during coagulation is largely inactivated by the built-up fibrin. Finally, thrombin is inhibited in its activity by other substances in the plasma (e. g., antithrombin III, heparin). Some coagulation factors need calcium to effect coagulation. If, for instance, citrate or oxalate ions are added to blood that has been drawn, they bind calcium ions and inhibit coagulation of the blood.

In congenital classical hemophilia (*hemophilia A*), normal clotting does not occur, owing to a deficiency in a coagulation factor (factor VIII). Consequently, even minor injuries can be accompanied by considerable bleeding. Similarly, a lack of thrombocytes (thrombocytopenia) leads to impairment of clotting and hence to an increased bleeding tendency (*hemorrhagic diathesis*).

The coagulability of blood can be reduced by medications such as heparin or dicumarol (e. g., Dicumarin, warfarin). While heparin inhibits coagulation indirectly by inactivating thrombin (see above), dicumarol acts in its capacity as vitamin K antagonist (displaces vitamin K at its site of action) and so inhibits the vitamin K-dependent synthesis of various coagulation factors (e. g., prothrombin) in the liver. For this reason, bedridden patients for whom the danger of thrombosis (formation of thrombi because of the greatly slowed blood flow in some veins) is increased, e. g., by prolonged bed rest, are heparinized or, in the case of prolonged treatment, given dicumarol (*anticoagulant therapy*). There is always a danger that a thrombus, e. g., in a pelvic vein, can float free in the blood (embolus) and reach the lungs by way of the right heart, causing occlusion of a pulmonary vessel (pulmonary embolus). On the other hand, with an overdose of heparin or dicumarol, coagulation of the blood can be severely impaired, leading to hemorrhages that are difficult to control.

■ The Immune System

The immune system, an effective network of immune cells (leukocytes), soluble proteins, and organs, is responsible for the ability of the human organism to defend itself against bacterial infections, viruses, fungi, and parasites. It can instantly react to and combat invading pathogens, foreign materials, or degenerated cells (e. g., tumor cells). The immune system is supported by external protective systems (skin and mucous membranes) that prevent the invasion of most infectious agents before they can penetrate. Should pathogens nevertheless invade the body, they must be rendered harmless by the immune system. The immune defenses are divided into a nonspecific and a specific immune system. Both systems include cells (*cellular immunity*) and soluble (*humoral immunity*) factors distributed throughout the body.

Nonspecific Immunity

Nonspecific immunity is the first line of defense. Its mechanisms are innate.

Cellular Immunity

The most important cells included here are neutrophils, monocytes, and macrophages (see The Cells of the Blood above), the first to reach the site of attack, e. g., the infective focus, or to be attracted there by chemotaxis. They are designed to phagocytose foreign material and render it harmless. This process results in typical signs of infection, namely redness, swelling, heat, and pain. There follows the formation of pus, consisting of cellular debris, dead bacteria, and necrotic granulocytes.

■ **Natural Killer Cells (NK Cells).** Natural killer cells are immune cells specialized to defend against pathogens (e. g., viruses, bacteria) and tumor cells. They include special large lymphocytes (about 5 % of leukocytes) that are attracted by *interferons* liberated by virus-infected cells. They perforate cell membranes with the aid of special proteins (perforins). The infected cell dies and the virus cannot multiply without the enzyme apparatus of its host cell. T-killer cells (*cytotoxic T cells, CTL*) function more precisely, killing cells infected by viruses as part of specific immunity (see below).

Humoral Immunity

Monocytes and macrophages also produce a number of soluble factors (cytokines) that lead to the infiltration and activation of other cells of the nonspecific immune system. They are supported by the so-called *complement system*, a system of about 20 soluble plasma proteins, which are a part of an enzymatic cascade (*complement cascade*) that are activated either by the carbohydrates of bacterial cell walls (alternative pathway) or by definite antigen–antibody complexes (classical pathway). In the final stage, some of the plasma proteins (factors C6–C9) form a so-called *membrane attack complex*, which perforates the bacterial cell wall. At the same time, *lysozyme* (an enzyme that splits carbohydrates in the plasma, the lymphatic fluid, and the saliva among others) breaks down the bacterial cell walls enzymatically.

Specific Immunity

Specific immunity comprises mechanisms that are always directed against a specific agent. This type of immunity is not innate but is acquired or "learned".

Antigen Presentation by Macrophages

Macrophages are a link between nonspecific and specific immunity. After phagocytosing and digesting a pathogen, they combine specific proteins of the pathogen (e. g., virus fragments) with autologous proteins (MHC,[1] HLA I, HLA II) and incorporate them in their membranes. By this

---

[1] MHC (major histocompatibility complex), in the human also called HLA class I and class II proteins = human leukocyte antigen. These tissue-compatible proteins alow the immune system to recognize foreign cells. The formation of these proteins is regulated by a total of six genes. A consequence of their numerous combinatory possibilities is that even close relatives rarely possess the same set of MHC proteins. In tissue or organ transplantation, foreign MHC proteins act as tissue antigens and elicit the formation of antibodies. The tissue is rejected. The immune system learns the difference between autologous and foreign material at birth. The substances it touches at that time it recognizes normally throughout life as autologous (*immune tolerance*), while everything arriving later is foreign. When this distinction fails, the results are autoimmune diseases, in which antibodies are formed against autologous proteins.

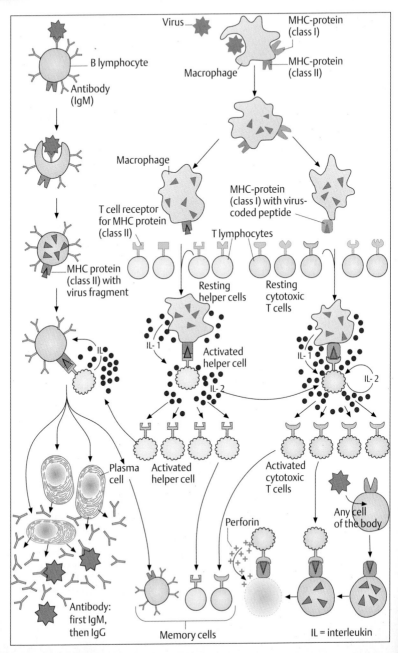

means they present the antigen proteins (antigen presentation) to the T lymphocytes (T-helper and T-killer cells, see below) (Fig. 6.**6**).

T Lymphocytes (Cellular Immunity)

The soluble factors and the cells of nonspecific immunity do not always succeed in destroying the invading pathogens completely. Moreover, granulocytes, monocytes, and macrophages are not always in a position to adapt their reaction to the various pathogens or to recognize them after repeated invasion of the organism. This is the point where the specific immune system intervenes. It consists of the T and B lymphocytes (cellular immunity) (see Cells of the Blood, The Leukocytes above) and the soluble antibodies (humoral immunity) produced by the B lymphocytes.

In order to reach their immune competence, the lymphocytes must undergo a process of maturation. The T lymphocytes receive this stamp in the thymus (T = thymus). The lymphocytes are then extruded into the secondary lymphoid organs (see The Lymphoid Organs [Immune Organs] below). T lymphocytes create the specific cellular immunity; they include the following types.

- **T-helper cells** (T$_H$, stimulate the immune system). Certain T helper cells bind to the MHC–antigen fragment complex of the antigen-presenting macrophage (activated T-helper cell). The T cells carrying the corresponding receptor secrete a signaling substance (interleukin) to accelerate their *clonal proliferation* (clonal selection). At the same time, the activated T-helper cell binds to the B lymphocyte, which, after contact with the antigen, also presents the antigen fragment to the MHC protein on its surface. This leads to the selection of individual lymphocytes and their selective proliferation. Stimulated by interleukins (produced by T-helper cells), these B cells mature into *antibody-producing plasma cells* (see B lymphocytes below, and Fig. 6.**6**).
- **T-suppressor cells** (T$_S$, inhibit the immune system). These terminate the immune reaction. The T-helper and T-suppressor cells produce and secrete cytokinins that regulate their interaction. This interaction

◁ Fig. 6.**6** **Simplified schema of the immune response.** (Modified from Koolman and Röhm)

is disturbed e.g., in the acquired immune deficiency syndrome (AIDS). The AIDS virus affects T_H cells, but not T_S cells, so that the immune-inhibiting T_S cells predominate.

■ **T-killer cells** (T_K, cytotoxic cells): these destroy autologous virus infected or degenerated (tumor) cells by direct contact. Their selective proliferation and activation is triggered in exactly the same way as the T-helper cells (Fig. 6.**6**). Like the natural killer cells, they destroy infected cells by perforin. However, their reaction is directed against a specific antigen, i.e., an antigen–antibody reaction. They are effective because the clonal proliferation of the T-killer cells makes antibodies available almost instantly.

B Lymphocytes (Humoral and Cellular Immunity)

B lymphocytes undergo maturation in the bone marrow (B = bone marrow). Antibodies of the IgM group (first antibodies) are attached to the surface of B lymphocytes and bind to the corresponding antigen. B lymphocytes take up an antigen–antibody complex (cellular immunity) and present an antigen fragment attached to a MHC protein at their surface. T-helper cells, activated by macrophages that also present antigen, bind to these B lymphocytes and, by releasing interleukins, stimulate their selective clonal proliferation and their transformation into antibody-producing plasma cells (Fig. 6.**6**). These processes take place predominantly in the secondary lymphoid organs (see below). For every antigen there are B lymphocytes that recognize it exclusively and form antibodies against it. The antibodies (immunoglobulins IgA, IgD, IgE, IgG, IgM; see Plasma Proteins) are released into the plasma and the surrounding body fluids (humoral immunity). Their function is to neutralize the antigens, to mark them as foreign materials for the nonspecific immune cells ("opsonization"), and to activate the complement system (see p. 283). Immunoglobulins cannot destroy pathogenic agents directly, only inactivate them. The elimination of the antigen–antibody complexes is again accomplished nonspecifically (by the complement system or by eosinophil granulocytes; see above The Leukocytes).

On contacting an antigen, the plasma cells first form IgM type antibodies (primary response). The early forms are attached to the surface of plasma cells, the later ones are secreted into the plasma. The primary response develops relatively slowly and does not last long. As the response proceeds, the plasma cells switch to IgG production (secondary response, faster and more lasting). The IgG are present in the plasma in the greatest amounts and are the only immuno-globulins that can cross the placenta, that is, that can be passed on to the fetus.

Memory Cells

Some of the lymphocytes (B lymphocytes, and T-helper and T-killer cells) when stimulated by antigens are transformed into so-called memory cells. These leave the blood and wander into the lymphoid tissues and organs. Here they circulate for long times, sometimes decades, until they meet the specific antigen again. Immunity rests on these memory cells. On repeated contact with the same antigen, the organism can react more rapidly and effectively than on first meeting, so that the disease does not recur or takes a more benign course (e. g., chickenpox, German measles). Active immunization occurs when the organism itself forms the antibo-dies during an interaction with a pathogenic agent. This can also be achieved if the organism is given attenuated, nonpathogenic agents (an-tigens) (active immunization). Such acquired active immunity can at times be maintained for years. *Passive immunization* is the administra-tion not of antigens but of ready-made antibodies prepared by active im-munization of another organism. Such passive immunization, however, usually only lasts a few weeks, since the antibodies are degraded by the organism.

■ The Lymphoid Organs (Immune Organs)

The surveillance of the body by immune cells and their rapid deploy-ment presupposes not only a finely meshed transport system (blood and lymph vessels) but also the organization of cells in lymphoid organs. With the exception of the thymus (see below) the specific immune sys-tem in the form of lymphoid organs is localized at the danger sites, the entry portals of pathogens.

The lymphoid organs are divided into two types by their functions (Fig. 6.**7**):

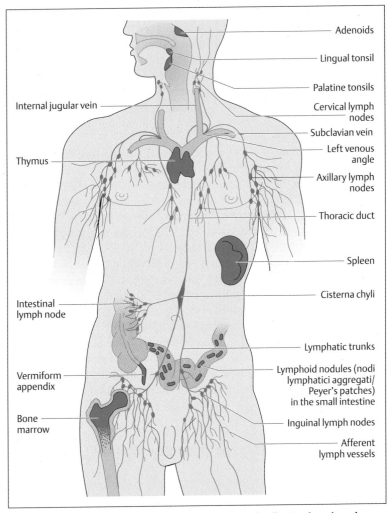

Adenoids

Lingual tonsil

Palatine tonsils

Cervical lymph nodes

Internal jugular vein

Subclavian vein

Left venous angle

Thymus

Axillary lymph nodes

Thoracic duct

Spleen

Cisterna chyli

Intestinal lymph node

Lymphatic trunks

Vermiform appendix

Lymphoid nodules (nodi lymphatici aggregati/ Peyer's patches) in the small intestine

Bone marrow

Inguinal lymph nodes

Afferent lymph vessels

Fig 6.7 **Lymphoid organs, lymph vessels, and regional collecting lymph nodes**

- **Primary lymphoid organs,** which generate, develop, and mature the immune cells. In the adult this includes especially the thymus (to develop and mature the T cells) and the bone marrow (generates all immune cells, develops and matures the B cells).
- **Secondary lymphoid organs,** to which the immune cells migrate, including the spleen, the lymph nodes, and the lymphoid tissues of the mucous membranes (e.g., tonsils, Peyer's patches of the small intestine, appendix).

The basic framework of all secondary lymphoid organs is a meshwork of reticular connective tissue, in which numerous lymphocytes are deposited. In places they form round collections of cells, the *lymphatic follicles*. These may be regarded as the functional units of the secondary lymphoid organs. About 98 % of all lymphocytes are found there and in the connective tissue, while only about 2 % are in the blood. A large proportion of the lymphocytes recirculate between the lymphoid organs and the blood (lymphocyte recirculation; see Gut-Associated Immune System below). The lymphocytes leave the bloodstream in *postcapillary venules* (transitional vessels between capillaries and veins) within the lymphoid organs, pass through the lymph vessels, and after a certain time return to the peripheral blood, e.g., by the thoracic duct (see Chapter 5: The Lymph Vessels). Under special circumstances, e.g., in inflammations, the lymphocytes can also leave the blood vessels outside the lymphoid organs.

The lymph vessels are a drainage system of the connective tissue. They return to the venous blood tissue fluid that has left the blood vessels and reached connective tissue while transporting substances (see Chapter 5: Substance Exchange between Blood and Tissues). They thus form a parallel pathway to the venous limb of the circulation. Into their course lymph nodes are inserted as "*biological filters*" where, for example, antigens meet with immune cells. Having proliferated, the lymphocytes leave the lymph nodes and return to the bloodstream and other parts of the body by way of the lymph vessels (see below).

The Thymus

The thymus lies behind the sternum and is especially well developed in the newborn and the growing child (Fig. 6.**8**). The surface of the infantile thymus is divided into individual lobules, in which a cortex covers a medulla. While the cortical areas show large deposits of lymphocytes, the medulla is filled with blood vessels and strikingly wide capillaries. After puberty, the thymus undergoes a process of gradual involution and is replaced by fatty tissue. At 60 years of age, next to no lymphoid tissue remains.

The thymus is an *overriding lymphatic organ* and is indispensable for the development of cellular immunity. This where especially the T (thymus) lymphocytes acquire their *immune competence* during embryonic development. From the bone marrow, where they are generated as precursor T cells, they enter the bloodstream to reach the thymus, where they become specialized. They learn to distinguish autologous from foreign structures. Additionally, the T lymphocytes mature into variously differentiated cells (T-helper cells, T-suppressor cells, and cytotoxic T cells) under the influence of substances (thymopoietin) released from the structural elements of the gland. These cells are now prepared to react to antigens in specific immunologically competent ways. After this process of specialization, maturation, and differentiation, the lympho-

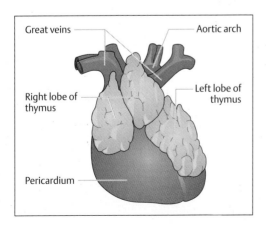

Fig. 6.**8**   **Thymus of a newborn.** The thymus lies in front of the pericardium and behind the sternum. (After Feneis)

Great veins

Aortic arch

Right lobe of thymus

Left lobe of thymus

Pericardium

cytes return to the bloodstream and settle in the secondary lymphoid organs such as tonsils, lymph nodes, and spleen. The B lymphocytes that produce antibodies acquire their life-long immune competence in the bone marrow.

The Lymph Nodes

Lymph nodes are *biological filters* inserted like pearls on a string into the course of the lymph vessels (Fig. 6.**7**). By their situation they monitor lymph coming from the periphery. Lymph nodes near organs that are the first to receive lymph from an organ or a circumscribed region are designated *regional lymph nodes*. Lymph nodes that occur beyond these points and receive lymph from several regional lymph nodes are *collecting nodes* (Fig. 6.**9**), but they are distinguished from regional lymph nodes only by their location.

In the lymph node, lymphoid tissue is completely surrounded by a solid connective tissue capsule, forming a bean-shaped body several millimeters in size. Several connective tissue septa run from the capsule inward and, together with the basic framework of reticular connective tissue, divide the lymph node into a loose meshwork where numerous *lymphatic follicles* are deposited (Fig. 6.**10**). Several afferent lymph vessels pierce the capsule on one side, while on the opposite side usually only one or two vessels leave the lymph node. These are also the sites where the blood vessels enter and leave.

While passing through the lymph node, the lymphatic fluid has considerable contact with the surface of the lymphatic tissue. Cells of the *macrophage system* monitor and phagocytose foreign bodies, pathogens, and cell debris. When inflammations affect the area they drain, lymph nodes swell, become painful, and are easily palpable. At the same time, the macrophages stimulate (antigen presentation, see p. 283) the lymphocytes to proliferate (divide) and form specific antibodies. Cancer cells also reach the lymph nodes through the lymph, and in this way can develop lymph node metastases. From the lymph node, the antibody-forming plasma cells reach other lymph nodes and eventually the bloodstream by way of efferent lymph vessels.

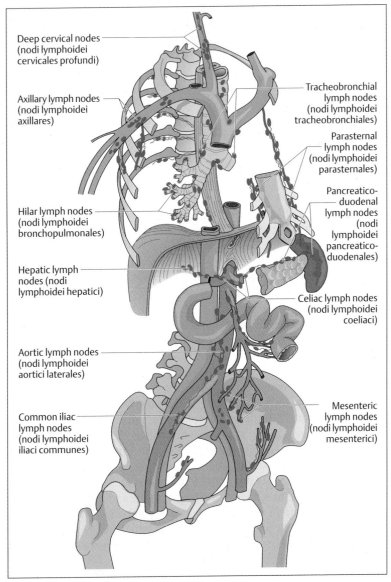

Deep cervical nodes
(nodi lymphoidei
cervicales profundi)

Axillary lymph nodes
(nodi lymphoidei
axillares)

Hilar lymph nodes
(nodi lymphoidei
bronchopulmonales)

Hepatic lymph
nodes (nodi
lymphoidei hepatici)

Aortic lymph nodes
(nodi lymphoidei
aortici laterales)

Common iliac
lymph nodes
(nodi lymphoidei
iliaci communes)

Tracheobronchial
lymph nodes
(nodi lymphoidei
tracheobronchiales)

Parasternal
lymph nodes
(nodi lymphoidei
parasternales)

Pancreatico-
duodenal
lymph nodes
(nodi
lymphoidei
pancreatico-
duodenales)

Celiac lymph nodes
(nodi lymphoidei
coeliaci)

Mesenteric
lymph nodes
(nodi lymphoidei
mesenterici)

Fig. 6.**9** **Principal regional and collecting lymph nodes of the trunk**

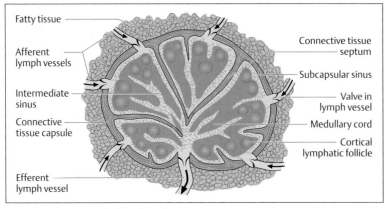

Fig. 6.**10** **Structure of a lymph node**

The Spleen (Splen, Lien)

The spleen is the only lymphoid organ in the bloodstream and can be regarded as an organ to *monitor and filter* the blood. It extracts aging erythrocytes, and provides immunological monitoring of the blood. It is soft, about the size of a fist (150–200 g), and is shaped like a coffee bean. The spleen lies in the left upper abdomen under the diaphragm (Fig. 6.**11**) and is normally well protected from the outside by the ribs.

If a fresh spleen is cut open, its gross structure can be seen by the naked eye to consist of red tissue (red pulp) interspersed with many small, white splenic nodules surrounded by a connective tissue capsule. The cut surface also reveals cut lymph vessel sheaths. Splenic nodules and lymphatic sheaths consist of lymphoid tissue (white pulp). Red and white pulp are embedded in a tough framework of septa of connective tissue that jut inward from the capsule (Fig. 6.**12a**, **b**). The red pulp (about 80 % of the splenic volume) consists of a framework of reticular connective tissue, traversed by a complex system of blood vessels. Each of the smallest branches of the blood vessels is a central vessel running through a splenic nodule. Inside the splenic nodules the lymphatic follicles are arranged in the form of lymphatic cords, where the B lympho-

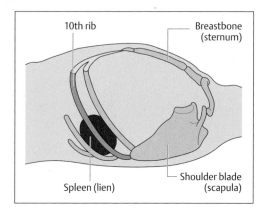

Fig. 6.**11 Position of the spleen in a recumbent patient (viewed from the left).** A normal-sized spleen is not palpable. It lies in the left upper abdomen with its longitudinal axis at the level of the 10th rib. (After Beske)

10th rib

Breastbone (sternum)

Shoulder blade (scapula)

Spleen (lien)

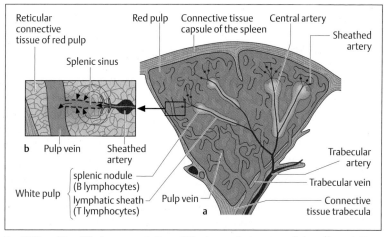

Reticular connective tissue of red pulp

Red pulp

Connective tissue capsule of the spleen

Central artery

Sheathed artery

Splenic sinus

b Pulp vein

Sheathed artery

Trabecular artery

White pulp { splenic nodule (B lymphocytes) / lymphatic sheath (T lymphocytes)

Pulp vein

Trabecular vein

Connective tissue trabecula

a

Fig. 6.**12 a Simplified representation of the internal structure of the spleen. b** Magnification of a section from **a**

cytes have settled. There are no lymphatic follicles in the lymphatic sheaths, where T lymphocytes predominate. The spleen's role as an immune organ in the immunological process is to form antibodies when antigens reach a lymphatic follicle through the bloodstream.

Numerous capillaries branch from the central artery, each surrounded by a spindle-shaped sheath (sheathed arteries) of densely packed macrophages. The capillaries then drain largely into the meshwork of reticular connective tissue (red pulp) surrounding every splenic sinus (open circulation). Aging erythrocytes are broken down as they pass through the reticular connective tissue. A few capillaries may drain directly into a sinus (closed circulation). The walls of the sinuses are lined with *reticular cells*, separated by more or less wide openings. At these points the erythrocytes must pass through narrow passages, which can only be surmounted by intact, pliable red cells. Unusable red cells are phagocytosed and broken down by the reticulum cells. In diseases that are accompanied by severe breakdown of blood (e. g., malaria), the spleen can enlarge markedly. Lastly, substances that can be used again can be stored here, e. g., iron from the breakdown of hemoglobin.

Lymphoid Tissues of the Mucous Membranes

The Tonsils

The faucial (palatine), adenoid (pharyngeal), and lingual tonsils together form Waldeyer's tonsillar (lymphoid) ring (p. 400). To this must be added the lymphatic tissue on the pharyngeal wall, the eustachian tonsil (tubal tonsil, tonsilla tubaria), which lies close to the eustachian tube (connection between the middle ear and the pharynx). The tonsils lie under the epithelium of the oral cavity and their framework is also composed of reticular connective tissue containing lymphatic follicles. In many places the epithelium juts deeply into the lymphatic tissues, thus increasing their superficial contact. By this means, antigens invading through the nose and mouth can make timely contact with immune cells and activate the specific defenses. For instance, in the presence of a massive bacterial invasion, the lymphatic follicles enlarge as a result of the marked increase of antibody-producing lymphocytes. The tension in the connective tissue capsule can become very painful (tonsillitis). In early childhood there is often enlargement of the adenoids (pharyngeal polyps, commonly known as nasal polyps) at the transition from the nose to the pharynx (choanae). This can make it difficult to breathe through the nose.

Gut-associated Lymphatic Tissue (e. g., Peyer's Patches)

Because of their large surface, the intestines play a central role in immunity. After all, 70–80% of all antibody-producing cells are situated in the intestinal wall, the rest being distributed among the other secondary lymphatic organs, the vascular system, and the connective tissue. Diffuse collections and loose associations of lymphocytes (lymphatic follicles) can be found throughout the gastrointestinal tract, which, because of its direct contact with ingested nutrients, is an ideal portal of entry for antigens.

Organized lymphatic tissue is present in the vermiform appendix and in the terminal portion of the small intestine (ileum), where it takes the form of Peyer's patches in the submucosa and the connective tissue of the mucous membrane (mucosa) of the ileum. These are collections of lymphatic follicles, lying in platelike strands of five to one hundred. They are 1–12 cm in diameter and lie parallel to the axis of the intestine, usually on the side opposite the mesentery (Fig. 6.**13a**). The number of patches varies between 15 and 50 (up to 250) according to the individual. They are developed before birth and can be demonstrated in the small intestine even late in old age. The areas of the lymphatic follicles are devoid of villi and crypts. Over the lymphatic follicles the connective tissue of the intestinal mucosa, covered with mucosal cells, arches like a dome (Fig. 6.**13a–c**).

Into the epithelium of the intestinal mucosa are dispersed specific cells that apparently selectively recognize and take up antigenic substances. These *M cells* stand out as folded surface structures (microfolded cells = M cells) jutting into the intestinal lumen. They are horseshoe-shaped, with their closed end toward the intestinal lumen, and appear to be the site where antigens are primarily recognized, as they take up microorganisms and other potentially pathogenic substances and initiate an immune reaction. In this way, the small intestine is protected against future absorption of these antigens.

The defense process may be described as follows. Under the M cell, flanked by its open limbs, embedded as it were in this horse-shaped membranous fold, are T and B lymphocytes and macrophages (Fig. 6.**13c**). The M cells take the antigenic substance from the intestine and pass it to the macrophages. The macrophages present it by way of the T lymphocytes (T-helper cells) to the B lymphocytes, thus activating them

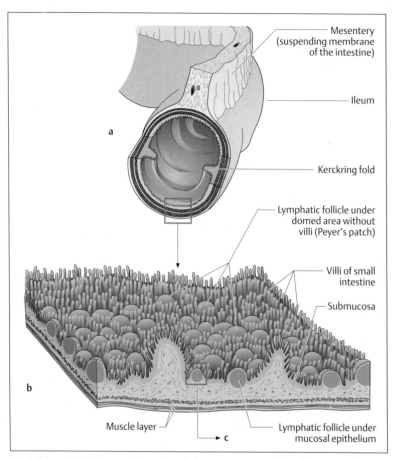

Fig. 6.13 a–c   Structure and function of the gut-associated lymphatic system
a Site of Peyer's patches in the ileum
b Lymphatic follicle under a domed area (magnification of a section from **a**)

(see above Specific Immunity). The B lymphocytes migrate through the lymph and blood vessel systems (lymphocyte circulation, which also takes place in the other lymphoid organs) and are transformed in part here already into antibody-producing plasma cells. The antibodies so

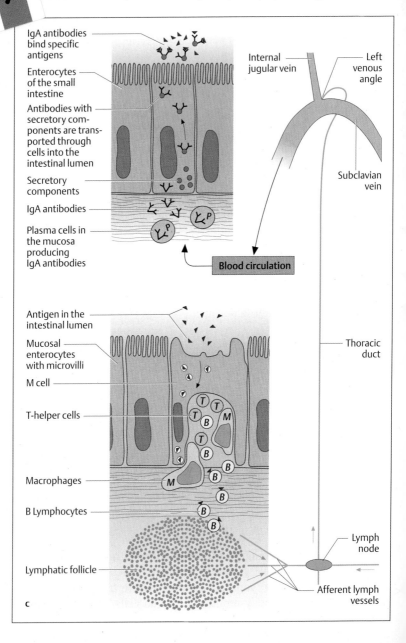

IgA antibodies bind specific antigens

Enterocytes of the small intestine

Antibodies with secretory components are transported through cells into the intestinal lumen

Secretory components

IgA antibodies

Plasma cells in the mucosa producing IgA antibodies

Internal jugular vein

Left venous angle

Subclavian vein

Blood circulation

Antigen in the intestinal lumen

Mucosal enterocytes with microvilli

M cell

T-helper cells

Macrophages

B Lymphocytes

Lymphatic follicle

Thoracic duct

Lymph node

Afferent lymph vessels

c

formed (IgA) are partly taken up by the liver cells and passed on to the bile, with which they reach the intestinal lumen. The antibodies so formed also reach other bodily secretions, including the mother's milk. This benefits the nursing infant, who receives with the mother's milk specific antigens against pathogens that the gut-associated immune system of the mother has already encountered.

The larger part of the B lymphocytes recirculate into the lymphatic follicles of the Peyer's patches, where they are transformed into IgA-producing plasma cells. The antibodies are passed on to the cells of the intestinal mucosa, provided with a layer of glycoproteins (secretory components) to protect them from digestive enzymes and passed into the intestinal lumen. These antibodies bind to the corresponding antigens, which cannot now be absorbed and are therefore excreted.

Summary **Blood, the Immune System and Lymphoid Organs**

■ **The Blood**

The blood (about 8 % of body weight) consists of plasma and cells: erythrocytes (red cells, red corpuscles), leukocytes (white cells), and thrombocytes (platelets).

Erythrocytes

Erythrocytes number 4.5–5.5 million per microliter (mm^3) of blood. Function: the transport of respiratory gases. The erythrocytes are formed (160 million per minute) in the bone marrow from nucleated stem cells, but later lose their nuclei and cell organelles. At this point they consist almost entirely of hemoglobin, which can bind oxygen reversibly. They are discoid and biconcave. Their lifespan is about 120 days and they are broken down in the spleen and liver.

In inflammations or increased tissue necrosis, erythrocytes tend to form clumps. In anticoagulated blood they therefore sediment more

◁ Fig. 6.**13 c**   Structure of the epithelium in the domed areas and the mechanism of intestinal mucosal immunity

rapidly (100 mm/h, otherwise 3–10 mm/h). A raised erythrocyte sedimentation rate is a nonspecific sign of illness.

Leukocytes (Granulocytes, Lymphocytes, Monocytes)

Leukocytes number 4000–8000 per microliter of blood (in inflammation well over 10 000/µl). Function: Together with the lymphoid organs they form the immune system. They can move autonomously by ameboid movement and so can migrate through the capillary walls (connective tissue immunity). As a rule, generation, maturation, and proliferation take place in the bone marrow (the exception is lymphocytes); they are subsequently washed into the blood. The cells are nucleated.

- *Granulocytes:* fine granules in the cytoplasm. (1) Neutrophils: 60–70% of leukocytes; phagocytosing cells of nonspecific immunity; decay in the process (forming pus). (2) Eosinophils: 2–3% of leukocytes; cells of nonspecific immunity that phagocytose antigen–antibody complexes; limit allergic reactions. (3) Basophils: 0.5–1% of leukocytes; elicit allergic reactions by histamine release; inhibit blood clotting by heparin.
- *Lymphocytes:* 20–30% of leukocytes; cells of specific immunity; they have a large nucleus and a cytoplasm rich in cell organelles. They are generated in the bone marrow, mature in the bone marrow (B lymphocytes) and thymus (T lymphocytes), and proliferate in the secondary lymphoid organs.
- *Monocytes:* 4–5% of leukocytes; the largest leukocytes; they leave the blood after 20–30 hours and outside the blood are transformed into macrophages. They are cells of nonspecific immunity (phagocytosis and digestion) but take part in specific immunity (antigen presentation).

Thrombocytes

Thrombocytes number 150 000–350 000 per microliter of blood. Function: hemostasis and triggering clotting of the blood. They are formed in the bone marrow by cytoplasmic extrusions from giant cells, and released into the blood as nonnucleated disks. Their lifespan is 5–10 days and they are broken down in the spleen.

Blood Groups

The heritable blood group antigens are glycolipids and glycoproteins in the cell wall of the erythrocytes that induce the formation of antibodies in foreign organisms:

- *The ABO system* with four blood groups: (1) blood group A (erythrocytes with antigen A), 44% of the population; (2) blood group B (erythrocytes with antigen B), 10% of the population; (3) blood group AB (erythrocytes with antigens A and B), 4% of the population; (4) blood group O (erythrocytes without antigens A or B), 42% of the population.
- *The Rh blood group system* (antigens = Rh factors C, D, E, mostly D): persons with the Rh factor are Rh-positive (Rh+, 85% of the population); persons without the Rh factor are Rh-negative (Rh–, 15% of the population).

From the first months of life, the plasma of each person contains the antibody against the missing antigen of the ABO system (in this case no contact with the foreign antigen is necessary): (1) for blood group A, anti-B; (2) for blood group B, anti-A; (3) for blood group AB, none; (4) for blood group O, anti-A and anti-B.

Antibodies against Rh antigens are formed only after contact with the antigen.

Blood Transfusions

During a blood transfusion, if blood incompatible with the recipient is given, the reaction of the ABO antigens with their corresponding antibodies leads to erythrocyte agglutination. To prevent mismatched transfusions, the following measures are taken before every transfusion:

- Test for ABO blood groups: serological compatibility testing (blood typing)
- Test for other antigens and antibodies (e.g., Rh factor): direct and indirect Coombs' test.

The Plasma

Plasma = blood without cells: 90% water, 10% dissolved substances (70% plasma proteins, 20% low-molecular-weight substances, 10% electrolytes).

Hematocrit = percent blood cells to volume of whole blood.
Serum = plasma without fibrinogen.

- **Plasma proteins:**

  1. *Albumins* (35–40 g/l plasma): maintain the colloid osmotic pressure; transport calcium ions, fatty acids, bilirubin, bile acids, a few hormones and vitamins.

  2. α_1-, α_2-, and β-Globulins: transport lipids (lipoproteins), hemoglobin, iron, vitamin B_{12}, adrenocortical hormones; constituent of fibrinogen and prothrombin. The lipoproteins are classified by decreasing size and increasing density. The proportion of fat declines with increasing density: very-low-density lipoproteins (VLDL, proportion of fat 90%), low-density lipoproteins (LDL), high-density lipoproteins (HDL, proportion of fat 50%). LDL transport lipids (especially cholesterol) from the liver to the tissues (risk of arteriosclerosis); HDL returns excess cholesterol to the liver. Hence high HDL combined with low LDL reduces the risk of arteriosclerosis.

  3. γ-Globulins (immunoglobulins, Ig): the antibodies of specific immunity produced by the B lymphocytes (plasma cells: mainly IgA (immune reaction of the mucous membranes, e.g., intestines); IgG (75% of all immunoglobulins, can cross the placental barrier); IgM (early antibodies); also IgD and IgE.

- **Low-molecular-weight plasma constituents:** nutrients, vitamins, trace elements, metabolic products, hormones, enzymes.

- **Plasma electrolytes:** extracellular (i.e., in the plasma) preponderance of sodium, calcium, and chloride ions; intracellular preponderance of potassium, magnesium, and phosphate ions. NaCl is the most important for osmotic regulation.

Blood Gas Transport in the Blood

- *Oxygen* is transported in the erythrocytes bound to hemoglobin (Hb). In the lung, four oxygen molecules are donated to the bivalent iron atoms of the four heme groups (oxygenation), transported by the blood to the tissues, and released there (deoxygenation). The Hb concentration is about 15 g/dl, so that about 200 ml O_2/l can be transported (without Hb, only 3 ml/l).

- 90% of *carbon dioxide* is transported in the plasma as soluble bicarbonate (generated from carbon dioxide with the aid of carbonic anhydrase in the erythrocytes), 10% as carbaminohemoglobin bound to hemoglobin and exhaled as carbon dioxide. These processes are linked to the oxygenation and deoxygenation of hemoglobin (buffer function of hemoglobin!).

Carbon monoxide has a higher affinity than oxygen for hemoglobin; 65% HbCO is life-threatening.

The Anemias

Erythrocyte or hemoglobin deficiency in the blood. Consequence: reduced availability of oxygen in the tissues (symptoms of pale skin and mucous membranes, easy fatigability).

- *Hypochromic anemia:* iron deficiency anemia, from chronic, mostly internal bleeding.
- *Hyperchromic anemia:* deficiencies in vitamin B_{12} (pernicious anemia), folic acid, or erythropoietin (a hormone generated in the kidney that regulates erythrocyte formation). Consequence: formation of fewer, much larger erythrocytes with increased hemoglobin content (macrocytes).
- *Aplastic anemia:* due to bone marrow aplasia (e. g., after treatment with cytostatics).
- *Hemolytic anemia:* due to increased erythrocyte destruction (e. g., transfusion reactions, Rh incompatibility)

Hemostasis and Coagulation of the Blood

1. *Arrest of bleeding (hemostasis):* begins immediately after injury. The sequence in order is: vasoconstriction—platelet deposition on the injured vascular walls (platelet plug)—agglutination of thrombocytes and release of the enzyme thrombokinase (= initiation of blood clotting).
2. *Coagulation:* in the presence of calcium ions, thrombokinase transforms prothrombin present in the plasma into the enzyme thrombin. By the action of thrombin, the fibrous substance fibrin is generated from fibrinogen in a sequence of several reactions in which, apart from fibrinogen, 12 other coagulation factors take part. Together with blood cells deposited at the site, fibrin forms the thrombus, which solidifies after coagulation is complete (retraction).
3. *Dissolution of the thrombus* in the course of wound healing: catalyzed by the enzyme plasmin, which is formed from plasminogen

dissolved in the plasma under the influence of activators in the blood and tissues.

A number of mechanisms and combinations provide a constant balance between activation and inhibition of coagulation of the blood (e.g., substances such as antithrombin and heparin in the plasma).

■ The Immune System

Divided into specific and nonspecific immunity. Nonspecific immunity is inborn; specific immunity is always directed against a definite pathogen and is acquired, i.e., learned. Both systems include cells (cellular immunity) and soluble factors (humoral immunity).

The Nonspecific Immune System

- *Cellular immunity:* this first immune process includes inflammatory phagocytosing cells (neutrophil granulocytes, monocytes, and macrophages) and killer cells specialized against viruses. In addition, macrophages present antigen proteins (antigen fragment + MHC protein: antigen presentation) to the T lymphocytes of the specific immune system, initiating specific immunity.
- *Humoral immunity:* this includes cytokines (generated by monocytes, macrophages), the complement system (enzyme cascade of ca. 20 plasma proteins, eliminating or perforating the walls of bacteria and antigen–antibody complexes) and lysosomes (break down bacterial cell walls enzymatically).

The Specific Immune System

- *Cellular immunity:* includes the T and B lymphocytes.
  1. *T-helper cells*—stimulate the immune system; bond first to the antigen-presenting macrophages, then to the antigen presenting B lymphocytes and stimulate their transformation into antibody-producing plasma cells by interleukins.
  2. *T-suppressor cells*—inhibit the immune system by terminating the immune reaction. (The balance between T-helper and T-suppressor cells is upset in AIDS.)
  3. *T-killer cells* (cytotoxic cells)—work similarly to natural killer cells, but each is directed against a particular virus.

4. *B-lymphocytes*—early antibodies (IgM) on B lymphocytes; bond to a specific antigen after ingesting it. Antigen fragment + MHC protein = antigen presentation.

5. *Memory cells*—B lymphocytes, T-helper cells and T-killer cells stimulated by antigens and so responsible for acquired immunity. With repeated contact with the antigen, the generation of antibodies is speeded up.

- *Humoral immunity:* This consists of antibodies IgA, IgD, IgE, IgG, and IgM produced by plasma cells derived from B lymphocytes. The antibodies inactivate the antigens by forming antigen–antibody complexes, which are then eliminated by nonspecific mechanisms (complement system, eosinophil granulocytes).

■ The Lymphoid Organs

These are divided into primary lymphoid organs, in which generation, development, and maturation of immune cells takes place (thymus, bone marrow), and secondary lymphoid organs, to which immune cells migrate and in which in the course of an immune reaction lymphocytes proliferate and antibodies are formed (spleen, lymph nodes, lymphid tissues of the mucous membranes); 98% of lymphocytes are found there. The lymphocytes recirculate between secondary lymphoid organs and the blood (lymphoid organ—blood—lymph vessels—thoracic duct—blood—lymphoid organ).

Structure of secondary lymphoid organs: collections of lymphocytes (lymphatic follicles) in reticular connective tissue.

Primary Lymphoid Organs

- *Thymus:* the thymus is the overriding immune organ. This is where cellular immunity develops during embryonic development (e. g., generation of T lymphocytes; differentiation of T-helper cells, T-suppressor cells, and T-killer cells). The thymus gradually involutes throughout life.
- *Bone marrow:* here all immune cells are constantly being generated. B lymphocytes attain their final form in the bone marrow.

Secondary Lymphoid Organs

- *Lymph nodes:* lymph nodes are biological filters inserted into the course of the lymph vessels throughout the lymph vascular system and evenly distributed. Secondary lymphoid organs are therefore specific immune defenses localized at nearly every danger point in the body.

- *The spleen:* the spleen is the regulatory and filtration organ of the blood, since it is the only secondary lymphoid organ inserted into the bloodstream.

- *Lymphoid organs of the mucous membranes:* include the tonsils (Waldeyer's tonsillar ring of pharyngeal, palatine, and lingual tonsils), the lymphatic tissue on the pharyngeal wall, and the gut-associated lymphatic system. Because of its large surface area, the intestinal mucosa is of special significance for immunity; 70–80% of all antibody-producing cells are located there. Lymphatic follicles are distributed throughout the gastrointestinal mucosa and form organized lymphoid tissue in the vermiform appendix and the terminal small intestine (Peyer's patches)

7

The Endocrine System

Contents

The endocrine system comprises all the organs and cellular systems that secrete *signal or messenger substances* (hormones), which they either dispatch to distant sites by way of the bloodstream or the lymph or secrete into the interstitial fluid to reach neighboring cells (*paracrine secretions*). Hormones can also act on the very cells that secrete them (*autocrine secretions*). In this way, the endocrine system differs from the exocrine glands of the body (e.g., salivary glands, sweat glands), that send their secretions directly or through ducts to the external or internal surfaces of the body (skin, intestines) (Fig. 7.**1a–c**).

In its biological functioning, the endocrine system is closely allied with the autonomic nervous system and the immune system, acting as a sort of "wireless communication" system. It coordinates the functions of widely separated organs. It differs from the autonomic nervous system in that its action develops more slowly but is more long lasting, and this is important for reproduction, growth, and the homeostasis of life-preserving metabolic processes (water and electrolyte balance, energy metabolism). With all the variety of their individual tasks, the

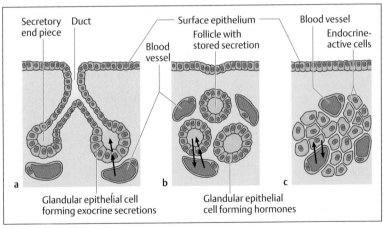

Fig. 7.**1a–c   Classification of glands by transport of the secretion**
a Exocrine gland
b Endocrine gland with follicle formation
c Endocrine gland without follicle formation.
The arrows indicate the direction of transport of the elements of secretion from the blood vessels and the direction of flow of the secretions

overarching goal of both systems is to adapt the body to the changing stresses of its surroundings. Impairment of the endocrine system, whether by deficiency or overactivity (see below) can lead to severe illnesses.

Hormones

Hormones are *chemical messengers* consisting of a variety of substances (e. g., proteins, peptides, steroids) that mostly act on their target cells in very small amounts. They can be relatively simple or quite complex molecules. Among other actions, hormones influence production and proliferation of certain enzymes in their target cells, thus coordinating and controlling the corresponding activities of the organism. Although the blood distributes hormones over the whole body, only certain cells, organs, or tissues respond to them. Hormones act on their target cells through *specific receptors*, that are localized either on the cell membrane or in the cytoplasm of these cells. A variety of hormone receptors on each cell usually ensures that different hormones can bind to it. The sensitivity of a cell for a particular hormone depends in part on the number of available receptors. The hormone is inactivated after it is bound or after its specific activity has been deployed.

Mechanisms of Hormonal Action

From a biochemical point of view, hormones can be divided according to their mechanism of action into those with *affinity for fat* (*lipophilic*) and those with *affinity for water* (*hydrophilic*) (Table 7.**1**). For instance, almost all steroid and thyroid hormones belong to the class of lipophilic hormones, while hydrophilic hormones are usually amino acid derivatives or have an amino acid structure (e. g., proteins, peptides) (Table 7.**1**).

Hydrophilic hormones mostly bind to their specific receptor on the external surface of the target cell. This results in a succession of defined reactions in the cell membrane, followed by the enzymatic release of a hormone called a "second messenger" inside the cell. The intermediary action of such a messenger substance (e. g., cyclic adenosine mono-

Table 7.**1** **Important sites of formation of hormones and similar substances**

Chief site of formation	Hormone/hormone-like substances	Properties: hydrophilic/lipophilic
Classic endocrine glands		
Pituitary gland (hypophysis)	ACTH (adrenocorticotropic hormone, corticotropin)	Hydrophilic
	TSH (thyroid-stimulating hormone, thyrotropin)	Hydrophilic
	FSH (follicle-stimulating hormone, follitropin)	Hydrophilic
	LH (luteinizing hormone, lutropin)	Hydrophilic
	GH (growth hormone, somatotropic hormone)	Hydrophilic
	MSH (melanocyte-stimulating hormone, melanotropin)	Hydrophilic
	PRL (prolactin)	Hydrophilic
	Oxytocin (generated in the hypothalamus and released by the neurohypophysis)	Hydrophilic
Pineal gland	Melatonin	Hydrophilic
Thyroid gland	Thyroxine and triiodothyronine	Lipophilic
C cells of the thyroid (parafollicular cells)	Calcitonin	Hydrophilic
Parathyroid glands	Parathormone	Hydrophilic
Adrenal glands (suprarenal glands)	Mineralocorticoids and glucocorticoids	Lipophilic
	Androgens	Lipophilic
	Epinephrine and norepinephrine (adrenaline and noradrenaline)	Hydrophilic
Pancreatic islet cells (islets of Langerhans)	Insulin, glucagon, and somatostatin	Hydrophilic
Ovary	Estrogen and progesterone	Lipophilic
Testes	Androgens	Lipophilic
Placenta	Chorionic gonadotropin, progesterone	Hydrophilic, lipophilic

Table 7.**1**   (continued)

Chief site of formation	Hormone/hormone-like substances	Properties: hydrophilic/lipophilic
Tissues and individual cells secreting hormones		
Central and autonomic nervous system	Neurotransmitters	Hydrophilic
Parts of the diencephalon (e. g., hypothalamus)	Releasing hormones (liberins, statins)	Hydrophilic
System of gastrointestinal cells	Gastrins, cholecystokinin, secretin	Hydrophilic
Atria of the heart	Atrial natriuretic peptide (ANP)	Hydrophilic
Kidneys	Erythropoietin, renin	Hydrophilic
Liver	Angiotensinogen, somatomedins	Hydrophilic
Immune organs	Hormones of the thymus, cytokines, lymphokine	Hydrophilic
Tissue hormones	Eicosanoids (e. g., prosta-glandins), histamine, bradykinin	Hydrophilic

phosphate) may, for instance, influence transport or enzyme systems and consequently certain metabolic pathways. In general, a hormone that evokes this reaction is called a *first messenger*, while the corresponding substance it induces is the *second messenger*. Hydrophilic hormones primarily influence the activity of a cell.

In contrast to hydrophilic hormones, steroid and thyroid hormones can penetrate the cell membrane relatively easily because of their lipid solubility. This enables them to bind to their specific receptor in the cytoplasm, and possibly directly in the nucleus. The hormone–receptor complex then migrates into the nucleus, where it activates a gene and so initiates the formation of messenger RNA, which in turn stimulates protein synthesis (see Chapter 1: The Cell Nucleus). Thus lipophil hormones have a direct effect on cell growth and multiplication.

Major Sites of Hormone Formation

The endocrine system is divided into classic endocrine glands (Fig. 7.**2**), the cells of which are exclusively concerned with hormone secretion, hormone-secreting tissues, and individual cells that secrete hormones but predominantly have other functions. These also secrete hormone-like substances such as tissue hormones, neurotransmitters and synthesized immune products. The most important sites of their formation are detailed in Table 7.**1**.

Such a classification of hormones and messenger substances by their main site of secretion must be viewed with some reserve, since a major part of peptide hormones are synthesized outside the corresponding peripheral endocrine organs, e. g., in the CNS, the autonomic nervous system, and the immune cells. Hence the messenger substances in the endocrine system are designated as *hormones*, those in the CNS and autonomic nervous system as *neurotransmitters* and *neuromodulators*, and those produced by the immune system (immune organs) as *cytokines*, *lymphokines*, and *monokines*.

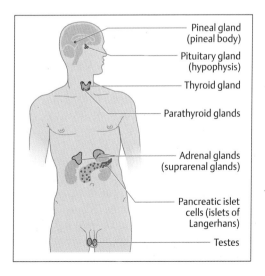

Fig. 7.**2** **Endocrine glands in a male**, (After Leonhardt)

Pineal gland (pineal body)

Pituitary gland (hypophysis)

Thyroid gland

Parathyroid glands

Adrenal glands (suprarenal glands)

Pancreatic islet cells (islets of Langerhans)

Testes

Regulation of Hormone Secretion

In order to maintain a constant hormone level in the blood, hormones must constantly be formed anew. Constant blood levels are achieved by complex *regulatory mechanisms* (feedback mechanisms). When the blood hormone level declines, more hormone is secreted. If there is an excess of hormone, the secretion must be reduced. Increased hormone release from the endocrine glands is in many instances initiated by the central nervous system. The CNS regions essential for such regulation are located in the hypothalamus, a part of the diencephalon (see Chapter 13: Diencephalon). The *function* of the hypothalamus is *closely tied* to that of the pituitary gland. It acts as an *overriding organizational control*, which regulates hormone secretion in the peripheral endocrine glands (hypothalamic–pituitary axis).

■ Hypothalamic-Hypophyseal Axis

The hypothalamus is connected to the hypophysis lying directly beneath it by numerous nervous pathways and blood vessels. The secretion and release of hormones in the pituitary gland is initiated by certain releasing hormones (called "liberins" and "statins"), which are formed in nerve cells in the hypothalamus and reach the pituitary through their axons or in the blood. These may either have a direct effect on the target organ (*somatotrope hormones*) or act first on the peripheral endocrine glands. The latter in their turn secrete hormones that reach their site of action via the bloodstream. *Chemoreceptors* in the hypothalamus constantly measure the concentration of hormones circulating in the blood. Depending on the hormone level more or less regulatory hormone will then be released. In this way the blood hormone concentration is kept constant or adapted to need (feedback system) (Fig. 7.**4**).

■ Pituitary Gland (Hypophysis)

The hypophysis weighs about 1 g and is the size of a pea. It lies at the base of the skull in the sella turcica above the sphenoid sinus. It consists of two parts, which differ in function and development: a nervous part, the *posterior lobe* (*neurohypophysis*), and a glandular part, the *anterior lobe* (*adenohypophysis*). Both are connected to the hypothalamus by the pituitary stalk (infundibulum) (Figs. 7.**3** and 7.**4**).

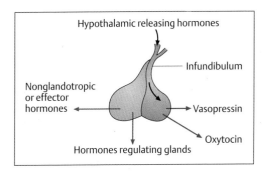

Fig. 7.**3** **Hormones of the anterior and posterior lobes of the pituitary gland** (anterior lobe, pink; posterior lobe, blue)

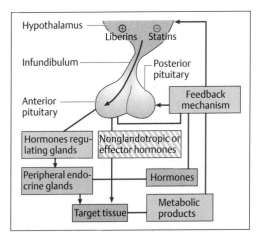

Fig. 7.**4** **Feedback mechanism of the anterior lobe of the pituitary (adenohypophysis)**

Neurohypophysis (Posterior Lobe of the Pituitary Gland)

The neurohypophysis consists of a meshwork of glia cells with numerous capillaries. It does not itself secrete hormones but is solely the storage and releasing organ for hormones formed in the hypothalamus, *antidiuretic hormone* (*vasopressin*) and *oxytocin*. These reach the posterior pituitary through nervous pathways (axons)—a process called *neurosecretion*—and are then released into the bloodstream. Oxytocin contracts smooth muscles (e.g., it promotes uterine contractions during labor), while vasopressin promotes the reabsorption of water in the collecting tubules of the kidney and so raises the blood pressure (increase in blood volume).

Posterior Pituitary Deficiency

In disorders of hormonal release from the posterior pituitary gland, one disease predominates: *diabetes insipidus*. It should not be confused with diabetes mellitus (see below: Islet Apparatus of the Pancreas). The lack of vasopressin leads to insufficient reabsorption of water in the kidney, resulting in daily urine volumes of 15–30 liters.

Overactivity of the Posterior Pituitary Gland

Increased release of vasopressin raises water reabsorption, which increases blood volume, almost always leading to raising of the blood pressure.

Adenohypophysis (Anterior Lobe of the Pituitary Gland)

The anterior lobe consists of an irregular collection of glandular cells in an extensive capillary bed. Release of anterior pituitary hormones is promoted (liberins) or inhibited (statins) by the action of *hypothalamic releasing hormones* (see above), which reach the anterior lobe through the bloodstream (Fig. 7.**4**).

Some anterior pituitary hormones are *nonglandotropic* or *effector* hormones, i.e., they act directly on their target organs, rather than on a peripheral endocrine gland serving as a relay. For example, growth hormone, also called somatotropin (STH), stimulates bodily growth, while prolactin (PRL) stimulates cell division and secretion of milk by the mammary glands in late pregnancy and during the breastfeeding period.

The remaining anterior pituitary hormones stimulate subordinated peripheral endocrine glands to grow as well as secrete and release their hormones. These hormones may be divided into gonadotropins, which act on the gonads, and nongonadotropic hormones, which influence the activity of the adrenal and thyroid glands, for example.

The gonadotropins include *follicle-stimulating hormone* (*FSH, follitropin*) and *luteinizing hormone* (*LH, lutropin*). Both act on the gonads of men as well as women. FSH stimulates the maturation of the follicle in the ovary and promotes spermatogenesis (development of sperm) in men. LH acts on the interstitial cells of the ovary and the testes, initiating ovulation in women and enhancing testosterone secretion in men.

The nongonadotropic hormones include corticotropin or *adrenocorticotropic hormone* (*ACTH*) and thyrotropin or *thyroid-stimulating hormone* (*TSH, thyrotropin*). Whereas ACTH acts to stimulate the adrenal cortex, TSH stimulates the secretion of hormones by the thyroid gland.

Anterior Pituitary Insufficiency

Anterior pituitary insufficiency means reduced release of anterior pituitary hormones. Deficiency of hormones affecting other endocrine glands is especially serious, since it leads to malfunction of the peripheral glands depending on it. For instance, a deficiency in ACTH leads to *adrenocortical insufficiency* (see Adrenal Cortex), while a lack of thyrotropin leads to symptoms of hypothyroidism (see below: Thyroid Gland). Disorders in the secretion and release of gonadotropins lead to various disturbances in gonadal function in both men and women. A postpubertal woman then suffers from amenorrhea and does not ovulate; an adult man will suffer primarily from loss of potency and libido, as well as shrinking of the testes.

If the somatotrope growth hormone is deficient in childhood, the result is *hypophyseal infantilism* (pituitary dwarfism), in which the bodily proportions are maintained.

Overactivity of the Pituitary Gland

Overactivity of the pituitary gland often occurs as a consequence of a benign pituitary tumor (adenoma), and leads especially to increased growth hormone secretion. According to the time when the overactivity occurs (before or after completion of growth), the result may be *excessive growth* (gigantism), in which the bodily proportions remain normal, or continued growth of the distal parts of the body (acra), such as nose, chin, fingers, and toes (acromegaly). Gigantism occurs when the epiphyses have not yet fused, allowing further growth in length. Once the epiphyses have fused, not only do the distal parts grow, but there is thickening of the tongue and lips, as well as some internal organs (e. g., heart, liver).

■ Pineal Gland (Pineal Body, Epiphysis Cerebri)

The pineal gland is about the size of a corn kernel. It is a part of the diencephalon and lies above the midbrain. Its structure is lobular with connective tissue and numerous blood vessels. It plays an important role in the coordination of hormonal processes in the hypothalamus. The most important hormone of the pineal gland is *melatonin*, a serotonin derivative. The formation of melatonin is dependent on light (high blood concentration at night, low concentration by day), and in many cases is also dependent on the season of the year. For this reason the pineal gland is sometimes called the "*biological clock*" (*circadian rhythm*). In childhood, melatonin inhibits the release of gonadotropins, and so the development of the gonads. A number of other functions of melatonin have been discovered more recently, leading to its use as a medication in some countries. It not only regulates the day–night rhythm (e. g., it has been used to help sleep, especially for shift workers and "jet lag"), but is apparently also an effective antioxidant, that is, it eliminates damaging oxygen radicals. This property is believed to strengthen the immune system, prevent cardiac and circulatory as well as malignant diseases, and retard aging. Autologous melatonin secretion declines with increasing age and the gland undergoes degenerative changes with calcium deposition. Hence in radiographic images of the head it serves as a marker for orientation.

Pineal Insufficiency

Certain forms of precocious puberty may be due to pineal insufficiency.

■ Thyroid Gland

The thyroid gland weighs about 15–60 g. It consists of two lobes joined by an isthmus and lies below the larynx on each side of the trachea (Fig. 7.**5a**). The gland is enclosed in a connective tissue capsule and is divided into lobules by connective tissue. The lobules are made up of numerous *tubular spaces* (*follicles*) of varying size, lined with glandular epithelial cells, in which large quantities of hormone can be stored. When the need arises, the hormone can be taken up again by the epithelial cells of the gland and secreted into neighboring blood vessels.

The hormones secreted by the thyroid gland, *thyroxine* (T_4, tetraiodothyronine) and *triiodothyronine* (T_3) are distinguished by their iodine content. Their action is to stimulate cellular metabolism. Triiodothyronine is the actual active thyroid hormone, generated by the splitting of one iodine atom from thyroxine. T_3 and T_4 are necessary for normal growth. Secretion and release of both hormones are regulated by the action of TSH from the hypothalamopituitary system. If, for instance, a decline in blood thyroxine level is registered in the hypothalamus, the latter liberates a releasing hormone (thyrotropin-releasing hormone, TRH), which in turn induces the liberation of TSH in the anterior pituitary. TSH stimulates the thyroid, which releases thyroxine into the bloodstream.

Fig. 7.**5 a–c** **Anatomy and histology of the thyroid and parathyroid glands with their** ▷ **blood supply**
a Anterior view of thyroid gland
b Cross-section of left superior parathyroid gland and adjoining thyroid tissue
c High magnification of **b** (schematic histological section). Upper left, parathyroid cells; lower right, several thyroid follicles in various stages of activity. During the hormone storage phase, the follicular epithelium is low. During formation and release of the hormone, it is secreted into the follicle or through the epithelium into the bloodstream. Groups of C cells can be seen between the thyroid blood vessels

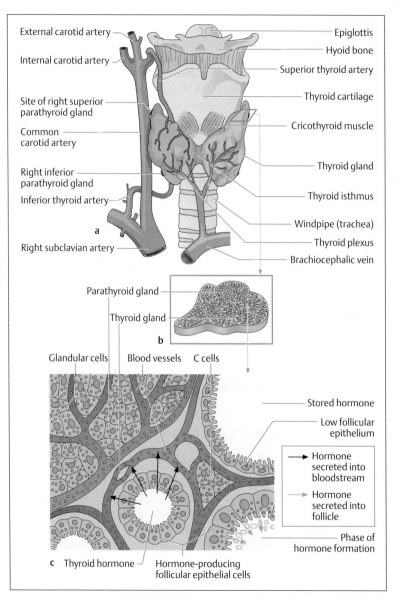

External carotid artery

Internal carotid artery

Site of right superior
parathyroid gland

Common
carotid artery

Right inferior
parathyroid gland

Inferior thyroid artery

a

Right subclavian artery

Epiglottis

Hyoid bone

Superior thyroid artery

Thyroid cartilage

Cricothyroid muscle

Thyroid gland

Thyroid isthmus

Windpipe (trachea)

Thyroid plexus

Brachiocephalic vein

Parathyroid gland

Thyroid gland

b

Glandular cells   Blood vessels   C cells

Stored hormone

Low follicular
epithelium

Hormone
secreted into
bloodstream

Hormone
secreted into
follicle

Phase of
hormone formation

c   Thyroid hormone

Hormone-producing
follicular epithelial cells

Overactivity of the Thyroid Gland

In thyroid overactivity (hyperthyroidism, Graves disease), cellular combustion increases (increased basal metabolism). This results in weight loss, raised body temperature, and acceleration of the heart rate. Often the eyeball protrudes from the orbit (exophthalmos), the pupils enlarge, and the condition may be accompanied by nervous excitability.

Thyroid Insufficiency

In thyroid insufficiency (hypothyroidism), metabolism, growth, and mental activity are all slowed. In addition, the skin thickens and swells (myxodema). The commonest cause of hypothyroidism is iodine deficiency in the diet (or drinking water), which induces increased release of TSH from the pituitary gland. This causes the thyroid gland to become enlarged, a condition called *goiter* (*struma*). Congenital goiter results in dwarfism and cretinism.

The C Cells of the Thyroid Gland

In addition to the two hormones thyroxine and triiodothyronine, another hormone, calcitonin, is secreted in cells called *parafollicular cells* (C cells). Calcitonin reduces the level of calcium in the blood and promotes bone formation (Fig. 7.**5c**).

Parathyroid Glands (Epithelial Bodies)

The four parathyroid glands, or epithelial bodies, lie on the posterior side of the thyroid gland. They are often enclosed in the thyroid capsule, in which case they are not visible from the outside (Fig. 7.**5a**, **b**). They are lentil-shaped, flat and oval. Reticular connective tissue and numerous capillaries surround the cells. The parathyroid hormone is also called *parathormone* and plays a part in calcium and phosphate metabolism. Among other actions, it stimulates osteoclasts to break down bone, raising the calcium level in the blood. In this action it is an antagonist of calcitonin.

Overactivity of the Parathyroid Glands

Overactivity increases phosphate excretion, bone breakdown (decalcification), and blood calcium level, leading to increased calcium deposition in the walls of the blood vessels.

Parathyroid Insufficiency

In parathyroid deficiency the extracellular calcium concentration falls, leading to increased excitability of the nervous system. The result is often increased muscular activity with cramps (tetany).

■ Adrenal Glands (Suprarenal Glands)

Each adrenal gland weighs about 5 g and sits on the superior pole of the respective kidney, like a cap. The glands are included in the fatty capsule of the kidney, and are noteworthy for their rich supply of nerves and vessels. A fresh postmortem section shows a vivid yellow cortex, making up about 80% of the organ, and a more reddish-gray medulla (Fig. 7.**6a**, **b**). The endocrine activities of the adrenal cortex and the adrenal medulla differ both in development and function.

Adrenal Cortex

The adrenal cortex can be divided both morphologically and functionally into three zones of different widths, all made up of hormone-secreting *epithelial columns*, between which connective tissue, blood vessels, and nerves run radially from the cortex toward the medulla (Fig. 7.**6c**). All three layers form steroid hormones, called corticosteroids, classified in three groups according to their function: *mineralocorticoids. glucocorticoids*, and *androgens* (*male sex hormones*).

The *outer zone* (*zona glomerulosa*) lies directly under the capsule and secretes the most important mineralocorticoid, *aldosterone*. This hormone is not governed by the hypothalamopituitary axis, but is regulated by the renin–angiotensin system (see Chapter 10). Aldosterone acts on the kidney and influences water metabolism through potassium excre-

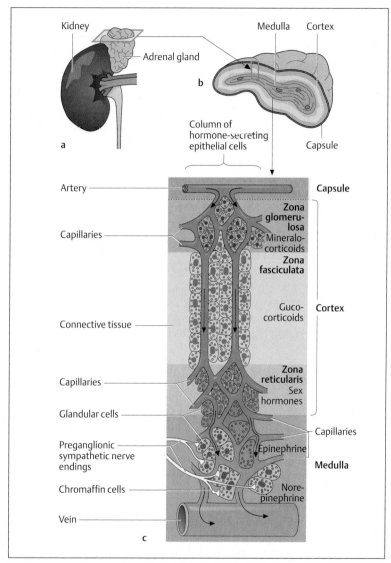

Fig. 7.**6 a–c** **Anatomy and histology of the adrenal glands with their blood supply**
a Right adrenal on the superior pole of the kidney
b Cross-section through the adrenal gland
c Schematic enlargement of a histological section from **b**. The hormone-producing epithelial columns can be seen in the adrenal cortex, extending to the adrenal medulla

tion and sodium reabsorption in the renal tubules. The enzyme ATPase in the distal renal tubule facilitates this action.

The *intermediate zone* of the adrenal cortex, the *zona fasciculata*, is the widest zone and it secretes glucocorticoids. It is deep yellow in color, giving the cortex its yellow coloration. *Cortisol (hydrocortisone)*, is the most important representative of the group, which regulates carbohydrate, fat, and protein metabolism. For instance, it regulates the blood level of glucose by a special metabolic process, gluconeogenesis, in which amino acids, derived from protein metabolism, are converted into glucose. Glucocorticoids also reduce the number of lymphocytes in the blood and inhibit the phagocytic activity of granulocytes and monocytes, limiting inflammation, but also inhibiting the immune system. The inhibition of immunity explains the effectiveness of glucocorticoids in the treatment of allergic disorders (allergy = excessive immune reaction), though the same process also delays wound healing. Glucocorticoids have a major role in dealing with extreme physical stress such as starvation, thirst, extreme temperature changes or other severe physical stress. They all lead to a rise in glucocorticoid concentration in the blood. Finally, it should be mentioned that the glucocorticoid blood level fluctuates during the course of the day (*circadian rhythm*), blood level being high between 0600 and 0900 and very low about midnight.

The *inner zone*, *zona reticularis*, secretes primarily male (*androgens*) and to a small extent female (*estrogens*) sex hormones, to the same extent in both sexes. These hormones are also formed as intermediate products during formation and breakdown of corticosteroids in the intermediate zone. Androgens stimulate protein metabolism and muscle build-up, an effect called *anabolism*. Derivatives of these hormones (anabolic steroids) are often used as performance-enhancing drugs to increase muscle mass in high-level athletics.

The intermediate and inner zones of the adrenal cortex are dependent on the hypothalamopituitary axis and their activity is influenced by ACTH. Hence increased or decreased ACTH release mainly affects the intermediate and inner zones

Adrenal Insufficiency

Bilateral adrenal cortical failure is also called *Addison disease (adrenal insufficiency)*. In the zona glomerulosa, the main hormones affected are the mineralocorticoids. Their insufficiency leads to disorders of ion and water metabolism. Lack of aldosterone due to disease leads to increased loss of sodium chloride and an increase in the potassium chloride content of extracellular fluid. Because of the elevated blood potassium level, these patients suffer from disturbances in cardiac rhythm, and they are weak and easily fatigued. Insufficiency of the zona fasciculata, on the other hand, results in a reduced blood sugar level (hypoglycemia) and other deficiencies.

Adrenal Overactivity

Adrenal cortical tumors (e. g., benign adenomata) or increased ACTH release from the anterior pituitary (constant stimulation of the adrenal cortex) lead to increased glucocorticoid secretion (e. g., cortisol), called *Cushing syndrome*, marked by "moon face" and increased fat deposition in the body (truncal obesity, "buffalo torso"). An elevated androgen blood level leads to precocious puberty, and in women to masculinization of secondary sexual characters (e. g., male type hirsutism).

Adrenal Medulla

The adrenal medulla has a special intermediate place between the autonomic nervous system and the endocrine system. The cells of the adrenal medulla are the equivalent of *postganglionic sympathetic neurons* without axons (see Chapter 14: Sympathetic Nervous System, Structure). They are supplied by preganglionic sympathetic nerve fibers of the autonomic nervous system. The granule-containing cells lie in clusters between capillaries and larger, muscular veins (Fig. 7.**6c**). They form the two hormones *epinephrine* (*adrenaline*) (80%) and *norepinephrine* (*noradrenaline*) (20%). Epinephrine and norepinephrine are released into the bloodstream during stress and they act on the whole organism by preparing it for increased energy use. Both hormones, for instance, activate the liberation of fatty acids from fat depots and liberate glucose from glycogen storage in the liver (producing a rise in the blood sugar level). They raise the blood pressure and stroke volume of the heart and may lead to vasoconstriction in certain defined areas.

■ Islet Apparatus of the Pancreas

The endocrine portion of the pancreas consists of about 1–2 million is-lets, called the islets of Langerhans. The round, sometimes oval, islets lie within the pancreatic tissue (see Chapter 9: The Pancreas) and consist of glandular cells surrounded by numerous capillaries (Fig. 7.**7**). The most important hormones secreted here are *insulin* (beta cells, B cells), *glucagon* (alpha cells, A cells), and *somatostatin* (delta cells, D cells). In-sulin and glucagon act in opposite (antagonistic) ways, while soma-tostatin has a paracrine function, inhibiting the liberation of both insulin and glucagon and thereby reducing the utilization of nutrients absorbed from the intestines. About 60% of islet cells secrete insulin, 25% glucagon, and 15% somatostatin.

Insulin and glucagon are the key hormones for the regulation of car-bohydrate metabolism. Insulin promotes the storage of the absorbed nutrients in the form of glycogen or fat, while glucagon mobilizes energy reserves during starvation or in stressful situations (see epinephrine and norepinephrine above). In addition, the two hormones regulate blood glucose concentration (blood glucose level), keeping it as constant as possible (60–100 mg glucose/100 ml blood). Insulin promotes glycogen synthesis in the liver and facilitates glucose uptake into the cells, thereby lowering the blood sugar level. The action of glucagon is to break down glycogen to glucose in the liver, raising the blood sugar level.

Pancreatic Islet Insufficiency

Inadequate physiological activity of the insulin secreted by the pan-creatic islet cells is the cause of diabetes mellitus, a very common metab-olic disease affecting some 5% of the population at large. Its two most common forms are called *type I* and *type II diabetes.* Type I diabetes (ca. 5% of all cases) usually begins in childhood and necessitates lifelong treatment with insulin, because the insulin-producing cells are de-stroyed by an autoimmune process. Type II diabetes (ca. 90% of all cases) appears later in life (at age 35 or older) and is due to an inadequate re-sponsiveness of peripheral tissues to insulin (insulin resistance). In dia-betes mellitus of either type, the diminished uptake of glucose from the bloodstream into the cells results in an elevation of the blood glucose

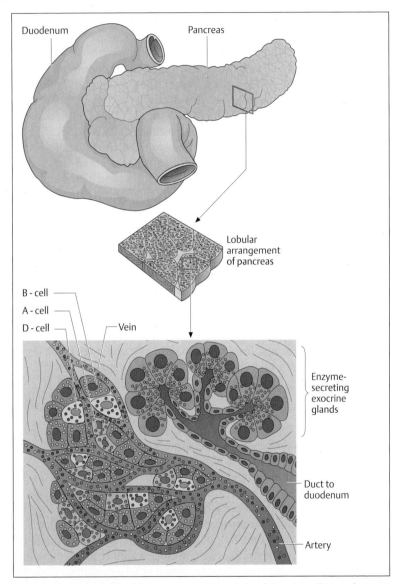

Fig. 7.7 **Pancreatic islet.** The hormone-secreting cells of the islets of Langerhans are embedded in the exocrine pancreatic tissue. A cells secrete glucagon, B cells secrete insulin, and D cells secrete somatostatin

concentration (*hyperglycemia*). Glucose can thus no longer supply the energy needs of the cells, and there is increased utilization of other energy carriers, such as fatty acids and endogenous proteins. The result is a disturbance of lipid metabolism in which fat is deposited in blood vessel walls (*diabetic macroangiopathy*), leading to the early onset and rapid progression of arteriosclerosis, which, in turn, causes ischemia in multiple organ systems. Another consequence of hyperglycemia is the excretion of excessive amounts of glucose in the urine (*glycosuria*). This, in turn, causes an osmotic diuresis, which manifests itself as an abnormally high volume of urinary output (*polyuria*), with considerable loss of fluid, leading to abnormally severe thirst and compensatory drinking of high volumes of fluid (*polydipsia*). In severe diabetes, acidic metabolic products, such as ketone bodies, can dangerously acidify of the blood (*diabetic ketoacidosis*). This, if untreated, can cause an acutely life-threatening condition characterized by slow, very deep breathing (Kussmaul respiration), convulsions, and impairment of consciousness, i.e., *diabetic coma*.

Diabetes mellitus is treated with strict dietary carbohydrate restriction and regular administration of insulin. If the blood glucose concentration is not adequately controlled, chronic hyperglycemia can lead to severe late complications, including *diabetic microangiopathy*, which affects small and very small blood vessels. This is due to hyperglycemia causing increased nonenzymatic glycosylation of proteins, which, in turn, leads to thickening of vascular basal membranes, as well as endothelial changes. The most damaging effects of diabetic microangiopathy are found in the retina (*diabetic retinopathy*) and kidney (*diabetic nephropathy*).

■ The Gonads

The hormones elaborated in the gonads serve the development of male and female sexual characteristics, growth, physical and emotional maturity, and reproduction (generation of germ cells, pregnancy, and lactation). They are steroid hormones and are formed by both sexes, though in different quantities and proportions. The most important female sex hormones are the estrogens (e. g., estradiol) and progesterone. The male sex hormones include testosterone and dihydrotestosterone.

Estrogens and progesterone in women are formed principally in the ovary and the placenta, and in men in small amounts in the testes. Androgens are formed in men principally in the testes, but also in the adrenal cortex, and in women partly in the ovary and also in the adrenal cortex (for action and regulation of male and female sex hormones see Chapter 11: The Reproductive Organs and Chapter 12: Reproduction, Development, and Birth).

■ Other Tissues and Single Cells Secreting Hormones

Messenger substances formed in the hormone-secreting tissues and in widely scattered single cells (Table 7.**1**) reach their target cells via the blood (e. g., erythropoietin is formed in the kidneys and acts on the maturation of red cells in the bone marrow). However, many of these substances act at their site of origin (paracrine and autocrine signaling). Paracrine signaling, for instance, is especially important in the regulation of gastrointestinal function and in the transmission of chemical signals in the synapses of the nervous system. Many tissue hormones, e. g., histamine and prostaglandin, also have paracrine effects. For their various actions, see relevant chpaters on the digestive system (Chapter 9), the heart and vascular system (Chapter 5), the kidneys (Chapter 10), the central and peripheral nervous system (Chapter 13), and the immune system (Chapter 6).

Summary   **The Endocrine System**

The endocrine system includes all hormone-secreting organs (endocrine glands) and cellular systems (hormone-secreting tissues and single cells).

■ Hormones
Hormones (chemical messengers) in general reach their target cells by way of the bloodstream or lymph channels (exceptions are paracrine and autocrine secretions, where the site of action is a neighbor-

ing cell or the secreting cell itself). Like the autonomic system, they coordinate the functions of widely scattered sites, but they do this "wirelessly," much more slowly, and over a more prolonged period. The target cells possess specific hormone receptors that respond only to their particular hormone. According to their mechanism of action they are classified as follows:

- *Hydrophilic hormones* (mostly proteins and peptides): these influence cellular activity. The hormone receptor is mostly on the cell membrane. The hormone ("first messenger") generates a "second messenger", which can influence certain metabolic processes in the cell.
- *Lipophilic hormones* (steroids and thyroid hormones): directly influence cell growth and multiplication; the hormone receptor is in the cytoplasm or nucleus of the target cell. The hormone penetrates the nucleus and stimulates protein synthesis.

Hormone secretion in the endocrine glands is regulated by feedback mechanisms. The controlling mechanism resides in the hypothalamus (part of the diencephalon). In response to the blood hormone level it releases regulating hormones that act as inhibitors (statins) or activators (liberins) of hormone release in the anterior pituitary gland (hypothalamopituitary system). This gland in turn liberates substances that act either directly on the target tissue (somatotrope hormones) or on peripheral endocrine glands that in turn secrete the hormones that act on the target tissue.

■ Hypophysis (Pituitary Gland)

- *Posterior lobe of the hypophysis* (neurohypophysis, posterior pituitary): neural part; does not itself secrete hormones but is the storage and releasing organ of the active hormones secreted in the hypothalamus (transport via axons to the posterior pituitary = neurosecretion). (1) Antidiuretic hormone (ADH, vasopressin), promotes water reabsorption in the kidney; (2) oxytocin, promotes e. g., uterine contraction during labor.
- *Anterior lobe of the hypophysis* (adenohypophysis, anterior pituitary): glandular part, concerned with the secretion of hormones. Their release is regulated by hypothalamic releasing hormones.

- Hormones acting directly on tissue. (1) Growth hormone (GH, somatotropin); deficiency during childhood leads to dwarfism; excess secretion (usually by adenoma) in childhood leads to gigantism, or in adults acromegaly. (2) Melanocyte-stimulating hormone (MSH): among other functions regulates skin color. (3) prolactin (PRL): stimulates milk formation during lactation.
- Hormones stimulating glands: *gonadotropins.* (1) Follicle-stimulating hormone (FSH): stimulates maturation of the ovarian follicle in women and spermatogenesis in men. (2) Luteinizing hormone (LH): acts on the intermediate cells of the ovary (ovulation) and the testes (increased testosterone secretion). Gonadotropin insufficiency: amenorrhea, shrinking of the testes and potency problems.
- Hormones stimulating glands: *nongonadotropins.* (3) Adreno-corticotrophic hormone (ACTH): stimulates hormone secretion in the adrenal cortex, insufficiency: adrenocortical insufficiency. (4) Thyroid stimulating hormone (TSH): stimulates thyroid hormone secretion; insufficiency: thyroid insufficiency.

■ Pineal Gland (Epiphysis)

Part of the diencephalon. Its principal hormone is melatonin (a powerful antioxidant; regulates day–night rhythm); melatonin secretion reduced with advancing age.

■ Thyroid Gland

Endocrine gland with "storage function" below the larynx on each side of the trachea. The hormones are stored in sacs (follicles). Production and release are regulated by TSH secreted by the hypothalamo-hypophyseal system. The two hormones thyroxine and triiodothyronine (active form of thyroxine) are growth hormones (stimulate cell metabolism). Overactivity (hyperthyroidism) includes increased basal metabolic rate leading to weight loss, increased heart rate. In insufficiency (hypothyroidism, most often due to iodine deficiency), metabolism, growth, and mental activity are slowed; there is compensatory thyroid enlargement (goiter).

- *C cells:* a few parafollicular cells secreting the hormone calcitonin (lowers blood calcium level)

- *Parathyroid glands* (epithelial bodies): four small epithelial bodies on the back of the thyroid; secrete parathormone, which regulates calcium and phosphate metabolism. It is an antagonist of calcitonin (raises blood calcium level by breaking down bone). Overactivity: breakdown of bone, calcium deposition in vessel walls. Insufficiency: muscle cramps by overexcitability of nerves (reduction in extracellular calcium concentration).

■ Adrenal Glands

- *Adrenal cortex:* constitutes 80% of the organ; consists of three layers, all secreting steroid hormones (corticosteroids). (1) Outer zone (zona glomerulosa) secretes mineralocorticoids: includes aldosterone (acts on water metabolism by potassium excretion and sodium reabsorption in the kidneys). (2) Intermediate zone (zona fasciculata) secretes glucocorticoids: including cortisol (regulates carbohydrate, fat, and protein metabolism, e.g., raising the blood sugar level by gluconeogenesis in stress; inhibits inflammation and suppresses immune reaction). (3) Inner zone (zona reticularis) secretes principally androgens, but also estrogens, equally in both sexes. Androgens stimulate protein metabolism (anabolic effect). The intermediate and inner cortex are regulated by the hypothalamo-hypophyseal system (ACTH), the outer cortex by the renin–angiotensin system.

  Bilateral adrenal deficiency: Addison disease with disturbances in cardiac rhythm due to elevation of the potassium level. Overactivity: Cushing syndrome (e.g., by increased ACTH release or adrenal cortical tumors) with truncal adiposity due to raised glucocorticoid secretion. Increased androgen secretion: precocious puberty; in women, masculinization of secondary sexual characteristics.

- *Adrenal medulla:* connects the autonomic nervous system with the endocrine system, since its cells correspond to postganglionic cells without axons. Supplied by preganglionic sympathetic nerve fibers. Secretes the stress hormones epinephrine and norepinephrine (which activate fat depots and glycogen stores, and raise blood pressure and cardiac stroke volume).

■ The Pancreatic Islets

There are 1–2 million islets of Langerhans in the pancreatic exocrine tissue: beta cells (60%, secrete insulin), alpha cells (25%, glucagon), and delta cells (15%, somatostatin).

1. Insulin: lowers the blood sugar level by promoting glycogen synthesis and increased absorption of blood sugar into cells.
2. Glucagon: insulin antagonist, raises the blood sugar level by breaking down glycogen.
3. Somatostatin: inhibits both hormones and so reduces the utilization of nutrients absorbed from the intestines.

Insufficiency (most often affects the insulin-secreting beta cells): diabetes mellitus with raised blood sugar level by increased uptake of glucose into the cells.

■ Gonads

The sex hormones stimulate development of sexual characteristics, growth, physical and mental maturation, and reproduction.

- *Ovary:* estrogens (estradiol) and progesterone
- *Placenta:* progesterone, choriogonadotropin
- *Testes:* androgens (testosterone, dihydrotestosterone)

■ Tissues and Single Cells Secreting Hormones

This category includes cells of the nervous system and in the immune organs that secrete messenger substances (transmitters in the nervous system, cytokines, lymphokines and monokines secreted by immune cells); regions or cells of the hypothalamus (liberins, statins); certain cells of the kidneys (erythropoietin, renin) and liver (angiotensinogen, somatomedins); cells secreting tissue hormones (e. g., prostglandins, histamine) among others.

8

The Respiratory System

Contents

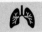

The organs of respiration ensure that, as conditions change, oxygen is made available to the organism, excess carbon dioxide is removed from the body, and, in conjunction with the kidneys, acid–base balance is maintained (see also Chapter 6: CO_2 Transport and Chapter 10: The Na^+-K^+ Pump). The organs of respiration can be divided into *air passages* (*upper* and *lower airways*) and the *alveoli* in the lungs where the exchange of gases between air and blood takes place. In the lower airways, the inhaled air leaves the windpipe and enters the bronchial tree, which is considered a part of the lung. The bronchi divide into ever smaller branches, of which the terminal branches (bronchioles) end in the alveolar ducts, from which the alveoli are suspended.

■ The Path of Oxygen to the Cell: External and Internal Respiration

The human body gains most of its energy through the combustion (oxidative degradation) of nutrients and therefore depends on a constant supply of oxygen (O_2) to every single cell of the organism. During oxidative breakdown carbon dioxide (CO_2) is formed, and this must be released into the surrounding atmosphere. These combustive processes of metabolism are called "*internal respiration*" or *cellular respiration*. By contrast, the gas exchange in the lungs between the organism and its surroundings is known as "*external respiration*."

Since, in contrast to monocellular organisms, most cells of our body are far removed from the surrounding air, the respiratory gases must be transported over long distances by convection (transport through the air passages and the circulation of the blood) and diffusion through thin boundary surfaces (gas exchange in the pulmonary alveoli and the tissues). Thus *oxygen transport* from the outside air to the individual cells of the body can be divided into *four successive steps*:

1. O_2 transport into the alveoli by ventilation
2. Diffusion of O_2 into the pulmonary capillaries
3. O_2 transport by the blood to the systemic capillaries
4. Diffusion of O_2 from the systemic capillaries to the neighboring cells.

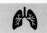

The removal of carbon dioxide from the individual cells to the outside takes place in the reverse sequence.

■ Organs of the Air Passages

The air passages (Fig. 8.**1**) include the **upper** (**nasal and oral cavities, nasal sinuses, pharynx, larynx**) and **lower air passages** (**trachea and bronchial tree**). They are the means of transportation of the inspired and expired air, and they warm it, humidify it, purify it, and regulate it (sense of smell). By its ability to close and create sounds, the larynx makes vocalization possible.

The air passages, with few exceptions, are lined by a *mucous membrane* consisting of *stratified ciliated columnar epithelium*. Mucus from numerous *goblet cells* and *seromucous glands* in the mucosa maintains the moisture of the mucous membrane. The *epithelial cilia* beat towards the pharynx in almost all sections and so transport mucus and its contained particles outward.

Nasal Cavity and Paranasal Sinuses

The two *nasal cavities* are separated by a *dividing wall* (*nasal septum*) consisting partly of bone, partly of cartilage (Fig. 8.**2b**). The surface of the side walls of the nasal cavity is significantly enlarged by the *superior, middle*, and *inferior nasal conchae*. The *nasal conchae* (*turbinates*) are bony projections covered by a mucous membrane, each enclosing a nasal meatus (Fig. 8.**3**). The floor is formed by the hard and soft palate. The nasal cavities open to the outside through the *nostrils* (*nares*). Inside each nostril sits a ring of short hairs that guard against foreign bodies. The transition to the pharynx is formed by the *posterior nasal apertures* (*choanae*).

The *olfactory mucosa* (*olfactory region*) lies in the superior nasal concha and the upper portion of the nasal septum. It contains numerous *olfactory nerves* (*fila olfactoria*), that exit in the roof of the nose through the lamina cribrosa of the ethmoid bone. The mucosa covering the remaining parts of the nasal cavity (*respiratory region*) warms, moistens, and purifies the inspired air. The respiratory region contains numerous veins

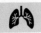

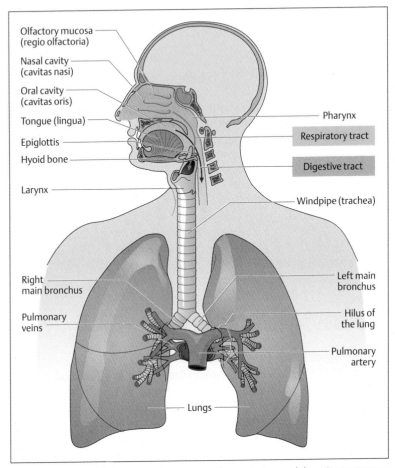

Fig. 8.**1** **Overview of the respiratory organs.** The respiratory and digestive tracts cross in the pharynx. (After Leonhardt)

and, especially around the turbinates, they form a cavernous plexus that, when full, can cause the mucous membrane to swell markedly (surface expansion).

The *paranasal sinuses* include the *frontal, maxillary, ethmoid* (with the ethmoid air cell), and *sphenoidal sinuses* (Fig. 8.**2a, b**). They are also

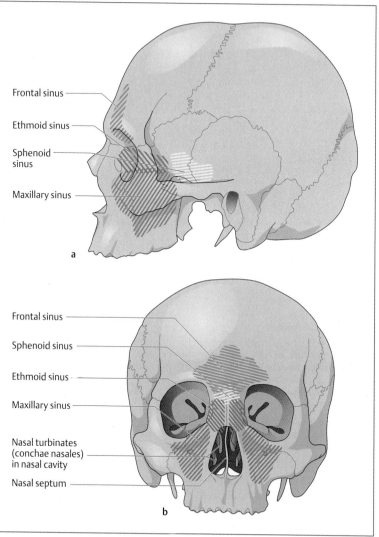

Fig. 8.**2 a, b The paranasal sinuses.** (After Platzer)
a Lateral view
b Anterior view

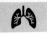

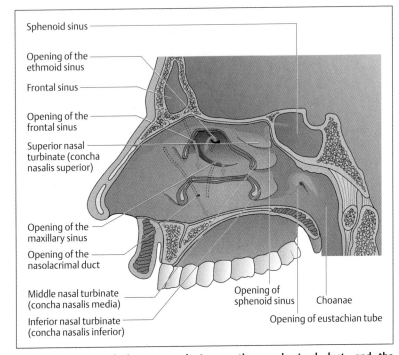

Fig. 8.3 Openings of the paranasal sinuses, the nasolacrimal duct, and the eustachian tube into the nasal cavity. View from inside toward the right wall of the nasal cavity; the nasal conchae have been partially removed. The blue arrows mark the openings of the paranasal sinuses, the eustachian tube, and the nasolacrimal duct. (After Leonhardt)

lined with mucous membrane and function mainly in the warming of inspired air and to create resonance in the voice. All paranasal sinuses are connected to the main nasal cavity. With the exception of the sphenoidal sinus, all paranasal sinuses open into the respective superior or middle meatus under the nasal chonchae (Fig. 8.3). The openings from the two maxillary sinuses are situated at the upper end of the sinuses, thus impeding drainage. They open below the middle nasal concha. The inferior nasal concha receives the *nasolacrimal duct*, which drains tears from the eye into the nose.

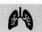

Pharynx

From the nasal cavity the air passage leads trough the choanae (Fig. 8.**3**) into the pharynx. The inspired air first reaches the nasopharynx (epipharynx), crosses the digestive tract in the oropharynx, and reaches the larynx in the throat (hypopharynx) (Fig. 8.**1**). Immediately behind the choanae on each side lies the opening of the *eustachian tube* (*tuba auditiva*) into the lateral pharynx (Fig. 8.**3**). It connects the air passages to the middle ear and its function is to provide air to the middle ear and equalize its pressure.

Larynx

The larynx can close the lower air passages (trachea and bronchi) from the pharynx, making it possible to raise the pressure in the thorax and abdomen, to strain and to cough. The larynx is also an important organ for vocalization. Its cartilaginous framework, covered with a mucous membrane, serves as origin and insertion for the laryngeal muscles. *Extrinsic laryngeal ligaments* also connect the larynx to the hyoid bone above and the trachea below (Figs. 8.**1** and 8.**4**). The *intrinsic laryngeal ligaments* connect parts of the larynx to each other.

Laryngeal Skeleton

The laryngeal skeleton consists mainly of hyaline (thyroid, cricoid, and arytenoid cartilages) and elastic (epiglottis) cartilage. In the male, the male sex hormones favor stronger growth of especially the thyroid cartilage. In both sexes *ossification* occurs to a varying extent, especially in the thyroid cartilage after puberty.

The *thyroid cartilage* with its two lateral walls projects like the prow of a ship in the middle of the neck, the so-called *Adam's apple* (Fig. 8.**4**). In the back, the thyroid cartilage is open. The back ends of the cartilaginous laminae (plates) extend upward as the superior horn (cornu superius) and downward as the inferior horn (cornu inferius) on both sides. The two inferior horns articulate with the *cricoid cartilage*, which consists of a ring in front and a (plate) lamina behind (signet-ring shape). At its top the lamina articulates with two pyramid-

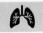

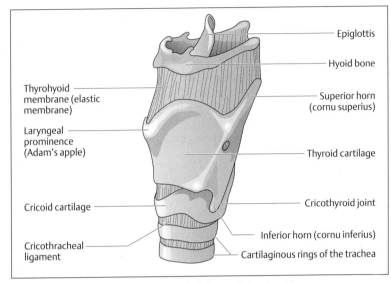

Fig. 8.**4** **Anterior view of the laryngeal skeleton.** (After Feneis)

shaped cartilages, the *arytenoids* (*arytenoid cartilages*), which have two processes, one pointing forward (vocal process) and one to the side (muscular process) (Fig. 8.**6b**). From each vocal process the *vocal ligament* (*vocal cord*) runs to the posterior surface of the thyroid cartilage. The vocal cords and vocalis muscle together form the vocal fold (plica vocalis, true vocal cord) (Fig. 8.**7a**, **b**). The vocal folds can be tensed by backward tilting of the cricoid cartilage. The two arytenoids can approach each other, separate and turn around a longitudinal axis. This narrows or widens the *glottis* between the vocal folds (Fig. 8.**5a**, **b**). The epiglottis is attached immediately above the attachment of the two vocal folds to the posterior surface of the thyroid cartilage. During swallowing, it descends to cover the larynx, preventing aspiration of food into the trachea (see Fig. 9.**11a**, **b** and Chapter 9: The Act of Swallowing).

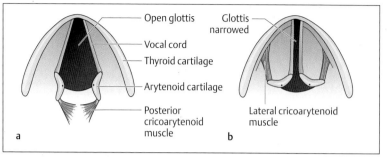

Fig. 8.**5 a, b   The glottis seen from above. a** The posterior cricoarytenoid muscle opens the glottis; **b** the lateral cricoarytenoid muscle closes the glottis. (After Schwegler)

Laryngeal Muscles

While the hyoid muscles (suprahyoid and infrahyoid muscles, see Chapter 4: Head and Neck) raise and lower the larynx, the intrinsic laryngeal muscles move parts of the larynx against each other (Fig. 8.**6a–d**). The striated, that is voluntary, laryngeal muscles can open and close the glottis as well as change the tension of the vocal cords. All laryngeal muscles are innervated by cranial nerve X (vagus nerve).

The posterior cricoarytenoid muscle is the only (!) *opener* (*abductor*) *of the glottis*, and it runs from the lamina of the cricoid posteriorly to the muscular process of the arytenoid. It opens the glottis for the passage of inspired air (Figs. 8.**5a**, 8.**6a–d**). All the other muscles narrow the glottis (lateral cricoarytenoid muscle, thyroarytenoid muscle, oblique and transverse arytenoid muscles) (Figs. 8.**5b** and 1.**8a–d**). The muscles determine the *position of the vocal cords during phonation*, controlling the formation of sounds and making *fine adjustment* in tension. Finally, the aryepiglottic muscle helps to close the laryngeal inlet.

Laryngeal Mucosa

The inner aspect of the laryngeal skeleton, the glottis and the laryngeal muscles, is lined with mucous membrane (Fig. 8.**7a, b**). Between the epiglottis and the arytenoid on each side, a mucosal fold (aryepiglottic

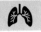

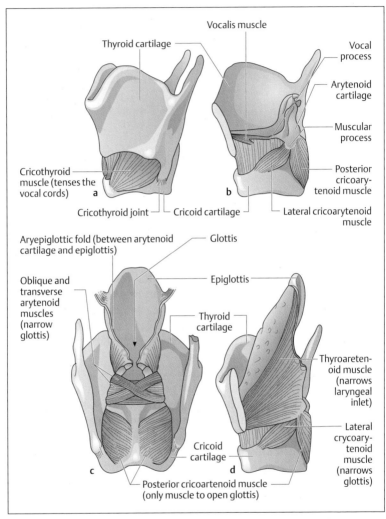

Vocalis muscle

Thyroid cartilage

Vocal process

Arytenoid cartilage

Muscular process

Cricothyroid muscle (tenses the vocal cords) **a**

Posterior cricoary-tenoid muscle

Cricothyroid joint — Cricoid cartilage — **b**

Lateral cricoarytenoid muscle

Aryepiglottic fold (between arytenoid cartilage and epiglottis)

Glottis

Oblique and transverse arytenoid muscles (narrow glottis)

Epiglottis

Thyroid cartilage

Thyroareten-oid muscle (narrows laryngeal inlet)

Lateral crycoary-tenoid muscle (narrows glottis)

Cricoid cartilage

c **d**

Posterior cricoartenoid muscle (only muscle to open glottis)

Fig. 8.**6 a–d** **The laryngeal muscles and their functions.** (After Leonhardt)
a Lateral view
b Lateral view with epiglottis and epiglottic muscles removed
c Posterior view
d Lateral view with left side of the thyroid cartilage removed

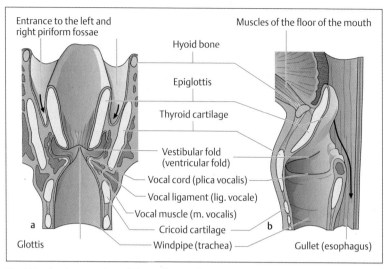

Fig. 8.**7 a, b** **Larynx viewed from the inside. a** Coronal section (anterior view) and **b** sagittal section through the larynx. The arrows indicate the path taken by a bolus of food. (After Leonhardt)

fold, *plica aryepiglottica*) forms the vestibule of the larynx (Fig. 8.**6c**). On each side of these folds runs a mucosal gutter, the *piriform fossa*, through which food bypasses the larynx to reach the esophagus. The laryngeal vestibules narrow below to a sagittal slit, bounded by two pocketlike folds, the vestibular folds, often called *false vocal cords*. Below the two vestibular folds, the space widens on both sides, to be narrowed again immediately below by two further sagitally placed folds, the *true vocal folds*. They bound the edges of the glottis (rima glottidis) and are formed by the *vocal cords* and the *vocal muscles* (Fig. 8.**7a, b**). Except at the vocal cords, the mucosa is applied relatively loosely to the underlying structures, creating the danger of swelling (glottal edema, angioneurotic edema of the larynx), which can lead to asphyxiation (e. g., as a consequence of an allergic reaction to an insect sting).

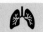

Voice Production

For voice production (phonation), the vocal cords are applied to each other and the pressure of air passing through them causes them to vibrate. For instance, a vowel can be sung at different pitches by voluntary changes in tension of the vocal cords. Vowels are formed by changes in the upper air passages (opening and closing of the glottis and changes in the tension of the vocal cords, Fig. 8.**5**), while consonants are formed by using the palate, the tongue, the teeth, and the lips. Loudness depends on the *strength of airflow*, pitch on the *frequency of the vibrations*. The pharyngeal and oral cavities, the nose, and the paranasal sinuses function as *resonators*.

The Windpipe and Bronchial Tree

The lower airways comprise the windpipe, the main bronchi (principal bronchi), the lobar bronchi, and the segmental bronchi (Fig. 8.**8a**, **b**). The bronchi are the parts of the lung that conduct air. They branch repeatedly and with their smallest divisions form the *bronchial tree*. At the blind end of the air passages lie the alveoli, where *gas exchange* takes place. The bronchi are accompanied by the blood vessels of the pulmonary circulation (pulmonary artery and vein) (Fig. 8.**9**), which form an extensive capillary network around the alveoli.

Windpipe (Trachea)

The windpipe is a tube, about 10–12 cm long and 2 cm wide, which is kept open by about 20 horseshoe-shaped cartilaginous tracheal rings, open to the rear (Fig. 8.**8a**, **b**). The cartilaginous rings are held together anteriorly and laterally by ligaments. Posteriorly, the ring is completed by connective tissue and muscle (tracheal muscle). The esophagus runs immediately behind the trachea. The internal surface of the trachea is lined by typical respiratory mucosa.

Bronchial Tree

At its *bifurcation* (*division*) (Fig. 8.**8 a**, **b**) the trachea divides into the right and left main bronchi, which pass into the lung. The right main bronchus

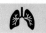

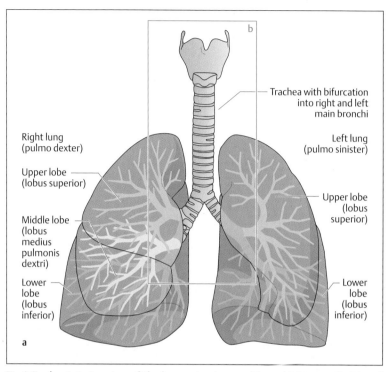

Fig. 8.8 a, b   Anterior view of the larynx, trachea, and bronchial tree. a Position of bronchial tree in the lungs; **b** section from **a**. The numbers in the circles mark the segments of the lung supplied by the corresponding segmental bronchi (see also Fig. 8.**11**) (in the left lower lobe there is no [medial basal] segment VII). Branches of the upper lobe are marked in red, of the middle lobe in yellow, and of the lower lobe in blue. The arrows show the direction of lymphatic drainage   Fig. 8.**8 b** ▷

is wider and directed more steeply downward than the left, and for this reason aspirated foreign bodies most often find their way into the right main bronchus (Figs. 8.**8** and 8.**9**). Above the left main bronchus runs the aortic arch and below it, in front of the left main bronchus, the pulmonary trunk divides into the left and right pulmonary arteries (Fig. 8.**9**). After a short course, each main bronchus divides into lobar bronchi, three on the right, two on the left. From the lobar bronchi on each side proceed 10 segmental bronchi although the 7th and 8th segmental bronchi on the left are usually combined (Fig. 8.**8**b). These divide in further steps into

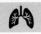

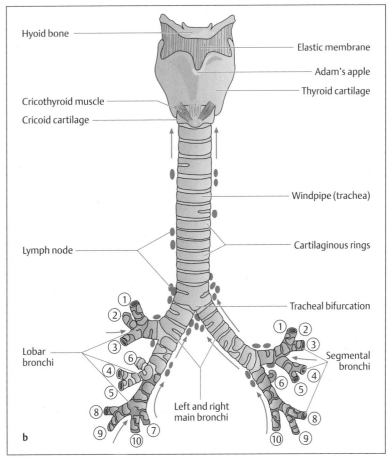

Hyoid bone

Elastic membrane

Adam's apple

Thyroid cartilage

Cricothyroid muscle

Cricoid cartilage

Windpipe (trachea)

Lymph node

Cartilaginous rings

Tracheal bifurcation

Lobar bronchi

Segmental bronchi

Left and right main bronchi

Fig. 8.**8 b**

ever finer branches. The terminal branches of the bronchial tree, the bronchioles, measure less than 1 mm in diameter (see Internal Structure of the Lung below). In contrast to the higher bronchial segments, which, like the trachea, contain cartilaginous rings to reinforce their walls, the bronchioles have no cartilaginous skeleton. They contain a profusion of smooth muscle fibers, and their lumen is kept open by the pull of *elastic fibers*.

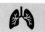

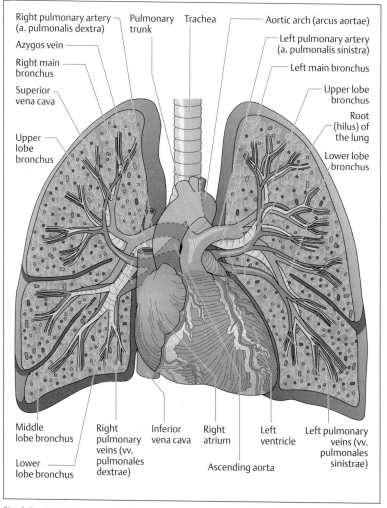

Right pulmonary artery (a. pulmonalis dextra)

Azygos vein

Right main bronchus

Superior vena cava

Upper lobe bronchus

Pulmonary trunk

Trachea

Aortic arch (arcus aortae)

Left pulmonary artery (a. pulmonalis sinistra)

Left main bronchus

Upper lobe bronchus

Root (hilus) of the lung

Lower lobe bronchus

Middle lobe bronchus

Lower lobe bronchus

Right pulmonary veins (vv. pulmonales dextrae)

Inferior vena cava

Right atrium

Ascending aorta

Left ventricle

Left pulmonary veins (vv. pulmonales sinistrae)

Fig. 8.**9**   **Anterior view of a heart–lung preparation.** The pulmonary vessels and the main bronchi enter the lung at the hilus. (After Netter)

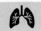

Mucous Membrane

The bronchial mucous membrane, like the other respiratory air passages, is lined with ciliated respiratory epithelium containing numerous goblet cells (see Chapter 3: Surface Epithelia). Additionally, many *endocrine cells* are scattered especially in the epithelium of the markedly branched part of the bronchial tree. These are said to regulate pulmonary perfusion and bronchial muscle tone.

■ Serous Cavities and Membranes of the Chest and Abdomen

The serous cavities of the chest and abdomen separate some of the organs of these spaces from the muscular and skeletal walls of the trunk, enabling the organs to glide against the walls of the trunk and against each other (Fig. 8.**10a**, **b**). They include the *pleural* (chest), *pericardial*(heart), and *peritoneal* (abdomen) *cavities*.

The *serous membrane* (*serosa*) is a thin, glistening, epithelial layer, connected to the wall of the trunk or to the organs by connective tissue. It permits an extensive exchange of fluid between the cavity and its surroundings and in many places can absorb large quantities of fluid from the serous cavities. On one side the serous membranes line organs and are called visceral linings, while on the opposite side they line the walls of the cavities as parietal linings (for example, in the case of the lung, *visceral pleura* = serous membrane around the lung, parietal pleura = serous membrane of the chest wall) (Fig. 8.**10a**, **b**).

■ Lungs (Pulmones)

The lungs are a pair of organs lying in the thorax on each side of the mediastinum, each in a pleural cavity. The mediastinum is the middle portion of the thoracic space lying between the two thoracic cavities. It contains the heart, the great vessels, the trachea, and the esophagus. It is bounded below by the diaphragm and above by the chest cage. The apices of the lungs reach above the first rib through the thoracic inlet.

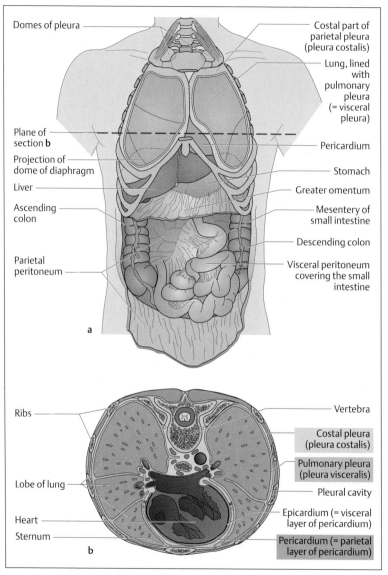

Domes of pleura

Plane of section **b**

Projection of dome of diaphragm

Liver

Ascending colon

Parietal peritoneum

a

Costal part of parietal pleura (pleura costalis)

Lung, lined with pulmonary pleura (= visceral pleura)

Pericardium

Stomach

Greater omentum

Mesentery of small intestine

Descending colon

Visceral peritoneum covering the small intestine

Ribs

Lobe of lung

Heart

Sternum

b

Vertebra

Costal pleura (pleura costalis)

Pulmonary pleura (pleura visceralis)

Pleural cavity

Epicardium (= visceral layer of pericardium)

Pericardium (= parietal layer of pericardium)

Fig. 8.**10 a, b   The serous cavities.** (After Frick et al)
a The pleura and peritoneal cavity have been opened. The pericardium is intact
b Horizontal section through the chest at the level of T8

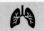

Visceral and Parietal Pleura

The pleural cavity is a *capillary cavity* with little fluid that lies between the visceral pleura that covers the lung and the parietal pleura that lines the inside of the chest wall (Fig. 8.**10b**). Because the pressure in the pleural cavity is below atmospheric pressure (intrapleural pressure), the lung must expand as it follows the inspiratory movements of the thorax and the diaphragm. The fluid in the pleural cavity prevents excessive friction between the two pleural layers. If an injury causes air to enter the pleural cavity, the lung collapses (pneumothorax, see Resistance to Breathing below).

External Structure of the Lung

Each lung is divided into lobes by deep fissures. The horizontal and oblique fissures divide the right lung into three lobes (upper, middle, and lower), while the oblique fissure divides the left lung into an upper and a lower lobe. In their turn, the *pulmonary lobes* can be divided into *pulmonary segments*, each supplied by a segmental bronchus (Figs. 8.**8** and 8.**11**). These segments, numbered I to X, are important both for radiological diagnosis and for surgical procedures. (the reader will find no segment labeled VII in Fig. 8.**11**, because the seventh and eights segments are usually combined.).

Hilus of the Lung

Bronchi, arteries, and autonomic nerves enter, and veins and lymph vessels leave the lung on its mediastinal side through the root of the lung (hilus) (Fig. 8.**9**). Important lymph nodes (hilar lymph nodes) that drain lymph from the lungs are located in the hilus. The parietal pleura and the visceral pleura meet at the hilus and the fold at their junction extends toward the diaphragm (pulmonary ligament).

Internal Structure of the Lung

Several small branches (*respiratory bronchioles*) leave the terminal branches of the bronchial tree (*terminal bronchioles*) and each of these

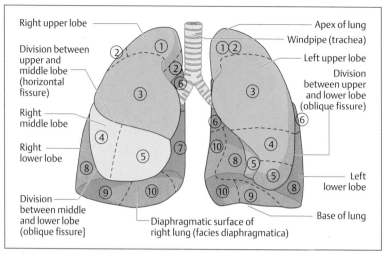

Right upper lobe

Division between upper and middle lobe (horizontal fissure)

Right middle lobe

Right lower lobe

Division between middle and lower lobe (oblique fissure]

Apex of lung

Windpipe (trachea)

Left upper lobe

Division between upper and lower lobe (oblique fissure)

Left lower lobe

Base of lung

Diaphragmatic surface of right lung (facies diaphragmatica)

Fig. 8.**11** **The segments of the lung viewed from in front.** The numbers in the circles indicate the segments of the lung I–X (segment VII of the left lower lobe is missing). The broken lines demarcate the segments

ends in two *alveolar ducts*. The alveolar ducts lead to the *alveolar sacs* (*sacculi alveolares*), in the walls of which alveoli are closely packed. These are the sites of gas exchange (Figs. 8.**12a**, **b** and 8.**13a**, **b**). All the *alveoli* supplied by one terminal bronchiole together form an *acinus* (containing about 200 alveoli), which may be regarded as the structural unit of the lung. Several acini form a *pulmonary lobule*. The lobules are bounded by connective tissue septa and can be seen on the surface of the lung as polygonal areas with sides of about 0.5–3 cm. The two lungs together consist of about 300 million alveoli, each with a diameter of about 0.2 mm. From these numbers, the total surface available for gas exchange after inspiration in an adult can be calculated to be about 100 m^2.

Pulmonary Vessels

The branches of the pulmonary arteries follow the bronchial tree to the alveoli, which are surrounded by a network of capillaries (Figs. 8.**12a**, **b** and 8.**13a**, **b**). The postcapillary veins run in the interlobular (between the lobules of the lung) and intersegmental (between the pulmonary

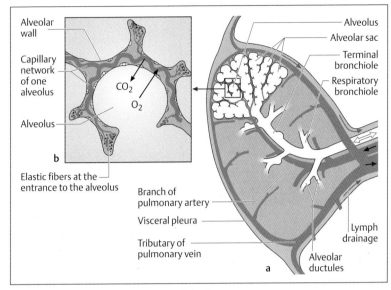

Fig. 8.12 a, b   Microscopic structure of the lung
a   Vascular supply of an acinus (the arrows show the direction of blood flow)
b   Schematic representation of an alveolus

segments) connective tissue and only the larger veins join the arteries and bronchi. The branches of the pulmonary artery and vein serve the gas exchange in the lungs.

Another vascular network supplies the pulmonary parenchyma: the bronchial arteries and veins supply the bronchi, pleura, and connective tissue structures of the lung. The arteries arise mainly from the aorta and branch in parallel with the bronchial tree. The bronchial veins drain mainly into the pulmonary veins.

Nerves and Lymph Vessels

Parasympathetic and sympathetic nerves run through the hilus of the lung to the muscles of the pulmonary vessels and bronchi. The lymph vessels originate in the loose areolar connective tissue under the visceral pleura, the connective tissue septa, and the connective tissue sheaths of

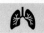

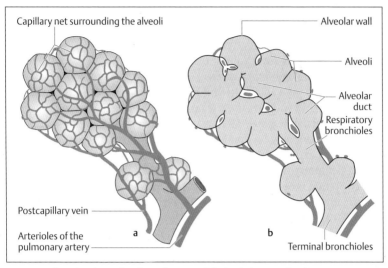

Fig. 8.**13 a, b   Blood supply of a pulmonary lobule.** (After Leonhardt)
a Lobule
b Longitudinal section through **a**

the blood vessels and bronchi. Their lymph drains into the regional hilar lymph nodes.

■ Ventilation of the Lungs

For gas exchange to occur between the alveoli and the blood, the lung must be *ventilated*. The rhythmic alternation between inhalation (inspiration) and exhalation (expiration) allows oxygen-rich fresh air to reach the alveoli and oxygen-poor air, enriched with carbon dioxide, to leave the alveoli and reach the ambient air. The driving forces accomplishing this exchange are the movements of the chest cage and the diaphragm, which expand and constrict the intrathoracic space (see The Mechanics of Breathing).

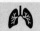

The Lung and Respiratory Volumes

The volume of a single breath, called the *tidal volume* (*volume of a normal breath*) is relatively small (about 0.5 liter) in quiet breathing when compared to the total volume of gases contained in the lungs (about 5.1 liters) (Fig. 8.**14**). Over and above the volume of a normal breath, however, considerably greater volumes may be taken in or expelled when breathing in or out respectively. Thus, after a normal inspiration another approximately 2.5 liters may be inhaled (called *inspiratory reserve volume*) and after normal expiration another approximately 1.5 liters more can be exhaled (*expiratory reserve volume*). This maximal amount of air available for ventilation is defined as the *vital capacity* (*maximal volume of a single breath*), which comprises the sum of the volume of a normal breath and normal inspiratory and expiratory reserve volumes (about 3–7 liters). This is a measure of the *ability of the lung and chest cage to expand* (difference between maximal inspiratory and maximal expiratory position), and it depends on age, sex, body build, and physical conditioning. But even with maximal expiration, a certain volume of gases remains in the lung and in the airways, called the *residual volume* (about 1–2 liters). The *total lung capacity* (*maximal lung volume*) is defined as the sum of the vital capacity and the residual volume.

With the exception of the residual volume, the respiratory and lung volumes can be measured with the aid of a spirometer (Fig. 8.**14**). Such an instrument consists essentially of a gas-tight chamber from which one can breathe in gases, and into which gases can be breathed out. By connecting the air passages of the person being tested with the spirometer, changes in lung volumes can be recorded in a spirogram as changes in respiration over time. These measurements are now made by more sophisticated instruments.

Minute Volume and Respiratory Frequency

The *respiratory minute volume* is defined as the volume of air breathed in (or, equivalently, out) per minute. It thus equals the volume of a single breath, multiplied by the number of breaths per minute (*respiratory frequency*). At rest, the minute volume is ca. 7.5 l/min (0.5 l/breath × 15 breaths/min). With physical exercise, it can rise to more than 100 l/min,

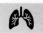

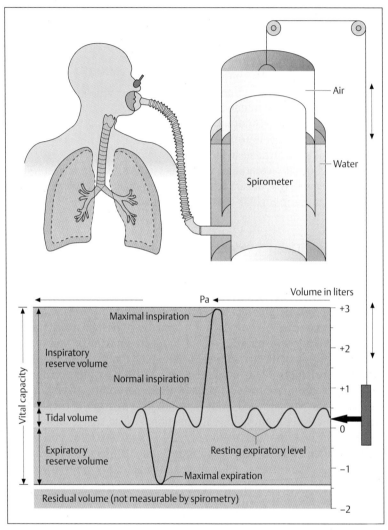

Fig. 8.**14   Measurement of the lung volumes.** The spirometer consists of a cylinder over which a bell has been inverted, sealed by water. The closed gas space has been connected to the air passage of the test subject. The volume of gases in the spirometer is shown by the position of the bell, which has been standardized in volumetric units (liters). Changes during inspiration and expiration are recorded on a drum. (After Silbernagl and Despopoulos)

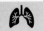

through a simultaneous increase of both the tidal volume (to 2 liters or more) and the respiratory frequency (to as high as 50/min). Maximal voluntary ventilation (*MVV, maximal breathing capacity, MBC*) is the maximal volume of gas that can be breathed in one minute (120–170 l/min). It amounts to about 20–25 times the vital capacity.

While the normal respiratory frequency in adults is 15/min at rest, higher rates are found in newborns (40–50/min), in small children (30–40/min), and in older children (20–30/min).

An increase in respiratory rate over the normal resting rate (*eupnea*) is usually called *tachypnea*, a decrease *bradypnea*. Difficulty in breathing (*dyspnea*) is usually combined with a subjective feeling of respiratory distress. Dyspnea that occurs when lying flat is called *orthopnea*, while a prolonged pause in regular breathing is called *apnea.*

Alveolar and Dead Space Ventilation

Only a part of the resting minute volume of 7.5 l/min reaches the alveoli, where gas exchange takes place (alveolar ventilation). The rest remains in the air passages (*anatomical dead space*). With a mean anatomical dead space of about 150 ml in an adult (oral cavity, nasopharynx, trachea, and bronchi) and a respiratory rate of 15 breaths/min, dead space ventilation takes up about 30% (150 ml × 15 breaths/min = 2.25 liters) and alveolar ventilation about 70% (5.25 liters). Dead space must be borne in mind in certain pulmonary diseases, where a part of the alveoli may be ventilated but not perfused, and so cannot take part in the exchange of gases. This creates a physiological (functional) dead space, which must be distinguished from the anatomical dead space described above.

Since after a normal quiet expiration about 3.5 liters of air remain in the lung, i.e., the residual volume plus the expiratory reserve volume, every breath mixes about 350 ml of fresh air (500 ml tidal volume – 150 ml dead space air) with about ten times that amount of air in the alveoli. The great advantage of this constant mixing lies in the relatively constant oxygen concentration in the alveoli, which changes little during inspiration and expiration.

The concentration of respiratory gases in the alveolar space diminishes rapidly, however, when an apparently normal minute volume of about 7.5 l/min is the result of rapid shallow breathing (e. g.,

220 ml tidal volume and 34 breaths/min during an acute state of shock). In such a case, ventilation is almost completely confined to the anatomical dead space (150 ml), while only a fraction of the inspired fresh air (70 ml) reaches the alveolar space beyond it. Consequently, dead space ventilation is markedly increased (150 ml × 34 breaths/min = 5.1 liters) at the expense of alveolar ventilation (70 ml × 34 breaths/min = 2.4 liters). Hence, whenever breathing deepens, alveolar ventilation improves.

■ Gas Exchange and the Blood–Air Barrier

The actual gas exchange in the lung takes place in the alveoli. Each alveolus is surrounded by numerous capillaries. Some capillaries are always open, while others open during periods of increased oxygen demand. The alveolar wall is made up of small alveolar cells (type I pneumocytes) that lie on a basement membrane and to the outside of which the capillaries are closely applied. Additionally, the alveolar wall contains scattered large alveolar cells (type II pneumocytes). These produce a substance called surfactant, a surface-active substance made up of phospholipids, which coats the interior of the alveoli and by reducing surface tension ensures that they do not collapse during expiration.

Gas Exchange in the Lung

Partial Pressures of the Respiratory Gases.

The dry atmospheric air we breathe in is composed of 78.1 % nitrogen, 20.9 % oxygen, and traces of carbon dioxide (0.03 %) and rare gases (e. g., argon). This composition is largely independent of elevation above sea level. Atmospheric pressure diminishes with increasing altitude from an atmospheric pressure at sea level that corresponds to a mercury column 760 mm high (760 mmHg).

In a mixture of gases, the sum of the partial pressures of the individual gases always equals the total pressure of the mixture of gases, where the relative proportion of the volume of each gas to the total

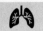

Table 8.1   Composition of dry air and partial pressure of its gases

Gas	Vol. % (F)		Partial pressure (mmHg (kPa)	
Oxygen (O_2)	20.9	(0.209)	158.8	21.17
Carbon dioxide (CO_2)	0.03	(0.0003)	0.23	0.03
Nitrogen (N_2) + rare gases	79.1	(0.791)	601	80.1
Dry air	100	(1.0)	760	101.3

volume (or the fractional concentration) determines the partial pressure of that gas. The fraction of a gas present in the total volume is usually defined in vol.% (ml/100 ml). It may be expressed in the new SI units as a *fractional concentration* (symbolized F), i.e., a fraction instead of a per cent value; for example, 0.209 instead of 20.9% oxygen. The composition of dry air and the partial pressures of the individual respiratory gases at sea level are given in Table 8.**1**.

In what follows, the percentage presence of gases will continue to be given in vol. % for the sake of clarity and simplicity. For the same reason, the pressures will continue to be given in mmHg. The SI values, the fractional concentration (F) for the fraction of a gas in the total volume and kilopascals (kPa) for pressure are given in parentheses.

Composition of Alveolar Air

While passing through the upper and lower respiratory passages, the inhaled air is saturated with water vapor. As a consequence, the partial pressure of water vapor in the alveoli at 37 °C rises to a maximal value of about 47 mmHg (6.27 kPa). The partial pressures of oxygen and nitrogen are reduced correspondingly. In an adult, the oxygen uptake at rest averages 300 ml/min and the carbon dioxide given off averages 250 ml/min. When the uptake and release of these gases is taken into account, the *composition of alveolar air* is 14% O_2 (100 mmHg = 13.3 kPa) and 5.6% CO_2 (40 mmHg = 5.3 kPa). The remaining gas is made up of water vapor (47 mmHg = 6.27 kPa), nitrogen, and a small fraction of rare gases (in total 573 mmHg = 76.37 kPa).

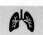

Table 8.2 O_2 and CO_2 contents of inspired, alveolar, and expired air

	Gas	Vol. %	Partial pressure (mmHg)
Inspired air (dry)	O_2	20.9	158
	CO_2	0.03	0.23
Alveolar air	O_2	14.0	100
	CO_2	5.6	40
Expired air	O_2	16.0	114
	CO_2	4.0	29

Since expired air contains an admixture of dead space air, its oxygen content is slightly higher at 16% (114 mmHg = 15.2 kPa) and its carbon dioxide content is lower at 4% (29 mmHg = 3.9 kPa) compared to the composition of alveolar air (Table 8.**2**).

Diffusion of Respiratory Gases

The exchange of gases in the lung transforms deoxygenated (poor in oxygen) venous blood that is rich in carbon dioxide into oxygenated (rich in oxygen) arterial blood with low carbon dioxide content (Fig. 8.**15**). The driving forces for the diffusion of respiratory gases are essentially the *partial pressure differences* between the alveoli and the blood. The partial pressures of O_2 (PO_2) in venous blood is about 40 mmHg (5.3 kPa) and that of CO_2 (PCO_2) 46 mmHg (6.13 kPa), creating a pressure gradient both from the alveolar partial pressure of O_2 of 100 mmHg (13.3 kPa) and the alveolar partial pressure of CO_2 of 40 mmHg (5.33 kPa). From alveolus to capillary this gradient is about 60 mmHg (100–40 mmHg) for oxygen and in the opposite direction for carbon dioxide about 6 mmHg (46–40 mmHg). After equalization of the partial pressures in the alveolar spaces and blood (see below), the partial pressure of oxygen in the arterial blood is 100 mmHg (13.3 kPa) and that of carbon dioxide is 40 mmHg (5.33 kPa) (Fig. 8.**15**).

Oxygen combines loosely with the four iron atoms in hemoglobin (Hb), and easily dissociates from it in an atmosphere low in oxygen. The amount of oxygen bound to hemoglobin depends on the partial pressure of oxygen (PO_2): the higher the PO_2, the more oxygen is carried by the blood. When

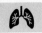

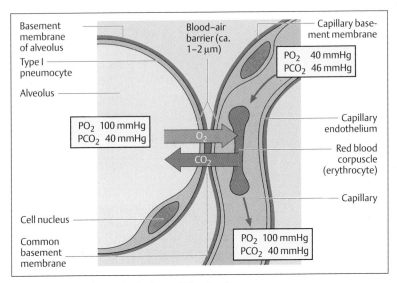

Basement membrane of alveolus

Type I pneumocyte

Alveolus

PO$_2$ 100 mmHg
PCO$_2$ 40 mmHg

O$_2$

CO$_2$

Blood–air barrier (ca. 1–2 μm)

PO$_2$ 40 mmHg
PCO$_2$ 46 mmHg

Capillary basement membrane

Capillary endothelium

Red blood corpuscle (erythrocyte)

Capillary

Cell nucleus

Common basement membrane

PO$_2$ 100 mmHg
PCO$_2$ 40 mmHg

Fig. 8.**15** **Gas exchange in the lung.** (After Kurz)

all the hemoglobin in a blood sample is combined with oxygen, the hemoglobin is said to be 100% saturated. The relationship between PO$_2$ and Hb saturation is given by the oxygen–hemoglobin dissociation curve. This curve, shown in Fig. 8.**16**, is S-shaped. The steep part of the curve lies in the range met in venous blood, and it shows that considerably more oxygen dissociates from Hb in oxygen-poor tissues than in an oxygenated lung. This facilitates the delivery of oxygen from lung to tissue, which is further enhanced by a shift of the curve to the right in an atmosphere rich in CO$_2$ and at a low pH (see insert in Fig. 8.**16**), the conditions found in the tissues. The shallow part of the curve near the top shows that even at a relatively low PO$_2$ (e. g., 70 mmHg) Hb is still nearly 90% saturated.

Carbon monoxide (CO) has a much greater affinity for Hb than oxygen, and it dissociates very little even at a low PO$_2$. Hence very little carbon monoxide can displace a great deal of oxygen from Hb, preempting the transport of O$_2$, and because of the shape of its dissociation curve most of the CO remains attached to Hb even in the tissues. Since carboxyhemoglobin is as red as oxyhemoglobin, carbon monoxide poisoning can be difficult to spot.

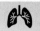

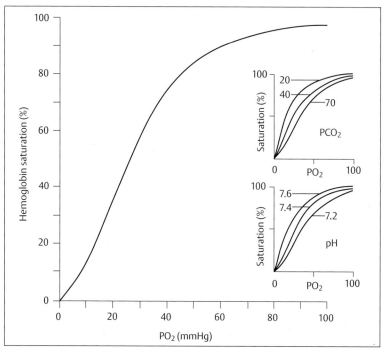

Fig: 8.**16**   **The oxygen–hemoglobin dissociation curve and its response to variations in PCO$_2$ and pH.** (Modified from F van den Berg (ed.), *Angewandte Physiologie, 2, Organsysteme verstehen und beeinflussen.* Georg Thieme, 2000, p. 63)

The Blood–Air Barrier (Alveolocapillary Membrane)

Effective diffusion requires a *large surface for exchange*, a *short diffusion path*, and a *sufficiently long time of contact* between the individual erythrocyte and the alveolar gas mixture. These conditions are met in the lung in an almost ideal fashion: the respiratory gases diffuse over a surface of close to 100 m² through a blood–air barrier (alveolocapillary membrane) that is about 1 µm (1/1000 mm) thick (capillary endothelium, alveolar wall, and the intervening basement membrane) in less than 0.3 seconds (Fig. 8.**15**). This relatively brief time of contact is

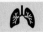

quite sufficient to fully equalize the partial pressures of the respiratory gases in the blood and the alveoli. Since the *diffusion resistance* of the blood–air barrier for CO_2 is much smaller than that for O_2, the relatively small partial pressure difference of 6 mmHg for CO_2 (see above) is quite enough to make effective CO_2 excretion in the lung possible.

Apart from unimpaired gas exchange through the blood–air barrier, the degree of "*arterialization*" of the blood also depends on alveolar ventilation and adequate perfusion of the capillaries. A further condition for optimal oxygenation of pulmonary venous blood is the even distribution of this arterializing effect in the segments of the lung. Thus, well-oxygenated blood from well-ventilated segments can mix with moderately oxygenated blood from poorly ventilated segments, and this can lead to incompletely oxygenated blood reaching the left heart.

While the partial pressure of arterial oxygen in healthy youths is about 95 mmHg (12.6 kPa), it is about 80 mmHg (10.6 kPa) in a 40-year old and about 70 mmHg (9.3 kPa) on average in a 70-year-old. Despite these low partial pressures in older people, the O_2 saturation of the red blood pigment is adequate, because the oxygen–hemoglobin dissociation curve is very flat at higher partial pressures of oxygen.

Oxygen Deficiency (Hypoxia, Anoxia)

Deoxygenated blood, in contrast to the bright red color of oxygenated blood, has a rather dark bluish-red color. Hence, oxygen deficiency in the blood (*hypoxia*) causes a purplish discoloration, especially in the skin and lips (cyanosis). If the oxygen content of the blood is insufficient to provide the cells' need for oxygen, the condition is called *anoxia*. This may have a number of different causes (e. g., a defect in O_2 uptake in the lung and the blood, disorders of O_2 transport in the blood, diminished capillary perfusion, disorders of O_2 utilization in the cells). The various organs, tissues, and cells respond to anoxia in different ways. The brain is especially sensitive to anoxia, for unconsciousness sets in after only 15 seconds of anoxia. Even after 3 minutes of anoxia, parts of the brain are damaged irreparably. As a rule, brain death supervenes after 5 minutes without oxygen.

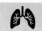

Artificial Respiration

The need for artificial respiration arises, for instance, when spontaneous respiration is inadequate while the heart continues to function. In case of respiratory arrest, mouth-to-mouth or mouth-to-nose resuscitation must be instituted if necessary. First, however, patency of the upper air passages must be ensured. They may be obstructed, for instance, by blood, foreign bodies, vomitus, or backward displacement of the tongue. Hence the mouth and pharynx must first be cleaned out, and possible airway obstruction by the tongue avoided by extending the head at the neck and at the same time lifting the jaw forward.

When air is blown into the nose or the mouth, the intrathoracic pressure rises above the atmospheric pressure acting on the chest cage, allowing the lung and the thorax to expand (inspiration). When the nose and mouth are freed, air leaves passively owing to the *elastic properties* of the lung. Inspiration and expiration can easily be followed by observing the movements of the chest (rising and falling). Since expired air still contains 16 % oxygen by volume (see above), breathing at about 5-second intervals lead to 90 % O_2 saturation of the arterial blood.

■ The Regulation of Breathing

Central Regulation of Breathing

The regulation of respiration is a centrally controlled mechanism that is constantly adapted to the needs of the organism by feedback of respiratory stimuli (see Chemical Regulation of Breathing). The respiratory movements of chest and diaphragm are coordinated by rhythmic excitation of nerve cells in the medulla oblongata (see Chapter 13: Medulla Oblongata). The neurons responsible for inspiration (*inspiratory neurons*) send nerve impulses to the inspiratory muscles (e. g., external intercostal muscles, diaphragm) by way of the spinal cord, increasing the volume of the thoracic cavity and expanding the lungs. This movement stimulates certain sensory cells (stretch receptors) in the lung, and these send nerve impulses to the respiratory centers, inhibiting the inspiratory nerve cells and at the same time stimulating those responsible for expiration (expiratory nerve cells).

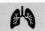

Chemical Regulation of Breathing

The overriding role in respiration, however, is taken by changes in the arterial blood gases (partial pressure of CO_2 and O_2) and the arterial pH (blood hydrogen ion concentration). Hence, the chemical regulation of breathing subserves a homeostatic function, allowing breathing to adapt to the metabolic activity of the organism. These respiratory stimuli originate in chemoreceptors in the aorta (aortic bodies, glomera aortica), the two carotid arteries (carotid bodies, glomus caroticum), and centrally near the respiratory center, from which they provide feedback (self-regulation) through nerves to the respiratory center. While the peripheral chemoreceptors measure mainly decreases in arterial PaO_2 the central chemoreceptors react to a rise in $PaCO_2$ and the fall in pH in the blood and the cerebrospinal fluid connected with it. When the arterial PaO_2 falls or the CO_2 concentration rises, with a decrease in the arterial pH below 7.5, respiration increases (increase in the minute volume) until enough O_2 has been taken up or CO_2 breathed out.

Of the three respiratory stimuli—carbon dioxide, hydrogen ion, concentration and oxygen, carbon dioxide has by far the greatest effect. For this reason, the drive for an increase in minute volume is not so much a decrease in the O_2 concentration of the blood as the rise in CO_2. If, for instance, the $PaCO_2$ rises from 46 mmHg to 70 mmHg, the ventilation increases 8–10-fold (corresponding to a minute volume of 75 l/min). Should the $PaCO_2$ increase further, however, the respiratory center is paralyzed (respiratory arrest). If a person breathes as rapidly and as deeply as possible (hyperventilation), respiration may also stop, because the blood is deprived of carbon dioxide to such an extent that the drive to breathe is absent. Hyperventilation can be especially life-threatening for divers who dive without tanks. In order to stay under water as long as possible, they hyperventilate for a considerable time beforehand. They then use up their oxygen stores while under water without realizing it, because their blood CO_2 has not yet reached the level that would activate the respiratory center. Consequently, these divers suddenly lose consciousness from lack of oxygen because the stimulus to take a breath, that is to surface, has not been activated.

Although lack of O_2 usually does not play a role in driving the respiratory center, it becomes vital when the respiratory center is no longer re-

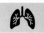

sponds to the CO_2 stimulus because the partial pressure of CO_2 is too high (respiratory failure). At this point the respiratory center is driven only by a relative lack of oxygen. Hence the administration of oxygen must be carefully controlled, in order not to extinguish the hypoxic respiratory drive. Paradoxically, in respiratory failure due to hypercarbia (PaO_2 > 50 mmHg), giving even a little too much oxygen can lead to respiratory arrest and death.

Nonspecific Respiratory Stimuli

While chemical respiratory stimuli may regulate breathing by feedback, nonspecific respiratory stimuli influence the respiratory drive without feedback. Thus, breathing may be increased by pain and temperature stimuli, psychological excitement (e. g., anxiety), arterial pressure stimuli from arterial pressure receptors (e. g., after a blood pressure drop), muscular work, and hormones (e. g., when the blood progesterone level is elevated during pregnancy).

■ The Mechanics of Breathing

Intrapulmonary Pressure

The driving forces for gas exchange between the alveoli and the ambient air are the pressure differences. If the outside pressure (atmospheric pressure) that acts on the chest cage is assumed to be zero, the pressure in the alveoli (intrapulmonary pressure) must be lower than the outside pressure during inspiration, and higher during expiration. In order to create these pressure differences, the volume of the lungs must be increased during inspiration and decreased during expiration. By expanding the thorax, air is sucked into the lungs (inspiration) and by contracting it, air is expelled (expiration) (Fig. 8.**17a**, **b**). Because the pressure in the pleural cavity is negative, the lung follows these movements passively (Fig. 8.**18a**, **b**). The diaphragm takes the principal role in this process. *Diaphragmatic respiration* is supplemented by *thoracic respiration*. In quiet respiration about 75 % of the intrathoracic volume changes are due to diaphragmatic breathing.

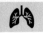

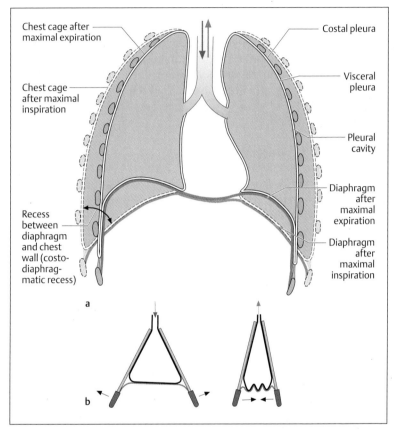

Chest cage after maximal expiration

Chest cage after maximal inspiration

Recess between diaphragm and chest wall (costo-diaphragmatic recess)

Costal pleura

Visceral pleura

Pleural cavity

Diaphragm after maximal expiration

Diaphragm after maximal inspiration

a

b

Fig. 8.**17 a, b The mechanics of breathing**
a Coronal section of the lung in inspiratory and expiratory position (blue superimposed on pink). The costodiaphragmatic recess expands during inspiration
b Equating the lung with a bellows. When the space expands, air rushes in; when it is reduced, air is pushed out

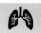

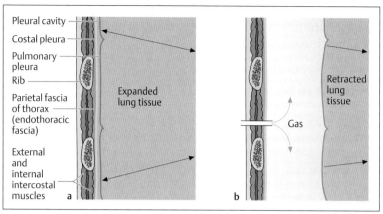

Fig. 8.**18 a, b**   **The pleural cavity**
a   Normal state
b   Pneumothorax (e. g., from a chest wall injury)

Inspiration

During inspiration, the diaphragmatic muscles contract, the central tendon (see Chapter 4:The Muscles of the Trunk, Fig. 4.**22**) moves down and
the space between the diaphragm and the chest wall (costodiaphragmatic recess, Fig. 8.**17a**) unfolds. The space thus created is filled by the
lung. In thoracic respiration, the chest cage is actively elevated by the external intercostal muscles and expanded by the action of the obliquely
placed ribs. During forced breathing, the chest cage is further elevated by
the scaleni and other accessory respiratory muscles (e. g., sternocleidomastoid, pectoralis major).

Expiration

During expiration, the diaphragm relaxes and is pushed up by the intra-
abdominal pressure. The muscles of the abdominal wall may enhance
this movement by pressing on the abdomen (see Chapter 4: The Diaphragm). Because its structure is elastic, the chest cage returns to its *re-*

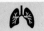

sting position passively after expiration. It is depressed actively by the internal intercostal muscles only during forced expiration. The latissimus dorsi muscle enhances this movement by reducing thoracic volume.

Resistance to Breathing

Because of its internal elasticity (stretching of its elastic fibers) and its surface tension, the lung tends toward reduction of its volume. This creates *negative pressure* in the pleural cavity (intrapleural pressure), and since the fluid in the *pleural cavity* cannot expand, the lung remains closely applied to the inside of the chest wall (Fig. 8.**18a**, **b**). If the chest wall or the surface of the lung is breached by an injury, air enters the pleural cavity (pneumothorax), and shortening of the elastic fibers causes the lung to collapse toward its root (hilus).

While elastic resistance to respiration need normally only be overcome during inspiration, the so-called *viscous resistances* (resistance to flow and resistance due to friction) act on expiration as well as inspiration. The resistance to flow depends largely on the diameter and the length of the respiratory passages leading into and out of the lung. Resistance increases as the diameter decreases. Even a slight narrowing of the bronchi can lead to a marked increase in resistance (by the Hagen–Poiseuille law, p. 246). For instance, allergic hypersensitivity to certain foreign substances in the air (bronchial asthma) may result in mucosal swelling in the smallest branches of the bronchial tree, the bronchi, and bronchioles. At the same time, increased mucus is secreted and the smooth muscles of the bronchial wall contract. All of this leads to narrowing of the air passages and considerable increase in resistance to breathing. This results in a reduced tidal volume, and expiration is obstructed more than inspiration. Blood CO_2 content rises and respiratory distress results.

The Work of Breathing

The respiratory muscles must perform physical work to overcome the resistance to breathing, that is, work against the *elastic forces* in the lung and chest wall, as well as the *flow* and *friction resistances*. The elastic

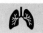

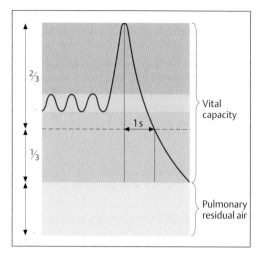

Fig. 8.**19** **Tracing of a single forced expiration.** At least 2/3 of the vital capacity should be expired in one second after a maximal inspiration

forces only play a role in inspiration, since they actually reinforce expiration. The work against flow and friction resistances, on the other hand, acts equally during inspiration and expiration.

Pulmonary Function Tests

Every increase in resistance to flow makes ventilation of the lung more difficult and leads to an increase in the work of breathing. Patients experience this as dyspnea (see Minute Volume and Respiratory Frequency above). One way of detecting the presence of such a restriction is by pulmonary function testing. A clinically useful test is the timed forced expiratory volume, or forced expiratory volume in 1 second (FEV_1). The patient is asked to inspire as deeply as possible, and expire as rapidly as possible; the FEV_1 is the volume of air expired in the first second of expiration (Fig. 8.**19**). The volume is given as a percentage of the vital capacity (see The Lung and Respiratory Volumes above). If, for instance, 3.5 liters of a vital capacity of 5 liters were expired in the first second, the FEV_1 would be 75%, which is a normal value. A smaller value, on the other hand, suggests a ventilatory problem and indicates, for instance,

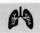

internal narrowing of the airways on the inside (increased mucus in chronic bronchitis or bronchial asthma) or outside (thyroid enlargement). This obstructive pulmonary condition is distinguished from restrictive conditions, in which the expansion of the lung and thorax are limited (e.g., due to adhesion of the two pleural layers) or the surface available for gas exchange is reduced (e.g., in pulmonary edema or pulmonary fibrosis). Since ventilation in restrictive lung disease is undisturbed, these patients have a normal FEV_1.

Summary   **The Respiratory System**

The respiratory organs may be divided into ventilatory organs (upper and lower air passages) and those subserving the exchange of gases between air and blood (alveoli).

Oxygen, with the generation of carbon dioxide, is needed for the oxidative breakdown of nutrients in every cell of the organism (internal respiration). Oxygen is taken up from the surrounding atmosphere into the lungs, while carbon dioxide is released (external respiration). After gas is exchanged between air and blood in the alveoli, the oxygen is transported by the bloodstream to the cells of the body. Here oxygen is given up in exchange for carbon dioxide, which is then transported in the reverse pathway.

■ Organs of the Air Passages

The upper air passages—nasal and oral cavity with paranasal sinuses, pharynx, larynx; lower air passages—trachea, and bronchial tree.

With the exception of the oral cavity, the mesopharynx, and the hypopharynx, the mucosa of the ventilatory respiratory passages is lined with respiratory ciliated epithelium with numerous goblet cells.

Nasal Cavity and the Paranasal Sinuses

- *Two nasal cavities* (separated by the nasal septum). External opening: nostrils (nares). Pharyngeal opening: choanae. Floor: hard and soft palate. Surface of side-walls is increased by bones (nasal conchae) lined with mucosa. On each side a superior (olfactory region, lined with olfactory mucosa), a middle, and an inferior concha

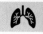

(respiratory region, warms and cleans the inspired air) form the boundary of the nasal passage.

- *The paranasal sinuses* are lined with mucous membrane; they pre-warm the inspired air and form a cavity for resonance. One frontal sinus, two maxillary sinuses, two ethmoid sinuses with ethmoid air cells, two sphenoid sinuses, all draining into the nasal cavity.

Pharynx

Superior pharyngeal space: nasopharynx (transition from the nasal cavities through the choanae). Middle pharynx: oropharynx (crossing of the digestive tract). Inferior pharynx: hypopharynx (next to the larynx).

Larynx

Function: can close the trachea to the pharynx, separating the respiratory and digestive passages, enabling increase in pressure in the thorax and abdomen, allowing straining and coughing; voice production.

Structure: Cartilaginous skeletal elements covered with mucous membrane (hyaline cartilage: thyroid cartilage, cricoid cartilage, two arytenoid cartilages; elastic cartilage: epiglottis). external (connect to the hyoid bone and the trachea) and internal (connect skeletal elements) laryngeal ligaments; muscles.

- *Thyroid cartilage:* Cartilage open posteriorly, anteriorly forms the Adam's apple; posterior border with two processes, one superior, one inferior; the inferior share a joint with the cricoid cartilage.
- *Cricoid cartilage:* A ring in front, posteriorly a lamina (plate) sharing a joint with the arytenoids.
- *Arytenoid cartilages:* include the vocal processes, from which the vocal cords run to the posterior side of the thyroid cartilage. The vocal cords and the vocal muscles form the vocal folds; the space between the vocal folds is the glottis.
- *Epiglottis:* attached to the posterior side of the thyroid cartilage by an elastic membrane. It closes the laryngeal opening during swallowing.
- *Muscles:* superior and inferior hyoid muscles elevate and depress the larynx; striated laryngeal muscles move the parts of the larynx on each other, and produce the voice by opening (one muscle only)

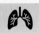

and closing of the glottis and changes in the tension of the vocal cords.

Windpipe (Trachea)

A tube formed by about 20 cartilaginous rings lined by a mucous membrane, about 10–12 cm in length and 2 cm in diameter; at the bifurcation divides into left and right bronchi.

Bronchial Tree (Bronchi = Pulmonary Air Passages)

Left and right main bronchi branch into lobar bronchi (three right, two left): each divides into 10 segmental bronchi supplying the segments of the lung, each continuing to divide until they reach the terminal bronchi, which no longer have cartilaginous reinforcements in their walls.

■ Serous Cavities and Membranes of the Chest and Abdomen

- *Pleural cavity* (contains the lungs). Serous membranes: visceral pleura and parietal/costal pleura.
- *Pericardial cavity* (contains the heart). Serous membranes: epicardium (visceral pericardium) and pericardium (parietal pericardium).
- *Peritoneal cavity* (contains the abdominal organs). Serous membranes: peritoneum with visceral and parietal layer (visceral and parietal peritoneum).
  Visceral layers cover the organs, parietal layers line the walls of the serous cavities. Fluid in the cavities allows the organs to move against the walls of the trunk.

■ Lungs

Location: in the thorax left and right of the mediastinum, each in a pleural cavity. The pressure in the pleural cavity between the visceral and parietal pleura is negative, ensuring that the lung follows the inspiratory movements of the thoracic wall and the diaphragm.

External Structure

Division into lobes: (right lung: upper, middle and lower lobe; left lung: upper and lower lobe). Each lung is also subdivided into 10 segments, corresponding to the distribution of the segmental bronchi. The root of each lung is located on the medial side (hilus—entry of the

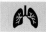

bronchi, arteries, autonomic sympathetic and parasympathetic nerves, exit of the veins and lymph vessels).

Internal Structure

The respiratory bronchioles branch off the terminal bronchioles, each leading into two alveolar ducts. These lead into the alveolar sacs, which contain the alveoli (300 million in the two lungs, corresponding to a gas exchange surface of $100 \, m^2$).

Acinus: all the alveoli (about 200) supplied by one terminal bronchiole; one lung lobule: several acini.

Pulmonary vessels: (1) those subserving gas exchange in the alveoli—capillary net supplied by branches of the pulmonary arteries and veins surrounding the alveoli; (2) those subserving the nutrient needs of the tissues of the lungs—bronchial arteries and veins.

▩ Ventilation of the Lungs

- *Total lung volume* = volume of gas in the lungs (ca. 5 l)
- *Tidal volume* = normal volume of one breath at rest (ca. 0.5 l)
- *Inspiratory reserve volume* = additional amount of air that can be taken up after a normal inspiration (ca. 2.5 l)
- *Expiratory reserve volume* = additional amount of air that can be exhaled after a normal expiration (ca. 1.5 l)
- *Vital capacity* = maximal respiratory volume: tidal volume plus inspiratory and expiratory reserve volume (ca. 3–7 l); depends on age, physical condition, etc.
- *Residual volume* = volume of gas remaining in the lungs after maximal expiration (ca. 1–2 l)
- *Total lung capacity* = vital capacity + residual volume

All these volumes and capacities (except residual volume) can be measured with a spirometer.

- *Timed respiratory volume* = volume of gases inspired and expired per unit time: tidal volume × breaths/min (respiratory rate) = minute respiratory volume; at rest ca. 7.5 l/min (0.5 l × 15 breaths/min); during strenuous work up to 100 l/min.
- *Maximum voluntary ventilation* = maximal breathing capacity: the maximum volume that can be ventilated in 1 minute (120–170 l/min).

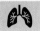

- *Alveolar ventilation* = the part of the tidal volume that actually reaches the alveoli and takes part in gas exchange (70% of 7.5 l = 5.25 l).
- *Anatomical dead space volume* = part of the ventilated air that does not take part in gas exchange because it remains in the air passages (ca. 150 ml).
- *Dead space ventilation* = the part of the minute volume that remains in the air passages (150 ml × 15 breaths = 2.25 l = 30%).

Mixing of the ventilated air: after quiet expiration about 3.5 liters of gas remains in the lung (residual plus expiratory reserve volume) and this mixes with only 350 ml (1/10 the amount) of fresh air (500 ml tidal volume – 150 ml dead space).

■ Gas Exchange and Blood–Air Barrier
Gas exchange takes place in alveoli surrounded by a capillary network (some always open, some open only during increased demand). Structure: small (type I pneumocytes) and large (type II pneumocytes) alveolar cells (produce surface-active "surfactant").

Partial Pressure of the Respiratory Gases
The sum of the *partial pressures of the respiratory gases* equals the total pressure (atmospheric pressure). This decreases with increasing elevation above sea level, while the composition of respiratory gases in the atmosphere is relatively constant: 78.1% nitrogen, 20.9% oxygen, 0.03% carbon dioxide and traces of rare gases (atmospheric pressure at sea level = 760 mmHg or 101.3 kPa).

Composition of Alveolar Gases
The *composition of alveolar gases* (condition during gas exchange) is: 14% oxygen (100 mmHg), 5.6% carbon dioxide (40 mmHg), water vapor (47 mmHg, added during passage of the gases over the moist mucous membranes of the upper and lower air passages), nitrogen, and traces of rare gases.

Since the expired air mixes with dead space air, its oxygen concentration is somewhat higher than that in alveolar air (16%), and the carbon dioxide content is somewhat lower (4%).

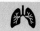

Diffusion of Respiratory Gases through the Blood–Air Barrier

Gas exchange in the lungs changes oxygen-poor, carbon dioxide-rich venous blood into oxygen-rich, carbon dioxide-poor arterial blood. The driving force for the diffusion of respiratory gases is the partial pressure gradient of the gases between the alveoli (oxygen 100 mmHg, carbon dioxide 40 mmHg) and venous capillary blood (oxygen 40 mmHg, carbon dioxide 46 mmHg). After equalization of the partial pressures in blood and alveoli, the arterial capillary blood has a PaO_2 of 100 mmHg (PCO_2 40 mmHg).

The large gas exchange area of the sum of all the alveoli (100 m²) and the short diffusion path through the blood–air barrier (capillary endothelium, alveolar wall, common basement membrane: 1 µm = 1/1000 mm) result in an effective diffusion process (requirement: adequate alveolar ventilation, adequate perfusion of the pulmonary capillaries).

■ The Regulation of Breathing

Breathing is regulated by the respiratory center in the medulla oblongata.

Chemoreceptors connected by nerve fibers to the respiratory center sense the arterial PaO_2, $PaCO_2$, and pH (feedback stimulus).

- *Aortic bodies* (*glomera aortica*) (in the aorta), respond to reduction in arterial PaO_2.
- *Carotid body* (*glomus caroticum*) (in the carotid arteries), stimulated like the aortic bodies.
- *Central chemoreceptors* near the respiratory center respond to raised carbon dioxide concentration and the accompanying fall in blood pH.

The strongest chemical respiratory stimulus is a raised carbon dioxide content (not a diminished O_2 content!), which leads to an increased minute volume. Thus prolonged hyperventilation can lead to respiratory standstill, because it diminishes the blood carbon dioxide to the point where the respiratory drive is absent. Other respiratory stimuli (nonspecific, not part of feedback): e.g., pain and temperature stimuli, agitation, muscular work, hormones.

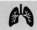

■ Mechanics of Breathing

The driving forces for the exchange of gases between the alveoli and the ambient air are pressure differences, generated as follows:

- *Inspiration*: active expansion of the chest cage, the lungs following passively because of negative pressure in the pleura; the diaphragm contracts (diaphragmatic breathing = 75%), the external intercostal muscles raise and expand the thoracic cage, air is sucked in; pressure in the alveoli is lower than ambient pressure. In forced inspiration additional muscles used are the accessory respiratory muscles (e.g., scalene muscles).
- *Expiration:* passive contraction of the chest cage, air is pushed out. Pressure in the alveoli is greater than ambient pressure, diaphragm relaxes, muscles of the abdominal wall can add to upward pressure on the diaphragm (straining). Accessory muscles during forced expiration include the internal intercostal muscles.

Inspiration requires active work by the respiratory muscles against the elastic resistance to respiration (internal elasticity of the lung, especially noticeable when air enters the pleural cavity [pneumothorax]). Expiration is passive, aided by the elastic forces. Resistances to flow and friction (depend on diameter and length of the air passages) must be overcome during inspiration as well as expiration (e.g., inspiration and expiration are made more difficult by increased mucus production and bronchial narrowing in allergic asthma).

- *Dyspnea:* difficulty in breathing
- *Orthopnea:* difficulty breathing when lying flat
- *Tachypnea:* increase in the respiratory rate
- *Bradypnea:* decrease in respiratory frequency
- *Eupnea:* normal quiet respiration

9

The Digestive System

Contents

By taking up nourishment or nutrients (proteins, fats, carbohydrates, vitamins, minerals, and trace elements) the body can create energy by the "combustion" of nutrients to maintain its organization (structure, catabolic, or energy metabolism) and the functions derived from it (growth, renewal of cells, body temperature, mechanical and chemical work). The nutrients are degraded by the enzymes of the digestive glands in the various divisions of the digestive system, broken down into chemical combinations that can be absorbed, and taken up (resorbed) by the gastrointestinal mucosa. These energy-rich combinations (e. g., fatty acids, amino acids, or glucose) enter the bloodstream and next reach the liver by way of the portal vein (see Liver, Function below). Eventually they reach the cells of the body, where they are broken down oxidatively in the mitochondria to energy-poor combinations (CO_2 and H_2O) (biological oxidation). The energy thus liberated is stored in energy-rich ATP following a chain reaction (mitochondrial respiratory chain). ATP in its turn is made available to processes requiring energy (e. g., protein synthesis or muscular work). ATP splits off phosphate molecules to liberate energy (see Chapter 1: Mitochondria).

■ Metabolism, Energy Requirements and Nutrients

Metabolism

Metabolism, which includes all the biochemical processes needed to maintain life by building, transforming, and breaking down the organism, can be divided into *constructive* (*productive*, *anabolic*) and *energy transforming* (*catabolic*) *metabolism. Anabolism* (*constructive metabolism*) includes the production of cellular substances, i.e., the synthesis of endogenous (the body's own) substances (.e. g., proteins, carbohydrates, fats) involved in the growth of the organism.

In general we call processes in which substances foreign to the body are transformed into the body's own substances *assimilative* energy-consuming (anabolic) processes. In plants *assimilation* (photosynthesis) involves capturing energy from sunlight, by which energy-poor inorganic substances are transformed into energy-rich organic substances (*autotrophic organisms*). *Heterotrophic organisms*, such as humans and animals, acquire energy by taking up nourishment that already contains energy-rich substances formed by other organisms.

Energy-transforming metabolism (*catabolism*) involves the breakdown of energy-rich substances (e. g., fats, carbohydrates, proteins) into those containing less energy with the liberation of energy (= *dissimilation*). Dissimilative processes are breaking down or catabolic processes. One of the most important catabolic processes is the biological oxidation described above. The energy stored in ATP is used for anabolic as well as energy-transforming metabolism, that is, it serves the maintenance of processes needed to maintain life, such as the maintenance of body temperature, muscular work, absorption and transport at cell membranes, the transmission of nerve impulses, etc. In the course of these processes, a considerable amount of energy is lost, e. g., as heat. Since, unlike plants, humans and animals cannot build organic substances by photosynthesis, they must regularly take in food to make energy available.

Energy Requirements

The energy requirements and energy transformation of the human body depend on many factors such as age, sex, weight, ambient temperature, and physical activity and vary considerably even at complete rest (basal metabolism). Hence, metabolism may be divided into *basal metabolism*, measured under standard conditions (in the morning, fasting, resting quietly, normal body temperature, comfortable ambient temperature) and the excess metabolism of exercise measured under varying conditions.

Energy Content of Nutrients

The energy gained from metabolic processes depends among other things on the nature of the metabolized substances (proteins, fats, and carbohydrates). If, for instance, we want to measure the energy content of individual nutrient materials outside the body, we can burn them in a combustion chamber (calorimeter) and measure the heat or energy liberated (*physical caloric value*). The results can be given in calories (cal) or joules (J), though the unit most often used in practice is the calorie: 1 cal corresponds to 4.185 J. In nutrition, the old distinction between a "small calorie" and a "large calorie" has largely been abandoned in favor of the larger Calorie (1 Cal = 1000 small calories or 1 kcal), which is equivalent to the old large calorie. Such a measurement gives the following results for the three most important energy-providing nutrients: carbohydrates 4.1 kcal/g (17 kJ/g), fats 9.3 kcal/g (39 kJ/g) and proteins 5.3 kcal/g (22 kJ/g).

If the nutrients are "burnt" completely in the organism, i.e., broken down oxidatively to CO_2 and water, the energy available to the body (*physiological caloric value*) from fats and digestible carbohydrates approximates the physical caloric value (fuel value). During the breakdown of protein, however, urea is formed in addition to CO_2 and water. Since this would generate more energy if it underwent complete combustion, the fuel value of proteins is higher than the physiological caloric value. Hence, under physiological conditions, energy generated by the same amounts of different substances is:

1 g carbohydrate (e. g., starch):	4.2 kcal (17.6 kJ)
1 g fat (e. g., triglyceride):	9.3 kcal (38.9 kJ)
1 g protein (e. g., animal protein):	4.1 kcal (17.2 kJ)
1 g alcohol (e. g., ethyl alcohol):	7.1 kcal (30.0 kJ)

Energy Requirements at Rest (Basal Metabolism, Basal Metabolic Rate, BMR)

As already noted, the basal metabolic rate depends on a variety of factors. As a guide, the following facts may help: the value of the BMR in a grown man per kilogram body weight is about 1 kcal (4.2 kJ) per hour. For a weight of 70 kg this correspond to round 1700 kcal (7000 kJ) a day. The corresponding value for a woman of equal weight is lower by about 10–20 %. However, the body's energy metabolism depends on factors other than height, weight, age, and sex. For instance, intellectual activity, emotional reactions (joy, fear), fever, or thyroid overactivity (hyperthyroidism) increase metabolism, while sleep, anesthesia, or thyroid deficiency (hypothyroidism) lower it.

Energy Requirements during Physical Activity (Excess Metabolism of Exercise)

Physical activity increases metabolism (excess metabolism of exercise). As a result the metabolism developed during working hours exceeds that developed during leisure hours:[1]

- About 2760 kcal (12 000 kJ) during light work (e. g., desk work)
- About 3680 kcal (16 000 kJ) during moderately heavy work (e. g., mowing the lawn)
- About 4600 kcal (20 000 kJ) during very heavy work (e. g., moving furniture)

Exceptionally top-ranked athletes may attain 16 100 kcal (70 000 kJ) for brief periods (e. g., marathon runners, triathletes), but of course their daily metabolism is much lower.

Determination of Energy Metabolism

In order to determine energy metabolism, the total heat production of the body would have to be measured. It is, however, simpler to calculate the energy consumption of the body from the oxygen consumption (O_2 taken up in the lung). For instance 134 liters of oxygen are used in the complete combustion (oxidation) of 1 mole (=180 g) of a simple sugar (glucose), involving the generation of about 664 kcal (2,780 kJ) of energy, i.e., 4.95 kcal (20.7 kJ) energy is transformed for each liter of oxygen. This value is called the "*combustion equivalent*".

Since in each case the quantities of CO_2 produced and of O_2 consumed depend on the type of nutrient (carbohydrate, protein, or fat) being oxidized, the quotient of the two values (CO_2 production/O_2 consumption), called the "*respiratory quotient*" (RQ), gives information on the nature of the substance undergoing combustion. With approximately equal amounts of protein present, the RQ of a preponderantly carbohydrate diet is 1.0, while a preponderantly fatty diet has an RQ of 0.7, as can be determined from the following equations:

- Carbohydrate (glucose): $C_6H_{12}O_6 + 6\,O_2 = 6\,CO_2 + 6\,H_2O$ (RQ = 6/6 = 1)
- Fat (triglyceride): $2\,C_{51}H_{98}O_6 + 145\,O_2 = 102\,CO_2 + 98\,H_2O$ (RQ = 102/145 = 0.7)

---

[1] Energy metabolism developed during today's typical average leisure activity, i.e., without much movement.

Nutrients

In addition to proteins, carbohydrates, and fats, a balanced human diet should include vitamins, minerals, trace elements, and adequate water. Also desirable is a daily intake of fiber, i.e., substances derived from plants (e. g., cellulose) that are not digested and stimulate intestinal activity by their ability to swell.

The daily protein intake of a normal adult should account for 10–15 % of the total daily caloric intake (0.8 g per kg body weight, or about 56 g for a 70 kg man). Fat intake should account for a further 25–30 % (about 78 g of fat), and carbohydrate intake for the remaining 55–60 %. Carbohydrates are thus the body's main source of energy.

Proteins

The principal task of proteins is to provide the body with amino acids, which the body requires for the biosynthesis of its endogenous proteins. The human body cannot synthesize eight of the 20 naturally occurring amino acids that it needs to manufacture its own proteins. These amino acids are called "*essential amino acids*" and include leucine, lysine, methionine, phenylalanine, isoleucine, valine, threonine, and tryptophan. Other amino acids can be essential under special circumstances, e. g., tyrosine and cysteine in premature infants and in persons suffering from hepatic cirrhosis; histidine in uremic patients; and arginine in immunocompromised patients. Apart from lysine, which is absent or present only in insufficient quantities in many vegetable nutrients, both vegetable and animal proteins contain the essential amino acids.

Fats (Lipids)

Fats are dietary substances that are rich in energy (see Energy Content of Nutrients above) and they function primarily as energy providers, but they also store energy. They also include the *essential fatty acids* (polyunsaturated fatty acids occurring in vegetable oils, especially linoleic and linolenic acid). A diet lacking these substances leads to manifestations of deficiency. Lipids are present in high concentrations in the sex organs, for example, and form a large part of the lipids in the cell membrane. They also include cholesterol, which forms part of the structure of the cell (cell membrane) and is a hormone precursor. Finally, fats are solvents that allow the complete absorption of fat-soluble vitamins (e. g., vitamin A, vitamin E) from the gastrointestinal tract.

Triglycerides constitute the major portion of the fats included in the diet. These are neutral fats, each consisting of three fatty acids attached to the trivalent alcohol glycerol. Among the more frequently encountered fatty acids are palmitic, stearic, oleic, and linoleic acids. While animal fats are predominantly saturated fatty acids (exception: salt water fish), vegetable oils have a higher content of unsaturated fatty acids (exception: coconut oil).

Carbohydrates

Carbohydrates are the preferred sources of energy of many organisms. The combinations most important in the human diet are the *monosaccharides* (e. g., glucose = dextrose), *disaccharides* (e. g., *lactose = milk sugar*), and *polysacccharides* (e. g., starch). Our diet contains chiefly monosaccharides contained especially in honey and fruit, disaccharides in milk and in all foods sweetened with the common household sugar saccharose (sucrose, cane sugar), and polysaccharides in vegetable (starch) and animal (glycogen) products. Carbohydrates can only be stored in small quantities in the body. For instance, during starvation the total store of glycogen in the liver and the skeletal muscles (about 300–400 g) is used up in a day and a half. Because of their sweet taste, simple sugars (monosaccharides and disaccharides) are very popular and have multiple uses. They are also suitable for protecting food from deterioration and therefore for preserving. On the other hand, simple sugars put a considerable burden on the pancreas. The small molecules reach the bloodstream rapidly and the blood sugar level rises rapidly. The pancreas must secrete large quantities of insulin in order to lower the blood sugar level, which then sinks to such low levels that it evokes a strong sensation of hunger with fatigue. With renewed sugar intake, the level rapidly rises again. A diet rich in sugar entails strong swings in blood sugar level, with consequent variability in performance. Moreover, simple sugars have practically no nutritional value, they are "empty calories." Whole-grain products (starch + vitamins + fiber; see Fiber below) are more filling in the long run and avoid blood sugar peaks.

Vitamins

Vitamins are organic compounds that are indispensable for humans and animals and are synthesized insufficiently or not all in the body. Hence they must be ingested regularly in food or as supplements. In our diet they are present in quite variable quantities in the form of vitamins or vitamin precursors known as provitamins, that can be transformed into vitamins in the body. The best-known example of the latter is β-carotene, also known as provitamin A. On the other hand, vitamin D_3 can be synthesized from the provitamin 7-dehydrocholesterol, an intermediate metabolic product, by the effect of sunlight on the skin.

Vitamins do not play a role in the production of energy or in the structure of the body, but fulfill chiefly a catalytic or regulatory function. According to their solubility vitamins are divided into:

- **Fat-soluble vitamins:** vitamin A (retinol and others), vitamin D (ergocalciferol, vitamin D_2 or cholecalciferol, or vitamin D_3) vitamin E (α-tocopherol and others) and vitamin K (phytonadione or vitamin K_1, and menaquinone or vitamin K_2)
- **Water-soluble vitamins:** vitamin C (ascorbic acid), vitamin B_1 (thiamin), vitamin B_2 (riboflavin), niacin (antipellagra factor), pantothenic acid, vitamin B_6 (pyridoxine and others), folic acid, vitamin B_{12} (cyanocobalamin and others), inositol, and biotin. Inositol (a component of lecithin) is sometimes included among the B vitamins, even though it is synthesized in the body in quantities much greater than its dietary intake.

For practical purposes, water-soluble vitamins cannot be stored in the body. They circulate in the blood until they are needed for cellular reactions. Fat-soluble vitamins are chiefly contained in fatty foodstuffs and can only be absorbed in adequate quantities if fat digestion and absorption are intact. They can be stored in the liver and in fatty tissues.

Chemically, vitamins belong to several different types of substance and are defined according to their actions. By their function they can be divided into two major groups: vitamins of the B complex and vitamin K are components of coenzymes that catalyze carbohydrate, fat, and protein metabolism. Thus, by taking part in fundamental intermediary metabolic processes, they are indispensable for every living cell. Vitamins A, D, E, and C, on the other hand, can only be demonstrated at a more advanced stage of evolution, where the maintenance of specific organ functions is essential. These vitamins are highly specialized active substances coupled to certain cell and organ systems. Apart from vitamin A they are not components of coenzymes. In evolutionary history (phylogenesis), dependence on these vitamins can be found only in the more highly developed invertebrates, while the need for vitamin D is only found in vertebrates.

Age, sex, and physiological conditions such as pregnancy, physical stress, and nutrition influence vitamin requirements in humans. Vitamin deficiency (*hypovitaminosis*) can be due to such conditions as malnutrition, faulty nutrition (undiversified diet, e. g., in the elderly or alcoholics, a fast-food diet), or malabsorption in the gastrointestinal tract. Treatment with medications, e. g., those that damage the intestinal flora, may lead to vitamin deficiencies by eliminating bacterial vitamin synthesis (especially of vitamins B_{12} and K).

The following well-known severe illnesses are due to vitamin deficiencies: scurvy (vitamin C deficiency), beri-beri (vitamin B_1 deficiency), pellagra (niacin deficiency), and rickets (vitamin D deficiency). Moreover, vitamin A deficiency leads to night blindness, vitamin B_{12} deficiency to pernicious anemia, and vitamin K deficiency to clotting disorders.

Toxicity due to vitamin overdose (*hypervitaminosis*) occurs only with the fat-soluble vitamins A and D. This does not apply to the water-soluble vitamin precursor β-carotene. Normally, excess water-soluble vitamins are rapidly excreted in the urine.

Minerals (Macrominerals and Trace Minerals)

Minerals are classified according to their concentration in the body as *macrominerals* (>50 mg/kg body weight) or *trace minerals* (trace elements) (<50 mg/kg body weight). The recommended daily intake of the trace minerals is less than 100 mg/day. Iron is exceptional, in that it is present in high concentration in the body, and thus counts as a macromineral, but its recommended daily intake lies in the range of the trace minerals, because it is effectively recycled in the body, rather than being excreted. Trace elements are minerals the requirement of which is less than 100 mg/day. The total weight of all trace elements in the body is 8–9 g. They include chromium, iron, fluorine, germanium, iodine, cobalt, copper, manganese, molybdenum, nickel, selenium, silicone, vanadium, zinc, and tin. The significance of some others also present in the blood, such as aluminum, arsenic, barium, gold, and rubidium, is not entirely clear.

Adequate intake must be ensured especially for iron and iodine. The most important function of iron, which at 4–5 g is quantitatively the most important of the trace elements in the body, is as component of hemoglobin and myoglobin (daily requirement 10 mg for men, 15 mg for women). Iodine is part of the structure of the thyroid hormone thyroxin, and is contained especially in salt-water fish, iodized table salt, and drinking water (daily requirement 0.18–0.2 mg). Although fluorine is not necessary for life, daily use promotes remineralization of the teeth. The remaining trace elements are primarily components of important enzymes.

Calcium, magnesium, phosphorus, sodium, potassium, and sulfur belong to the *macroelements*. The most abundant of these is calcium with 1.5 kg (99% skeletal, 1% in bodily fluids and tissues). Minerals do not have a uniform biological function in the body. They take part in the structure, maintenance, and constant renewal of bones and teeth and in the activation of enzymes. They are responsible for the conduction of impulses in the nervous system, the functioning of muscles, the constant ion content of bodily fluids, and the regulation of water balance. They also take part in the maintenance of a constant osmotic pressure and pH in the blood and the other parts of the body.

Antioxidants (Free Radical Scavengers)

Vitamins A (β-carotene), E, and C, like the trace elements selenium, manganese, zinc, and molybdenum as well as several active plant ingredients (see below), possess anitoxidative activity, which gives them special significance. They inactivate free radicals that are metabolic by-products (e.g., superoxide anions, hydroxyl radicals) and so supplement the body's own antioxidative enzymes (e.g., glutathione peroxidase). Free radicals are molecules marked by high chemical reactivity, because they possess unpaired electrons (i.e., they are chemically unstable). Even oxygen, which is required for the oxidation of nutrients, is a radical in its basic configuration (a dioxygen radical, with unpaired electrons). The energy-creating (ATP) reaction in the cells (oxygen + hydrogen → water) is only possible because of the high reactivity of oxygen. The same process may create other reactive forms of oxygen that are not radicals (e. g., hydrogen peroxide), some of which are even more reactive and so aggressive that they can extract electrons from other molecules. The result is new radicals that oxidize other molecules as they try to become stabilized, producing damage to cellular structures:

- Damage to DNA in the chromosomes may entail mutations in the genes or uncontrolled cell division (cellular degeneration or cancer production).
- Oxidized LDL (see Chapter 6: Plasma Proteins) in the blood are deposited preferentially in damaged vascular walls (arteriosclerosis); antioxidants prevent the oxidation.
- Cell membranes are damaged when fatty acids in phospholipids are oxidized to peroxides (peroxidation of lipids). Premature senility may ensue (increased cell death, deposition of the products of oxidation). Antioxidants protect the cell membrane from oxidation and so prevent death of the cell or impairment of cellular function by the products of oxidation.

Extreme physical exertion and acute inflammation, as well as products that damage the environment (e. g., ozone, nitric oxide) and ultraviolet and radioactive radiation, lead to increased formation of free radicals during cell metabolism (oxidative stress).

Active Substances in Plants

As well as vitamins, minerals, trace elements, and fiber, fruit and vegetables contain a number of substances that protect them from dangerous components of sunlight, from pests, and from adverse environmental influences. Such substances also protect people from certain diseases. From a scientific point of view, the most interesting chemical compounds among the many thousand contained in every kind of fruit and vegetable are those that act as antioxidants or play a role in cancer prevention. Many of the active substances found in plants that have been studied are free radical scavengers; others show configurations that may deactivate carcinogenic (cancer-causing) substances or prevent their formation. These include:

- *p-Coumarins and quinic acid compounds* (found in tomatoes, pepperoni, strawberries, pineapple): inhibit the formation of carcinogenic nitrosamines.
- *Indoles* (found especially in broccoli, cauliflower, Brussels sprouts, kale, and cabbage): reduce estrogen synthesis and so reduce the risk of diseases due to hormone-dependent tumors. Moreover, they increase the activity of certain detoxifying enzymes in the liver that also break down carcinogens.
- *Allicins* (in alliums such as garlic, leeks, onions, chives): these have antibacterial activity. Alliums also contain organic sulfur compounds that activate enzymatic detoxifying systems in the liver.
- *Isocyanates* (all crucifers): activate detoxifying enzymes; inhibit reactions that alter DNA (phenethyl isocyanate). Sulforaphan is one of the very few active substances of which the activity has been studied in isolation, and which can be produced synthetically. The substance renders carcinogens harmless by activating certain detoxifying enzymes.
- *Flavonoids* and *isoflavonoids* (almost every fruit and vegetable contains its characteristic flavonoids): of the over 800 flavonoids known so far, many have antioxidative, antifungal (effective against fungi), anti-inflammatory (fighting inflammation), antiviral (fighting viruses), antiallergenic or anticarcinogenic effects or promote blood perfusion. For instance, substances such as catechin, nobiletin, hesperidin, quercetin, quercitrin, morin, robinin, myrecitin, rutin, kaemferol, and neoponcerin have antioxidative or anticarcinogenic properties. The isoflavonoid genistein (found in soy products) can inhibit tumor growth and prevent the development of metastases. Other flavonoids can guard against arteriosclerosis or reduce cholesterol synthesis. For instance, morin and sylimarin block oxidation of LDL and so prevent its deposition in vascular walls (antioxidative action).
- *Saponins* (found in soy products): prevent the synthesis of DNA in tumor cells.
- *Terpenes:* these include many aromatic vegetable oils, e. g., the limonene of citrus oil found in citrus fruit. All have marked antioxidative activity.

In contrast to vitamins, most active plant substances survive all processes used in preparation, industrial processing, and prolonged storage. Tomatoes alone contain 10 000 different active substances, of which only a fraction have been studied. Whether these substance continue to be active when they have been isolated from the other active substances in the plant (e. g., there might be interactions between the individual compounds), or if their action might then reverse has, with few exceptions, not yet been explored. Fruit and vegetables must continue to be included in the diet, especially in view of their fiber content.

Fiber

Fiber plays a special role in our diet. It includes indigestible plant carbohydrates such as cellulose and hemicellulose. Cellulose is a component of the cell wall of plants. Hence a diet rich in fiber includes fruit, vegetables, and whole-grain products. Substances rich in fiber not only promote intestinal activity, they also slow gastric emptying and are therefore more filling. This effect prevents blood sugar peaks. They have a high capacity for binding water and so stimulate intestinal activity, shortening the time of passage of materials through the intestines and so leading to regular emptying of the bowels.

■ The Digestive Organs

The digestive organs may be divided according to their function into the cephalic (foregut) and those of the trunk (midgut and hindgut). The cephalic digestive organs include the oral cavity with its salivary glands, the oropharynx, and the hypopharynx. The digestive organs of the trunk (Fig. 9.**1**) include the gullet (esophagus), stomach, small bowel (duodenum, jejunum, and ileum), large bowel (caecum, vermiform appendix, ascending, transverse, descending and sigmoid colon, and rectum) and the digestive glands (liver, pancreas).

The Oral Cavity

The oral cavity is bounded by the lips in front, the cheeks laterally, the muscles of the floor of the mouth below, and the hard and soft palate above. The back of the oral cavity (fauces) is formed by the oropharyn-

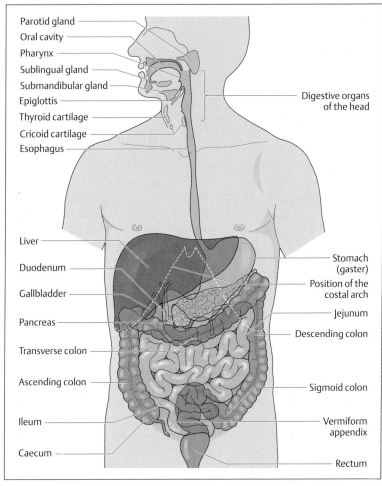

Parotid gland
Oral cavity
Pharynx
Sublingual gland
Submandibular gland
Epiglottis
Thyroid cartilage
Cricoid cartilage
Esophagus

Digestive organs
of the head

Liver
Duodenum
Gallbladder
Pancreas
Transverse colon
Ascending colon
Ileum
Caecum

Stomach
(gaster)
Position of the
costal arch
Jejunum
Descending colon
Sigmoid colon
Vermiform
appendix
Rectum

Fig. 9.**1** **Overview of the digestive organs.** (After Leonhardt)

geal isthmus, which comprises the anterior and posterior pillars of the fauces (palatoglossal arch and palatopharyngeal arch) and the uvula in the middle between them (Fig. 9.**2**). Between the two pillars of the fauces on each side sits the palatine tonsil. The oral cavity is primarily filled by

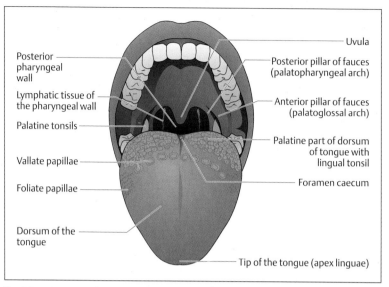

Uvula

Posterior pharyngeal wall

Posterior pillar of fauces (palatopharyngeal arch)

Lymphatic tissue of the pharyngeal wall

Anterior pillar of fauces (palatoglossal arch)

Palatine tonsils

Palatine part of dorsum of tongue with lingual tonsil

Vallate papillae

Foramen caecum

Foliate papillae

Dorsum of the tongue

Tip of the tongue (apex linguae)

Fig. 9.**2** **View into the oral cavity; the tongue is protruded.** (After Faller)

the tongue, and is lined on the inside by a mucous membrane that consists of stratified squamous epithelium.

Food is taken into the oral cavity, ground up mechanically, transformed into a semiliquid paste, and moved toward the pharynx. The teeth, lips, and tongue ingest the food and grind it. *Taste* and *smell receptors* sense and monitor its chemical constitution. The secretions of the salivary glands allow the food to glide smoothly, and in addition certain enzymes (e. g., amylase) contained in the saliva initiate the break-up of carbohydrates (e. g., starch).

The Tongue

The tongue is a *muscular organ* covered with a mucous membrane designed for the *transport of ingested material*. It aids in chewing and sucking and carries sensory organs for taste and touch. Beyond that, the tongue plays an important role in speech.

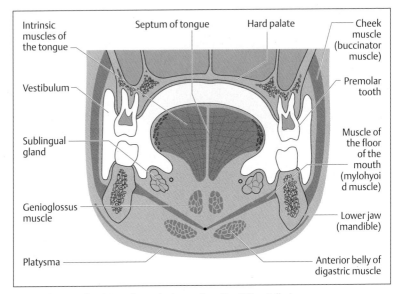

Fig. 9.**3** **Coronal section through the oral cavity.** (After Faller)

The muscles of the tongue are divided into intrinsic and extrinsic muscles (Fig. 9.**3**). The most important and strongest extrinsic tongue muscle is the *genioglossus muscle*, which takes its origin in the middle of the mandible and radiates fanwise from the tip of the tongue to its palatine end. It pulls the whole tongue forward and at the same time flattens the dorsum of the tongue. The intrinsic tongue muscles traverse the organ in all three directions. Their function is chiefly to deform the body of tongue.

Tactile and Taste Papillae

The dorsum of the tongue contains numerous papillae of various kinds, subserving the sensations of touch and taste (Fig. 9.**4**). The *filiform (threadlike) papillae* are distributed over the whole dorsum of the tongue and serve especially the perception of *touch*, *pressure*, *temperature*, and *pain*. The taste papillae include *fungiform (mushroom-shaped) papillae*, *vallate (walled) papillae* and *foliate (leaf-shaped) papillae*. They contain *taste buds* and can be found at specific locations on the dorsum of the

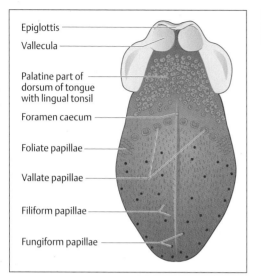

Epiglottis

Vallecula

Palatine part of
dorsum of tongue
with lingual tonsil

Foramen caecum

Foliate papillae

Vallate papillae

Filiform papillae

Fungiform papillae

Fig. 9.**4** **Papillae of the
tongue serving general
sensation and taste**

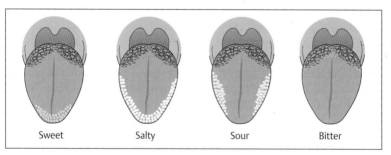

Sweet   Salty   Sour   Bitter

Fig. 9.**5** **Location of various taste sensations on the tongue.** (After Silbernagl and Despopoulos)

tongue (Fig. 9.**5**). The tongue can perceive four taste sensations: *sour*, *salty*, *bitter*, and *sweet*. However, individual tastes cannot be allocated to specific papillae, for the experience of taste is combined with the sense of smell. Hence, we cannot taste anything when the nose is blocked, as for instance when we have a cold. Behind the V-shaped arrangement of vallate papillae, the palatine part of the tongue is bounded by the *lingual* *tonsil.* In the midline, immediately behind the apex of the V, lies the *foramen caecum*, where the thyroid gland has developed.

The Teeth (Dentes)

The human dentition is arranged in two rows of teeth, the upper and lower dental arches, anchored in the upper and lower jaws. The first teeth formed are the milk (deciduous) teeth, replaced later by the permanent teeth. Human teeth have various shapes and have different functions. The incisors are the cutting teeth, the canines next to them help with tearing and fixing. Beyond these, the chewing surfaces of the premolars and molars grind and perform the major part of the work of chewing. Incisors and canines are also called the anterior (labial) teeth and the premolars and molars the posterior (buccal) teeth.

Structure of the Teeth

The tooth is divided into *crown*, *neck*, and *root*. The crown extends above the gum and is covered by *enamel* (Fig. 9.**6**). The root sits in an *alveolus* in the upper or lower jaw and is covered with *cementum* (*cement*). It is anchored in the bone by the *desmodontium* (*periodontal ligament, periodontal membrane*). The part of the tooth where cementum and enamel meet is called the neck of the tooth. The apex of the root is pierced by the root canal, through which nerves and vessels reach the *dental cavity* (*pulp cavity*). The dental cavity contains the *dental pulp*, a connective tissue structure containing blood vessels and nerves through which the tooth obtains its nutrition. The *odontoblasts*, dentin-forming cells, spread out like an epithelium, lie at the free border where pulp and dentin meet. They form dentin when needed and send processes into the dentin. These processes are accompanied by blood vessels and nerves that run in dental canaliculi (dental tubules) that give dentin a slightly wavy radial striation.

   Each tooth consists of three hard substances that resemble bone: *dentin* (*dentine*), *enamel*, and *cementum* (*cement*). Dentin forms the largest portion of the tooth and surrounds the dental cavity (Fig. 9.**6**). At the crown, dentin is covered by enamel, at the root by cementum. Dentin is sensitive to pain. Enamel is the hardest substance in the human body

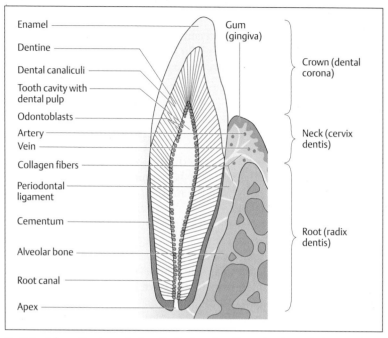

Fig. 9.**6**   **Schematic view of a longitudinal section through a lower incisor**

and consists of 97 % inorganic salts (chiefly hydroxyapatite). Dentin includes 70 % inorganic substances, cementum 65 %.

Support Structures of the Teeth (Parodontium)

The collagen fibers of the periodontal ligament (desmodontium) anchor the tooth elastically in its bony alveolus (Fig. 9.**6**). The collagen fibers (Sharpey's fibers) run between the alveolar wall and the cementum, and are mainly oriented toward the apex of the root. Because of this orientation, chewing puts pressure on them. The periodontal membrane, which covers and protects the *gum* (*gingiva*) to the neck of the tooth, contains a prominent vascular network and sensory nerves (sensitive to pressure). The support structures of the tooth include the alveolus, the edge of the gum, the periodontal ligament, and the cementum.

The Dental Formula

The human permanent dentition consists of 32 teeth (8 incisors, 4 canines, 4 canines, 8 premolars, and 12 molars). On each side of either jaw they have the following sequence from front to back (Fig. 9.**7a**, **b**)

- 2 incisors (dentes incisivi = I)
- 1 canine (dens caninus = C)
- 2 premolars (dentes premolares = P)
- 3 molars (dentes molares = M)

The number and sequence of the teeth can be expressed in brief by the *dental formula*. Where the structure is symmetrical, this is written for only one half of the mouth, with the maxillary teeth above the line and the mandibular teeth below, thus: $I^2/_2$ $C^1/_1$ $P^2/_2$ $M^3/_3$.

In dental practice the teeth are numbered in a particular order. The upper right third molar is given the number 1, and the teeth are then numbered in order along the upper alveolar margin from 1 to 16, 16 being the upper left third molar. The numbers then continue along the lower dental arch from left to right, the third left lower molar being 17, and the third right lower molar 32. The medial upper left incisor is 9, the medial lower left incisor is 24.

Left upper jaw	Right upper jaw
16 15 14 13 12 11 10 9	8 7 6 5 4 3 2 1

Left lower jaw	Right lower jaw
17 18 19 20 21 22 23 24	25 26 27 28 29 30 31 32

Shape of the Permanent Teeth

The crown of the incisors is shaped like a chisel, with a sharp horizontal cutting edge. The canines are the longest teeth and their crowns each have two cutting edges that come together in a point. The premolar teeth have a chewing surface and their crown has two cusps (bicuspids). Their roots are often bifurcated, particularly in the upper premolars. The molars are oriented in the direction of the masticatory muscles. Their chewing surfaces mostly form four cusps, and when the teeth are apposed the cusps of the upper molars are placed between those of the lower molars and vice versa. While the upper molars have three roots,

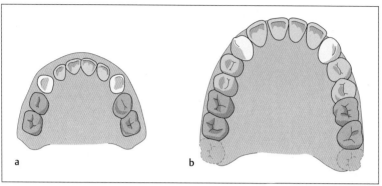

Fig. 9.**7 a, b   Deciduous (milk) and permanent dentitions** (both upper jaw)
a Deciduous dentition: incisors (blue), canines (yellow), deciduous molars (violet)
b Permanent dentition: incisors (blue), canines (yellow), premolars (green), molars (violet); the 3rd molars (wisdom teeth) not yet erupted

the lower mostly only form two. The third molars (wisdom teeth) vary in shape and sometimes do not develop.

Milk Dentition and the Eruption of Teeth

The *permanent dentition* must be distinguished from the *first* (*milk, deciduous*) *dentition*. The latter consists of 20 teeth (Figs. 9.**7a, b** and 9.**8**). With the exception of the premolar teeth, it is the same as the permanent dentition (8 incisors, 4 canines, 8 milk molars (deciduous molars). Between the 6th to 12th month of life the incisors are the first deciduous teeth to erupt. At 2 years the deciduous dentition is usually complete.

The first permanent teeth to erupt are the first molars. Since they appear in the 6th year of life they are sometimes called the *six-year-old teeth*. The last molar (wisdom tooth) often erupts late and may be malformed. The following are the times (years of life) of eruption of the permanent teeth:

Tooth:	I1	I2	C	P1	P2	M1	M2	M3
Eruption (year of life)	7	8	11	9	10	6	12	?

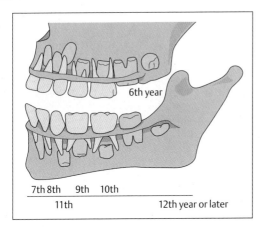

Fig. 9.**8** **Order of eruption of the permanent dentition.** Deciduous teeth in white. Germ of permanent dentition in green. The numbers indicate the time of eruption (the germ of the 3rd molar has not yet been laid down)

The Salivary Glands

The salivary glands are exocrine glands, that is, in contrast to endocrine glands, they discharge their secretions through ducts. The salivary glands of the mouth include small and large glands. The *small salivary glands* have short ducts and lie in the mucosa of the lips, cheek, tongue, and palate. The *large salivary glands* include the *parotid gland*, the *submandibular gland*, and the *sublingual gland* (Fig. 9.**9**). The parotid gland is the largest. It lies in front of the ear on the ascending ramus of the mandible. Its duct (*parotid duct*), 3 mm thick and 5–6 cm long, pierces the buccinator muscle and ends in the oral cavity at the level of the second upper molar. The submandibular gland is closely applied to the mandible and extends a fairly long process around the posterior border of the mylohyoid muscle. Its duct runs anteriorly and joins the duct of the sublingual gland, which lies laterally on the mylohyoid muscle under the tongue. The common duct ends in a small projection (*sublingual caruncle, caruncula sublingualis*) under the apex of the tongue. Several small accessory ducts from the sublingual gland open on each side of the sublingual papilla.

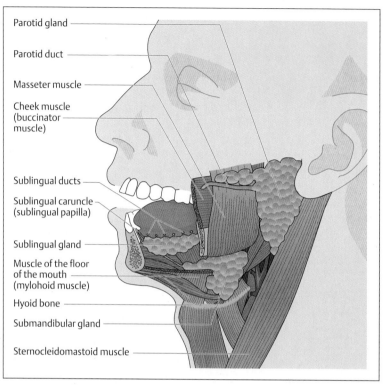

Parotid gland

Parotid duct

Masseter muscle

Cheek muscle
(buccinator
muscle)

Sublingual ducts

Sublingual caruncle
(sublingual papilla)

Sublingual gland

Muscle of the floor
of the mouth
(mylohoid muscle)

Hyoid bone

Submandibular gland

Sternocleidomastoid muscle

Fig. 9.**9** **The large salivary glands of the mouth**

All the salivary glands together secrete about 1–1.5 liters of saliva in
the course of a day. The saliva may be mucous or serous and the large and
small salivary glands secrete both kinds. Saliva increases the lubrication
of the food after chewing. Serous saliva begins the digestive process in
the mouth because it contains the sugar-splitting enzyme amylase. The
secretion of saliva is regulated by the autonomic nervous system, with
the parasympathetic promoting and the sympathetic inhibiting its formation.

The Throat (Pharynx)

The throat is the common portion of the respiratory and digestive tracts adjoining the nasal and oral cavities. It is a tube, about 12 cm long, attached to the base of the skull. The nasal cavity opens into the upper part (*nasopharynx, epipharynx*), the oral cavity into the middle part (*oropharynx, mesopharynx*), and the larynx and esophagus into the lower part (*hypopharynx*) (Fig. 9.**10**). The respiratory and digestive passages cross in the oropharynx. The tonsils of *Waldeyer's tonsillar ring* are situated where the nasal and oral cavities open into the pharynx (choanae). Their function is to attack pathogens as early as possible by

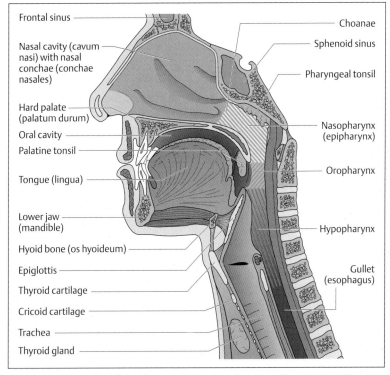

Fig. 9.**10** **Topography of the pharynx.** Sagittal section viewed from inside. (After Frick et al)

activating the specific immunity. They are named according to their location (Figs. 9.**2** and 9.**10**): midline pharyngeal tonsils (adenoids) in the roof of the pharynx, bilateral palatine tonsils between the two faucial arches, midline lingual tonsils on the palatine part of the tongue and the lymphatic tissue of the lateral pharyngeal wall, condensed around the entrance to the eustachian tube. The eustachian tube connects the pharynx with the tympanic cavity of the middle ear (see Chapter 15: Middle Ear).

The pharyngeal wall consists of mucosa, striated muscle, and a connective tissue fascia. The pharyngeal muscles include the muscles taking part in swallowing, namely, the *pharyngeal constrictors* and the *pharyngeal levators*. Whereas the pharyngeal constrictors are strong muscles that can narrow the pharynx and lift the larynx and hyoid bone (Fig. 9.**11**), the pharyngeal levators are rather weak. They raise and shorten the pharynx.

The Act of Swallowing (Deglutition)

The act of swallowing prevents the food from reaching the trachea. It includes a *voluntary* and an *involuntary* (*reflex*) *phase* (Fig. 9.**11a, b**). To begin the act of swallowing, the floor of the mouth is contracted voluntarily and the bolus is pressed against the soft palate. This action initiates the reflex (*swallowing reflex*), which includes the involuntary sealing of the respiratory passage. As the soft palate is lifted against the posterior pharyngeal wall (levator and tensor veli palati muscles) the upper respiratory passage is sealed from the digestive tract. The hyoid bone and the larynx are raised by the contraction of the floor of the mouth (pharyngeal constrictors and muscles of the floor of the mouth) and the epiglottis approaches the entrance to the larynx. During this action the glottis is closed and the breath is held. In this way the lower respiratory passages are also separated from the digestive tract. After the act of swallowing is complete, the infrahyoid muscles pull the larynx down again and so open the respiratory passages. This important and complex reflex is regulated by the *swallowing center* (*deglutition center*) in the medulla (medulla oblongata) in the brain.

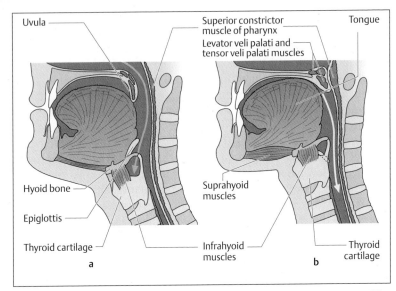

Fig. 9.**11 a, b** **Representation of the act of swallowing.** The respiratory passage (blue arrow in **a**) and the digestive passage (yellow arrow in **b**) cross in the oropharynx. The act of swallowing may be divided into a voluntary phase (contraction of the floor of the mouth and transport of the bolus to the soft palate) and a reflex securing of the respiratory passage (elevation of the soft palate, closure of the upper air passage, elevation of the hyoid bone and larynx with closure of the laryngeal inlet by the epiglottis). (After Leonhardt)

The Gullet (Esophagus)

The esophagus transports the bolus from the pharynx into the stomach. This transport is accomplished by waves of circular muscle contractions (peristalsis) that are normally directed toward the stomach. The esophagus is also subject to a longitudinal tension (fixed by the larynx above and the diaphragm below) that stabilizes its course and favors the passage of the bolus of food during swallowing. In the adult, the esophagus is about 25–30 cm long. It runs through the thorax behind the trachea and in front of the spine. Below, the esophagus penetrates the diaphragm through the *esophageal hiatus* to empty directly into the

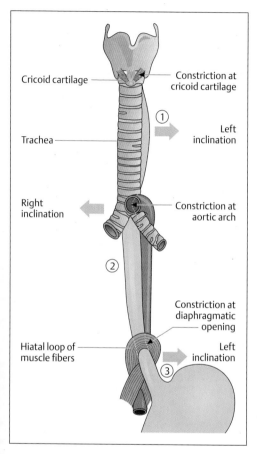

Fig. 9.12 Divisions, inclinations, and constrictions of the esophagus
1 Cervical part
2 Thoracic part
3 Abdominal part
Red arrows mark the inclinations; black arrows mark the physiological constrictions. The hiatus sling is part of the diaphragm.
(After Faller)

Within figure:
Cricoid cartilage
Constriction at cricoid cartilage
① Left inclination
Trachea
Right inclination
Constriction at aortic arch
②
Constriction at diaphragmatic opening
Hiatal loop of muscle fibers
Left inclination
③

stomach. The esophagus (Fig. 9. **12**) can be divided into a short *cervical part*, a *thoracic part*, and an *abdominal part*.

In certain places the esophagus is narrowed by *esophageal constrictions*. The highest constriction is at the cricoid cartilage; it is the narrowest with a diameter of about 14 mm. In the middle the closely related aortic arch causes a constriction. The lowest constriction corresponds to the diaphragmatic hiatus and is the site of a complex closing mechanism.

At this limited constriction, larger boluses can at times become wedged and cause severe pain.

The esophagus has the mural layers characteristic of the whole gastrointestinal tract (see The Small Bowel, Fig. 9.**17**). An inner *mucous membrane* (*tunica mucosa = mucosa*) is followed by a loose areolar *connective tissue layer* (*tunica submucosa = submucosa*), in which run larger blood and lymph vessels. Outside this is a *muscular layer* (*tunica muscularis = muscularis*), which consists of an inner circular layer and an outer longitudinal layer. By alternating the contractions of the circular and longitudinal muscles segment by segment (peristalsis), this arrangement of the muscles facilitates the transport of food toward the stomach. This, then, is the effective movement of the gastrointestinal tube, coordinated by the autonomic nervous system. Outside the muscle layer is a connective tissue layer (*tunica adventitia = adventitia*), which anchors the esophagus in its bed and allows some mobility.

The Stomach (Ventriculus, Gaster)

Function

By secreting gastric juice (pH 1.5–2, about 2–3 liters/day), consisting essentially of water, mucus, hydrochloric acid, and protein-splitting enzymes (pepsin), the stomach macerates and liquefies food chemically. The food forms a paste (chyme) that is moved back and forth and, after a delay of variable length (1–5 hours), transported into the small intestine in batches. Secretion of gastric juices occurs in three phases:

1. A **cephalic (reflex) phase**
2. A **local (gastric) phase**
3. An **intestinal phase**

Cephalic secretion is mediated by the vagus nerve (cranial nerve X) and initiated by sensory stimuli (taste, smell, sight). It may occur with an empty stomach. Gastric secretion is initiated by the food itself and begins when food reaches the stomach. It is triggered by substances resembling hormones (e. g., gastrin), which appear in the gastric mucosa near the outlet of the stomach under the influence of mechanical (e. g., distension) and chemical (e. g., amino acids) factors. Gastrin in turn reaches other parts of the stomach (body, fundus of the stomach, Fig. 9.**14**) through the bloodstream (endocrine activation) and triggers the formation of hydrochloric acid in the oxyntic cells. In the intestinal phase of gastric secretion the duodenum retroactively influences the secretion of gastric juice, in that hormones may inhibit (e. g., by secretin) or promote (probably also by gastrin) the composition and quantity of the chyme in the duodenum. In this way the duodenum adjusts the chyme coming from the stomach to the capacity of the small intestine.

Shape and Position

The stomach is located in the left upper quadrant of the abdomen under the diaphragm. Its shape and position may show wide variations (with degree of filling). The volume of the stomach is about 1200–1600 ml. It

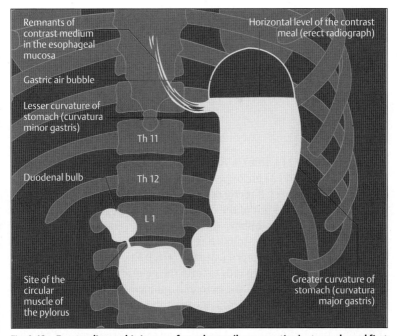

Fig. 9.**13**   **Erect radiographic image of esophagus (lower portion), stomach, and first part of duodenum after ingestion of contrast medium.**

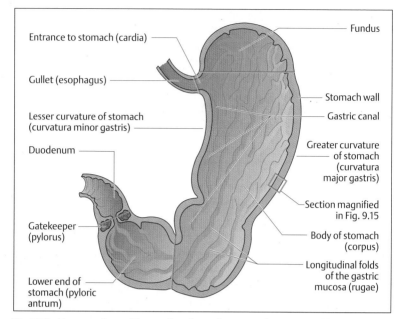

Entrance to stomach (cardia)

Gullet (esophagus)

Lesser curvature of stomach
(curvatura minor gastris)

Duodenum

Gatekeeper
(pylorus)

Lower end of
stomach (pyloric
antrum)

Fundus

Stomach wall

Gastric canal

Greater curvature
of stomach
(curvatura
major gastris)

Section magnified
in Fig. 9.15

Body of stomach
(corpus)

Longitudinal folds
of the gastric
mucosa (rugae)

Fig. 9.14 Topography and internal surface of a stomach cut open (blue lines represent notional lines marking the parts of the stomach)

consists of an *inlet* (*cardia*), a *fundus*, a *body* (*corpus*), a distal *chamber* (*pyloric antrum*), and a *gatekeeper* (*pylorus*). At the cardia, the esophagus opens into the stomach directly below the diaphragm. The fundus can be seen as a dome on the left of the cardia, where it is regularly outlined on radiographs by an air bubble (swallowed air) (Fig. 9.**13**). The upper border of the body of the stomach is formed by the *lesser curvature*, the lower border by the *greater curvature* (Fig. 9.**14**). Where the stomach meets the duodenum it expands to form the pyloric antrum and immediately behind it lies the pylorus, a circular sphincter muscle. On the outer surface the stomach is covered by peritoneum, allowing it to move against the other organs (see Chapter 8: Serous Cavities and Membranes of the Chest and Abdomen; and Relations of the Peritoneum and Mesenteries of the Abdominal Organs below, with Fig. 9.**25a, b**).

Mucosa and Muscular Layers

The mucosal surface shows numerous longitudinal folds (*rugae*), that form the *gastric canal* along the lesser curvature (Fig. 9.**14**). Small areas, about a millimeter in size, can be seen along the rugae. In these a magnifying glass will show densely concentrated punctiform *gastric pits* (foveolae gastricae), through each of which several gastric glands secrete hydrochloric acid and enzymes. To protect against digestion of the mucosa by hydrochloric acid, the cells secrete a viscous mucus that covers the mucosal surface. The gastric glands are especially numerous in the fundus and corpus of the stomach. They are stretched out and contain three types of cell (Fig. 9.**15**). The *mucous neck cells*, found mainly in the neck of the glands, form mucus and contain numerous mitoses (regeneration!). The *chief cells* and *parietal cells* are found farther down in the middle part of the glands. The chief cells form a precursor of the protein-splitting enzyme pepsin, pepsinogen, which is activated by hydrochloric acid formed in the parietal cells (see Protein Digestion below). Hydrochloric acid also has a bactericidal action, which kills a large portion of the bacteria ingested with the food. In addition, the parietal cells produce "*intrinsic factor*" that allows vitamin B_{12} to reach the ileum of the small intestine.

The smooth muscle of the gastric wall has an oblique muscle layer on the inside in addition to the circular and longitudinal layers (Fig. 9.**15**). At the pylorus the circular layer forms a strong sphincter muscle. When the stomach is full, peristaltic waves run from the fundus to the pylorus about every 3 minutes. Gastric emptying depends primarily on the pressure differences between the stomach and the small intestine and is regulated by tissue hormones.

The Small Bowel (Intestinum Tenue, Enteron)

Function

The actual digestion and absorption of nutrients takes place in the small bowel. The nutrients are broken down to easily absorbed components by pancreatic enzymes. During this process carbohydrates are broken down to simple sugars (monosaccharides), proteins to amino acids, and fats to fatty acids and glycerol (glycerin). The diges-

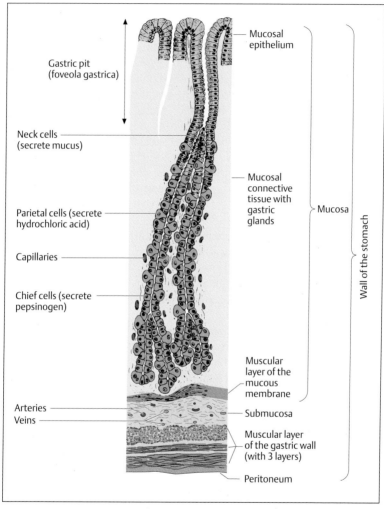

Gastric pit
(foveola gastrica)

Mucosal
epithelium

Neck cells
(secrete mucus)

Parietal cells (secrete
hydrochloric acid)

Mucosal
connective
tissue with
gastric
glands

Mucosa

Capillaries

Chief cells (secrete
pepsinogen)

Muscular
layer of the
mucous
membrane

Arteries
Veins

Submucosa

Muscular layer
of the gastric wall
(with 3 layers)

Peritoneum

Wall of the stomach

Fig. 9.**15** **Microscopic section of a gastric gland** (section from Fig. 9.**14**)

tion of fats requires bile acids. The chyme is propelled through the
small bowel toward the large intestine by *mixing* and *propulsive
movements.*

Shape and position

The small bowel begins distal to the pylorus and ends at the entrance to the large intestine (Fig. 9.**16a**, **b**). Depending on the state of contraction of its longitudinal muscle layer, it is 3–5 m long. It is divided into successive segments: the 25–30 cm (12 fingerbreadths) long *duodenum* (= *12-finger gut*), the *jejunum*, and the *ileum*. The duodenum is shaped like a 'C' embracing the head of the pancreas and is attached to the posterior abdominal wall. The *bile duct*, often joined with the main *pancreatic duct*, drains into a papilla (*papillla duodeni major*) that projects into its descending portion (see The Pancreas, Shape and Position below). The duodenum is followed by the ileum and jejunum, although there is no definitive transition between the two. The jejunum constitutes two-fifths and the ileum three-fifths of the combined coil. Both sections are attached to the posterior peritoneum by a *suspensory band*, the *mesentery* (Fig. 9.**16a** and **b** and 9.**19**). The mesentery contains the blood and nerve supply of the small intestine (see also Relations of the Peritoneum and Mesenteries of the Abdominal Organs below).

Movements of the Small Intestine

The small intestine is covered on the outside by the peritoneum (serosa). From this inward follows the smooth musculature consisting of an outer longitudinal and an inner circular layer (Fig. 9.**17**). The intestinal contents are mixed by alternating contraction and relaxation of the longitudinal and circular musculature (*pendular* and *segmentation movements*). The propulsion of the contents of the gut is accomplished by peristaltic waves, triggered by distension of the intestinal wall when the lumen is filled (see Chapter 14: Nervous System of the Intestinal Wall). These are circular contractions that advance along the gut and propel the intestinal contents forward.

Mucous Membrane of the Small Bowel

The mucosal surface, especially that of the jejunum, is considerably extended by *folds*, *villi*, and *microvilli* (Fig. 9.**18a**, **b**), thus facilitating the absorption of nutrients from the small intestine. Each of the about 600

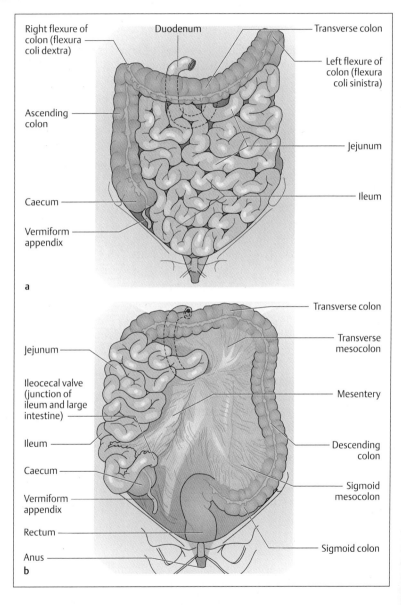

Right flexure of colon (flexura coli dextra)

Duodenum

Transverse colon

Left flexure of colon (flexura coli sinistra)

Ascending colon

Jejunum

Ileum

Caecum

Vermiform appendix

a

Transverse colon

Transverse mesocolon

Jejunum

Ileocecal valve (junction of ileum and large intestine)

Mesentery

Ileum

Descending colon

Caecum

Sigmoid mesocolon

Vermiform appendix

Rectum

Anus

Sigmoid colon

b

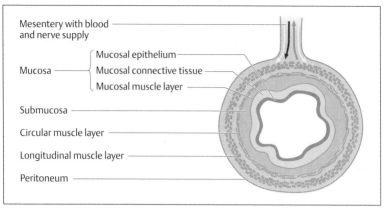

Fig. 9.**17** **Transverse section through the small intestine (structure of the layers).** (After Leonhardt)

circular folds (*Kerckring's folds*) projects about 1 cm into the submucosa and they enlarge the surface by about 1 m².

The intestinal villi are 1 mm high and 0.1 mm thick fingerlike projections from the mucosa into the intestinal lumen, giving the surface a velvety appearance. The pits between the bases of the individual villi are known as the crypts of Lieberkühn: 1 mm³ can carry up to 40 small intestinal villi (Figs. 9.**18a, b**). They expand the surface to about 5–6 m². Each villus contains a connective tissue framework with arterioles, venules, a network of capillaries (Fig. 9.**19**) and a central lymph vessel. The villi are lined by a simple columnar epithelium (enterocytes) containing mucus-secreting goblet cells (Fig. 9.**20**). The function of the enterocytes is absorption and they display a brush border (microvilli) on the cell membrane facing the intestinal lumen. Microvilli are projections from the plasma membrane (about 3000 for each cell, about 200 million per mm²) which gives the small intestine a total mucosal surface of over 120 m².

The villi of the small intestine are a functional entity concerned with absorption of the chyme. The nutrients (amino acids, sugars, free fatty

◁ Fig. 9.**16 a, b** **Position of the small and large intestine in the abdomen.** (After Leonhardt)
a Normal position
b With small intestine turned over to the right and the transverse colon turned upward

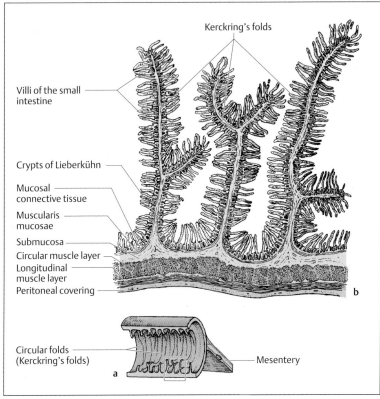

Kerckring's folds

Villi of the small intestine

Crypts of Lieberkühn

Mucosal connective tissue

Muscularis mucosae

Submucosa

Circular muscle layer

Longitudinal muscle layer

Peritoneal covering

b

Circular folds (Kerckring's folds)

Mesentery

a

Fig. 9.18 a, b   Longitudinal section through the jejunum
a Section through the small intestine; **b** magnified section of **a**

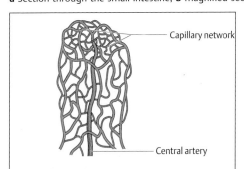

Capillary network

Central artery

Fig. 9.19   Villus of the small intestine injected to show blood vessels. A preparation of the vessels of a villus filled with a synthetic material, showing a central artery leading into a capillary network at the tip of the villus

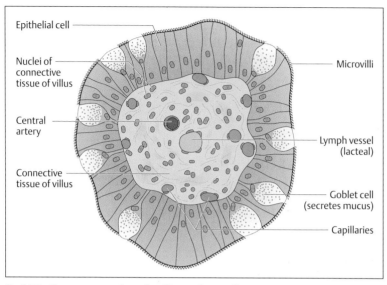

Epithelial cell

Nuclei of
connective
tissue of villus

Central
artery

Connective
tissue of villus

Microvilli

Lymph vessel
(lacteal)

Goblet cell
(secretes mucus)

Capillaries

Fig. 9.**20**   **Transverse section of a villus in the small intestine, greatly magnified**

acids, etc.) are taken up by way of the capillary network to reach the bloodstream and are transported by way of the portal veins to the liver. The fats (triglycerides) are resynthesized in the form of chylomicrons (see Fat Digestion below) in the epithelium of the villi and removed by way of a *central lymph vessel* (*cisterna chyli*) from which they reach the venous circulation through the *thoracic duct*.

The marked surface expansions of the mucosa of the small intestine decrease gradually toward the end of the small bowel, as less food and more water is absorbed. In the ileum, the folds fade and the villi project less.

Gut-associated Lymphatic Tissue (GALT)

Numerous lymphatic follicles can be found singly or grouped in the mucosa of the gastrointestinal tract. These, taken as a whole, together with diffusely distributed lymphocytes, form the gut-associated lymphatic tissue. It represents a part of the system of specific immunity that meets antigens in the intestine. The lymph follicles are especially closely packed in the *Peyer's patches* of the mucosa of the ileum and the vermiform appendix (see Chapter 6: Lymphoid Tissues of the Mucous Membranes, Gut-associated Tissue).

The Large Bowel (Intestinum Crassum)

Function

The chief task of the large intestine, which is composed of the caecum, colon, and rectum, is to reabsorb water and salts that have reached the gut with the digestive juices. The large intestine contains indigestible food remnants that bacteria decompose by fermentation and putrefaction.

Shape and Position

The ileum empties into the 1.5–1.8 m long large intestine at the *ileocecal valve* in the right lower quadrant of the abdomen (Figs. 9.**16b** and 9.**21**). The beginning of the large intestine, the caecum, pouches out below the ileocecal valve. The appendix (*vermiform appendix*), about 8 cm long and 0.5–1 cm thick hangs from the caecum; it has an important function in the human specific immune system (see Small Bowel, Gut-associated Lymphatic Tissue above). The colon continues from the caecum, framing the small bowel.

The colon begins on the right side as the *ascending colon* (*right colon*), which curves to the left below the liver (*right colic flexure*) and continues transversely to the left (*transverse colon*) (Fig. 9.**21**). At the *left colic flexure* it curves downward and runs along the lateral abdominal wall as the *descending colon* (*left colon*). At the level of the left ilium the large intestine curves into an S-shaped segment (*sigmoid colon, sigmoid*), that runs into the true pelvis. At the level of the 2nd to 3rd sacral vertebra (see Fig. 9.**23**), the sigmoid colon continues into the *rectum*, which is about 15 cm long, and which ends at the *anus* below the anal canal. In contrast to the sigmoid, caecum and transverse colon, the rectum lies outside the peritoneal cavity, in the true pelvis (extraperitoneal). Consequently, it has no mesentery (mesocolon). Similarly, the

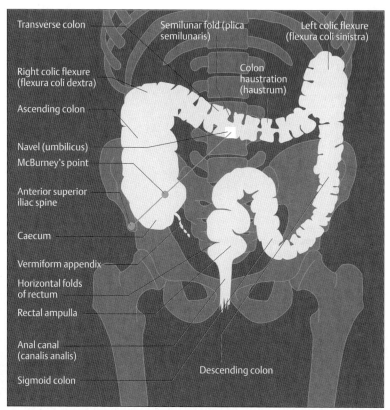

Fig. 9.21 Radiograph after a barium enema in the rectum and large intestine, anterior view. A square, radiopaque (i.e., white) marker overlies the umbilicus. McBurney's point, which lies one-third of the way from the anterior superior iliac spine to the umbilicus, is typically the most painful site in appendicitis

ascending and descending colon have no mesentery. They also lie outside the peritoneal cavity, but are retroperitoneal, i.e., they lie behind the peritoneum.

Externally, the large bowel is marked by a characteristic arrangement of longitudinal muscle bands, constrictions, sacculations, and fatty tags. The longitudinal muscular bands (*taeniae coli*) result from the tight bunching of the outer longitudinal muscle layer. They are divided into

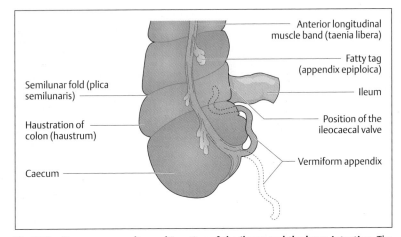

Anterior longitudinal
muscle band (taenia libera)

Fatty tag
(appendix epiploica)

Ileum

Position of the
ileocaecal valve

Vermiform appendix

Semilunar fold (plica
semilunaris)

Haustration of
colon (haustrum)

Caecum

Fig. 9.**22** **Caecum, appendix, and junction of the ileum and the large intestine.** The appendix lies behind the ileum; normal position shown by the broken line

the *taenia libera*, which can be seen along the whole length of the colon, and the *taeniae mesocolica* and *omentalis*, which are covered and so cannot be seen. Numerous fatty tags (*appendices epiploicae*) hang along the taeniae (Fig. 9.**22**). Contraction of the circular muscle layer forms numerous constrictions (*semilunar folds, plicae semilunares*) that project into the lumen of the large bowel. Between the semilunar folds, the intestinal wall bulges outward into pouches called *haustrations* (*haustra coli*) (Figs. 9.**21** and 9.**22**).

Mucosa of the Large Intestine

The mucosa of the large intestine is significantly less extended than that of the small intestine. There are no villi and the surface is enlarged only by deep depressions (*crypts of Lieberkühn*). The mucosal epithelium is composed overwhelmingly of mucus-secreting goblet cells and epithelial cells with a brush border, adapted to the extensive reabsorption of water. The mucosa includes numerous lymphatic follicles.

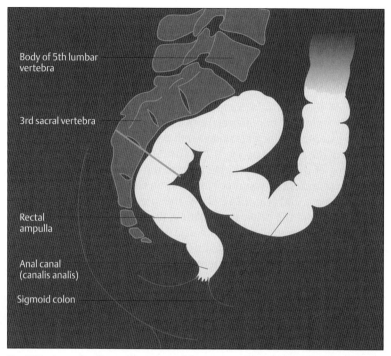

Body of 5th lumbar
vertebra

3rd sacral vertebra

Rectal
ampulla

Anal canal
(canalis analis)

Sigmoid colon

Fig. 9.**23**   **Lateral radiographic image of the rectum and sigmoid colon after contrast enema.** The junction of the sigmoid and rectum lies at the level of S3 (blue line)

Movements of the Large Bowel

The colon shows two types of movement: (1) Peristaltic waves, consisting of alternating contraction and relaxation of the circular and longitudinal muscular layers, run from the transverse colon in both directions and mix the contents. (2) By a few transporting movements in the direction of the rectum, the intestinal contents pass through the left colic flexure to reach the sigmoid colon and eventually the rectum. (mass movement). Evacuation begins with filling of the rectal ampulla (ampulla recti) (Figs. 9.**21** and 9.**23**). The rectal ampulla is a part of the rectum below the last right-hand horizontal fold (Figs. 9.**21** and 9.**24**), about 8 cm. above the anus. The horizontal fold is an orientation point during rectal examination (cancer prophylaxis).

Closure of the Anus

Closure of the anus is accomplished by two sphincters: the internal sphincter (*sphincter ani internus*) consisting of smooth muscle and the striated external sphincter (*sphincter ani externus*), as well as some of the muscles of the pelvic floor (Fig. 9.**24**). The internal sphincter consists of a thickening of the circular muscle layer of the large intestine, while the external sphincter has voluntary innervation and surrounds the internal sphincter like a cuff (Fig. 9.**24**). Above the internal and external sphincters lies a part of the pelvic musculature, the *m. puborectalis*, that forms an anterior loop around the rectum. The puborectalis is the most important of the sphincters, as injury to this muscle leads to rectal *incontinence* (inability to retain intestinal contents) more often than injury to either of the other sphincters.

Relations of the Peritoneum and Mesenteries of the Abdominal Organs

The *peritoneal cavity* is a space between serous membranes containing a scant amount of serous fluid (see Chapter 8: Serous Cavities and Membranes of the Chest and Abdomen). The organs of the peritoneal cavity fill it completely and are lined with the visceral layer of the peritoneum. These organs are often connected to the wall of the trunk by suspensory ligaments (e. g., mesentery of the small intestine, mesocolon, splenic ligaments; Fig. 9.**25**). These carry the nerves and vessels supplying the organs from connective tissue depots that lie outside the peritoneal cavity and are covered by the parietal layer of the peritoneum. At the origin of these ligaments the parietal layer of the peritoneum is reflected into the visceral layer (Figs. 9.**25a**, **b**). These organs are said to be intraperitoneal (e. g., stomach, liver, small intestine, caecum, appendix, transverse colon, sigmoid colon, and ovaries). Organs lying outside the peritoneal cavity are said to be *retroperitoneal* (e. g., kidneys, pancreas, parts of the duodenum, ascending colon, descending colon) when they are sit-

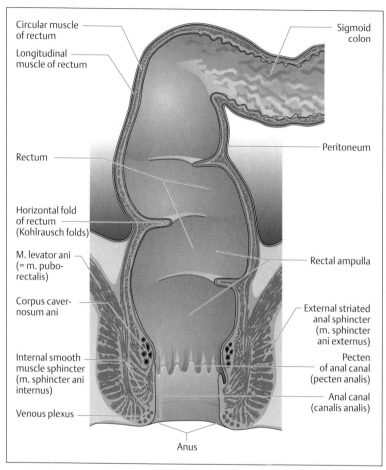

Fig. 9.**24 Coronal section through the rectum** (ventral view). (After Netter)

uated behind the peritoneum, and extraperitoneal when they lie in the true pelvis (e. g., rectum, urinary bladder, uterus, prostate) (Figs 9.**25a, b**). Organs lying outside the peritoneal cavity have no suspensory ligaments.

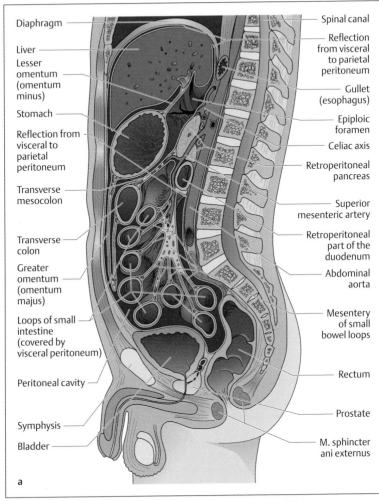

Diaphragm

Liver

Lesser
omentum
(omentum
minus)

Stomach

Reflection from
visceral to
parietal
peritoneum

Transverse
mesocolon

Transverse
colon

Greater
omentum
(omentum
majus)

Loops of small
intestine
(covered by
visceral peritoneum)

Peritoneal cavity

Symphysis

Bladder

Spinal canal

Reflection
from visceral
to parietal
peritoneum

Gullet
(esophagus)

Epiploic
foramen

Celiac axis

Retroperitoneal
pancreas

Superior
mesenteric artery

Retroperitoneal
part of the
duodenum

Abdominal
aorta

Mesentery
of small
bowel loops

Rectum

Prostate

M. sphincter
ani externus

a

Fig. 9.25 a, b   Diagrammatic representation of the relations of the peritoneum and the mesenteries of the abdominal and pelvic organs

a Sagittal section
b Transverse section at the level of the upper abdominal organs. (After Netter)

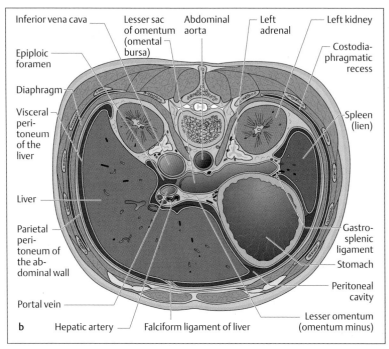

Fig. 9.**25 b**

The Pancreas

Function

The pancreas is the most important digestive gland. It is an exocrine gland (see Chapter 3: Glandular and Sensory Epithelia) and secretes about 2 liters of pancreatic juice a day. The endocrine islet apparatus secretes hormones that are instrumental in the regulation of the blood sugar level (see also Chapter 7: Islet Apparatus of the Pancreas). Pancreatic juice is alkaline, being remarkable for its high content of bicarbonate (HCO_3^- ions), which neutralizes the acid milieu of the duodenum. Pancreatic secretions contain numerous enzymes that digest fat (lipases; e. g., phospholipase A_2), proteins (proteases; e. g., trypsin, chymotrypsin), and carbohydrates (amylases). The enzymes reach the duodenum in the form of inactive precursors (e. g., trypsinogen) and are then activated.

The secretion and composition of pancreatic juice are regulated partly by the vagus, and partly especially by two mucosal hormones of the duodenum (*secretin* and *cholecystokinin* [*pancreozymin*]). Their secretion is triggered by fats and the low pH value of the chyme coming from the stomach.

Shape and Position

The pancreas lies behind the stomach at the level of L2. It is shaped like a horizontal wedge. The head of the pancreas lies in the C-shaped loop of the duodenum, and the body and tail of the pancreas reach the hilus of the spleen (see chapter 6: The spleen) in the left upper quadrant of the abdomen (Fig. 9.**26**). The pancreatic duct, about 2 mm thick, runs through the whole length of the gland and opens, often jointly with the common bile duct, at the duodenal papilla (sphincter of Oddi) into the

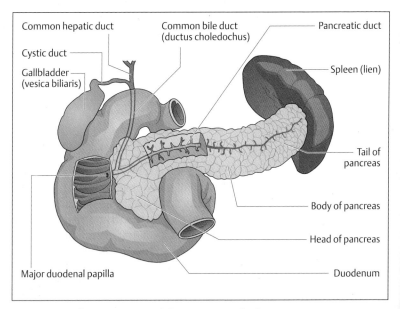

Fig. 9.**26**   **Duodenum, pancreas, bile passages, and spleen**

descending part of the duodenum (see above: Small Bowel, Shape and Position).

The Pancreatic Islets

The islets apparatus consisting of the islets of Langerhans forms the endocrine part of the pancreas (see Chapter 7: Islet Apparatus of the Pancreas).

The Liver (Hepar)

Function

The liver weighs 1500–2000 g and so is the largest gland in the human body. Because it secretes bile, it is an exocrine gland. The main components of bile are bile acids, which enable the absorption of fats in the intestine by emulsifying them. Bile pigments (e. g., bilirubin) are end products of hemoglobin formed during the breakdown of dead red blood cells. Numerous other substances (cholesterol, minerals) are excreted in the bile.

The liver is the largest metabolic organ and fulfills important functions in the metabolism of carbohydrates, proteins, and fats, as well as playing a part in detoxification. For this reason about 1.5 liters of blood flows into the liver through the *hepatic artery proper* every minute. Moreover, the nutrients absorbed in the intestine reach the *portal vein* and from there the liver through the portal circulation (see Chapter 5: The Venous System, Fig. 5.**26**). Within the liver, carbohydrates are stored as glycogen and are released again when needed. Fats and proteins are constantly transformed and broken down (e. g., fatty acid synthesis, amino acid breakdown, urea synthesis), and foreign substances such as medications or poisons are inactivated. The liver also takes part in the synthesis of numerous blood components (e. g., albumin, clotting factors).

Shape and Position

The liver lies in the right upper abdominal quadrant (Fig. 9.**1**), directly under the diaphragm, to which it is partly adherent (Figs. 9.**27a**, **b**).

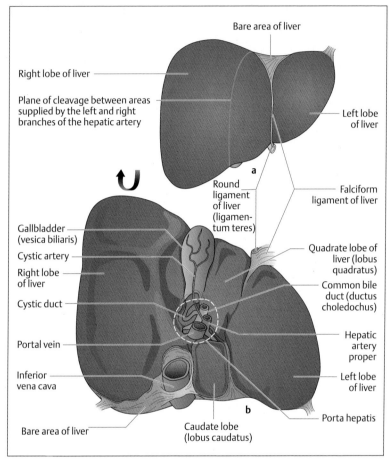

Bare area of liver

Right lobe of liver

Plane of cleavage between areas
supplied by the left and right
branches of the hepatic artery

Left lobe
of liver

a

Round
ligament
of liver
(ligamen-
tum teres)

Falciform
ligament of liver

Gallbladder
(vesica biliaris)

Cystic artery

Right lobe
of liver

Cystic duct

Quadrate lobe of
liver (lobus
quadratus)

Common bile
duct (ductus
choledochus)

Portal vein

Hepatic
artery
proper

Inferior
vena cava

Left lobe
of liver

b

Porta hepatis

Bare area of liver

Caudate lobe
(lobus caudatus)

Fig. 9.**27 a, b** **Anterior surface, visceral surface, and blood supply of the liver.** (After
Leonhardt)
a Liver viewed from in front
b Liver viewed from below (visceral surface)

Laterally, the lower border of the liver runs along the costal arch. The
right lobe of the liver extends to the anterior surface of the stomach. The
diaphragmatic surface of the right and left lobes of the liver is divided by

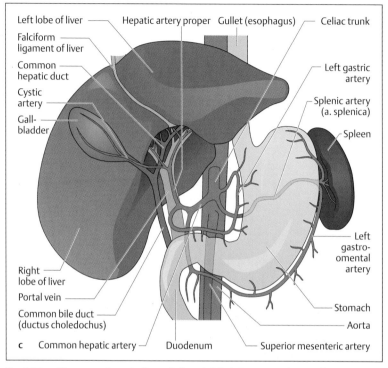

Fig. 9.**27 c   Liver seen from in front** (left and right lobes rotated upward)

a ligamentous structure (*falciform ligament*), which is attached to the inner surface of the abdominal wall. At its lower border runs the *round ligament* (*ligamentum teres*), which contains the remnant of what was once the fetal left umbilical vein (*vena umbilicalis sinistra*).

On the visceral surface of the liver (facing the intestines) lies the *porta hepatis* (liver gate), the entrance and exit of blood vessels (entering: portal veins, hepatic artery; exiting: bile duct, lymph vessels) and nerves. In front of the porta hepatis bulges the *quadrate lobe of the liver*, and behind it the caudate lobe (Fig. 9.**27b**). On the right side, the right lobe of the liver is bordered by a groove, in the front of which lies the gallbladder, while the inferior vena cava runs behind. To the left of the porta begins the left lobe of the liver, which functionally includes the quadrate and caudate lobes.

Fine Structure of the Liver

The dense capsule of the liver is covered by the peritoneum. Under it the blood vessels run in a delicate spongelike connective tissue framework. Hepatic tissue is subdivided into lobules about 1–2 mm in diameter (Figs. 9.**28a, b**). In cross-section they appear hexagonal with a *central vein* (Fig. 9.**28b**). Where several lobules adjoin there are connective tissue sheaths (Glisson's capsule), in each of which runs a branch of the portal vein, the hepatic artery and the biliary duct (*portal canals*). From the connective tissue capsules surrounding the lobules the epithelial cells of the liver (hepatocytes) are ordered in a stellate arrangement around the central vein. Between them run the tiny liver vessels called sinusoids, in which the peripheral blood runs to the central veins, which join the sublobular veins, which eventually drain into the hepatic veins. Finally, the blood flows through the hepatic veins into the inferior vena cava. The wall of the sinusoids consists of endothelial cells, which are lined by stellate Kupffer cells. These are immune cells with the capability of phagocytosis.

Drainage of the bile occurs in a direction opposite to the flow of blood, through the cholangioles (bile capillaries), which are dilated intercellular spaces between adjoining hepatocytes (Figs. 9.**28a, b**). They have no walls themselves and drain into the small biliary ductules of the portal canals. These join into larger ducts that transport the bile by way of the common hepatic duct into the cystic duct and the gallbladder (Fig. 9.**26**).

The Gallbladder (Vesica Biliaris) and Bile Duct

The gallbladder is a thin-walled pear-shaped sac with a capacity of about 30–35 ml. Its blood supply is the cystic artery, a branch of the hepatic artery proper (Fig. 9.**27b**). It lies on the visceral side of the liver and can be regarded as a reservoir for the bile (Fig. 9.**25b**). Bile is concentrated there (gallbladder bile) and when required released by way of the *cystic duct* into the common bile duct. The common bile duct formed by the

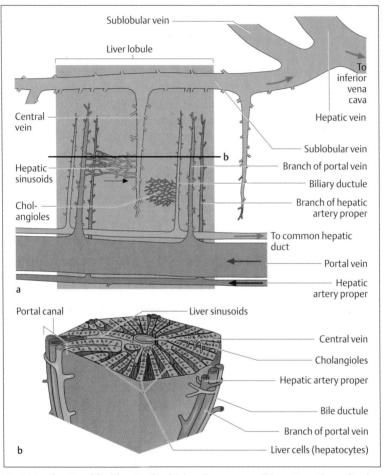

Fig. 9.**28 a, b** **Simplified longitudinal (a) and transverse (b) sections through a hepatic lobule.** Hepatic vessels and biliary passages are shown; the arrows represent the direction of flow

junction of the cystic duct and the common hepatic duct is also called the choledochous duct. The common bile duct is about 6–8 cm long and about the thickness of a pencil. It runs behind the duodenum in the direction of the head of the pancreas (Fig 9.**26**). In about 77 % of cases it joins the pancreatic duct and the ducts drain jointly into the major papilla of the duodenum (Fig. 9.**26**).

The muscle of the bile passages is smooth muscle. Just before its junction with the duodenum, the common duct has a circular sphincter (*sphincter of Oddi, m. sphincter ductus choledochi* and *m. sphincter ampullae hepatopancreticae*), that remains contracted during digestive quiescence, damming the bile back through the common duct into the gallbladder. The mouth of the bile duct opens shortly after food intake. Smooth muscle at the junction of the pancreatic duct as a rule prevents reflux of the bile into the pancreatic duct.

■ Overview of the Digestive Processes

Fat Digestion

Because fats are poorly soluble in water, the digestion and absorption of nutrient fats (lipids) presents some unique features (Fig. 9.**29**). Over 90 % of the fat ingested as food consists of neutral fats (triglycerides), while the remainder consists of cholesterol, cholesterol esters, phospholipids, and fat soluble vitamins. Before triglycerides can be absorbed in the small intestine, they must be split into free fatty acids and monoglycerides by fat-splitting enzymes called *lipases*. Together with a lipase formed in the palatine part of the tongue, fats reach the stomach, where 10–30 % of fats ingested with food are already split. The digestion of fats is continued in the duodenum and completed with the help of pancreatic lipase and phospholipase A_2.

For the fat-splitting enzymes to be presented with a large surface to attack, a prerequisite is emulsification of the fats (formation of small fat droplets in an aqueous milieu) by the bile acids formed in the liver and contained as bile salts in the bile. After enzymatic splitting of triglycerides, the split products (fatty acids, monoglycerides, cholesterol, phospholipids) form tiny globules called "*micelles*," which reach the epithelial cells of the small intestine by passive diffusion. These are partly transformed (by esterification, especially of the long-chain fatty acids and cholesterols) into *chylomicrons* (see Chapter 6: Plasma Proteins) in combination with phospholipids and proteins. These bypass the liver, reaching the thoracic duct and the bloodstream through the

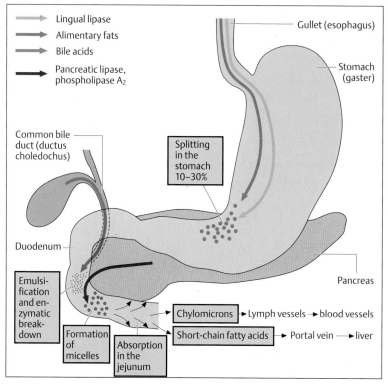

Fig. 9.**29**   **Diagrammatic representation of fat digestion**

lymph channels. From there the chylomicrons reach the tissues (e. g., muscle and adipose tissues) that take up the major part of the triglycerides. Short-chain fatty acids, on the other hand, pass through the portal vein and reach the liver directly to be metabolized there. The bile acids are also absorbed in the small intestine and reach the liver through the bloodstream, eventually passing back into the gallbladder (*enterohepatic circulation*). From there they are again passed into the small intestine with the bile.

Carbohydrate Digestion

The major part of the carbohydrates ingested in food consists of the polysaccharide starch. The remaining carbohydrates include animal glycogen, disaccharides such as sucrose (cane sugar) and lactose (milk sugar), and monosaccharides such as glucose (dextrose) and fructose (fruit sugar).

The digestion of carbohydrates begins in the mouth with the enzymatic splitting of starch into smaller fragments (oligosaccharides, disaccharides) by α-amylase (ptyalin) contained in saliva (Fig. 9.**30**). Admittedly this depends on the intensity of chewing and the consequent degree to which the food is mixed with saliva. In the small intestine, the

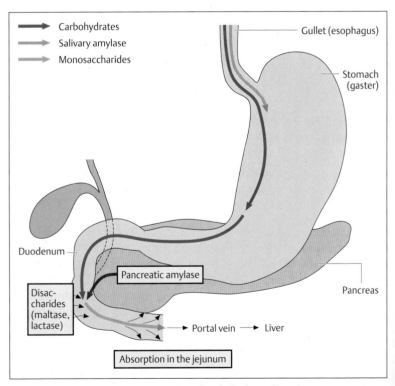

Fig. 9.**30** **Diagrammatic representation of carbohydrate digestion**

digestion of carbohydrates continues in the presence of another α-amylase (pancreatic amylase) as well as numerous other sugar-splitting enzymes (glycosidases, disaccharidases). After splitting by disaccharidases (e. g., maltase, lactase, saccharidase) the end products of carbohydrate digestion, the monsaccharides (e. g., glucose, galactose, fructose) are eventually absorbed by the epithelial cells of the small intestine by active and passive transport mechanisms. From there they reach the bloodstream and the liver (see The Liver, Function above). Often there is a deficiency of certain enzymes such as lactase, with the consequence that lactose cannot be split and so cannot be absorbed (*lactose intolerance*). This can lead to massive gas formation and diarrhea, since lactose retains water in the small intestine by osmosis.

Protein Digestion

In contrast to the digestion of fats and carbohydrates, the digestion of proteins does not begin until the food reaches the stomach (Fig. 9.**31**). The strongly acid gastric juices denature proteins, making them more suitable for processing by the protein-splitting gastric enzymes, which are formed as precursors (pepsinogen) in the chief cells of the stomach. The pepsinogens are transformed into active pepsin by the hydrochloric acid formed in the parietal cells. Pepsins, or endopeptidases, break down large protein molecules into smaller fragments (e. g., polypeptides, peptides).

When the fragments reach the neutral environment of the duodenum, they are further broken down by certain pancreatic enzymes (trypsin, chymotrypsin). These enzymes attack the polypeptide chains at their ends (exopeptidases) and split off dipeptides or tripeptides (small protein fragments with two or three amino acids). However, before individual amino acids or tripeptides or dipeptides can be taken up by the intestinal wall, other enzymes (carboxypeptidases, aminopeptidases) from the pancreas and the intestinal mucosa must split the greater part of the tripeptides and dipeptides into their respective amino acids. In contrast to the absorption of carbohydrates, dipeptide and tripeptide molecules and free amino acids are absorbed intact. Specific transport systems exist for dipeptides and tripeptides as well as the various amino acids (neutral, acid, and basic). They are

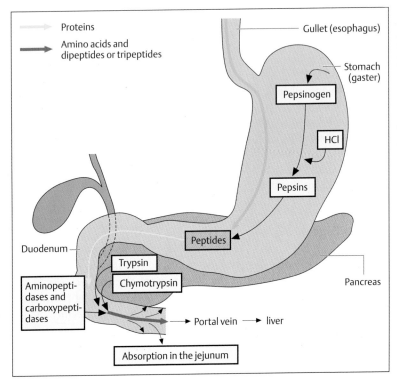

Fig. 9.**31** **Diagrammatic representation of protein digestion**

taken up actively into the epithelial cells of the small intestine and from there reach the bloodstream. About 10 % of the ingested proteins arrive undigested in the large intestine, where they are broken down by bacteria.

The Digestive System

■ Metabolism, Digestion, Energy Requirements

Nutrients (carbohydrates, proteins, fats) are split enzymatically in the various segments of the digestive tract into components that can be absorbed. They are then taken up by the mucous membrane of the small intestine. Through the bloodstream they reach the cells of the body, where in the presence of oxygen they undergo combustion in the mitochondria (biological oxidation). The energy liberated during this process is transmitted through a chain of reactions (mitochondrial respiratory pathway) to be stored in the form of the universal biological fuel ATP. From the mitochondria, ATP reaches the energy-consuming areas of the cell. ATP splits off phosphate molecules as required, liberating the stored energy.

- *Catabolism* or *metabolic degradation* (functional and energy metabolism): degradation of substances rich in energy into those with less energy (= dissimilation), e. g., biological oxidation, but also vital processes (e. g., muscular work, impulse conduction in nerve fibers etc.) requiring ATP (= hydrolysis of ATP).
- *Anabolism* or *metabolic synthesis* (constructive metabolism): synthesis of cellular substances; energy-consuming transformation of ingested foreign materials into endogenous substances (= assimilation).

Energy Equivalent (= Physiological Caloric Value) of the Most Important Nutrients

1 g carbohydrate:	4.2 kcal (17.6 kJ)
1 g fat:	9.3 kcal (38.9 kJ)
1 g protein:	4.1 kcal (17.2 kJ)

Energy Requirements of the Human Organism

- *Basal or resting metabolism:* the amount of energy required by the human body for maintenance of vital functions at complete rest in the morning, fasting, and at normal body and ambient temperature. For adult men, 1 kcal/kg body weight/hour: 70 kg body weight ≡ 1700 kcal/day. For women, 10–20 % less.
- *Leisure metabolism:* energy metabolism during average leisure activity, i.e., without much movement: about 2300 kcal/day.

- *Work metabolism:* energy requirement during physical labor; exceeds leisure metabolism to varying degrees.

The respiratory quotient ($RQ = CO_2$ production/O_2 consumption) provides information about the type of foodstuff metabolized: carbohydrate diet, $RQ = 1$; mixed diet, $RQ = 0.85$; fatty diet, $RQ = 0.7$.

■ Dietary Components

- *Proteins:* should make up about 15% of the daily energy requirement. They supply amino acids (for biosynthesis of endogenous proteins); of the 20 amino acids occurring in protein, 8 are essential (cannot be synthesized in the body). Other than lysine (which is not present in many vegetable foodstuffs), all the essential amino acids are present in vegetable and animal foodstuffs.
- *Fats:* should make up about 30% of the daily energy requirement. They supply and store energy, and supply cholesterol (cell membranes, precursors of sex hormones), essential fatty acids (in vegetable oils: linoleic acid, α-linolenic acid (components of membrane lipds). Intake usually includes more animal fats (mainly saturated fats) than vegetable fats (mainly unsaturated fats).
- *Carbohydrates:* should make up about 55% of the daily energy requirement. They are the most important source of energy: monosaccharides (glucose), disaccharides (cane sugar), and polysaccharides (starch). Simple sugars are "empty calories" and overload the pancreas, because the blood sugar rises rapidly to high levels. Whole-wheat products are better (starch + vitamins + fiber).
- *Vitamins:* cannot be synthesized by the body (exception: vitamin D_3). They do not supply energy and are not structural material but rather biocatalysts. They are classified into fat-soluble (A, D, E, K) and water-soluble (C, B_1, B_2, B_3, B_5, B_6, folic acid, B_{12}, biotin, and inositol) vitamins. Function: B vitamins and vitamin K are components of coenzymes for carbohydrate, fat, and protein metabolism (phylogenetically old, because they are indispensable for every cell), while vitamins A, D, E, and C are necessary to maintain certain organ functions (phylogenetically younger, demonstrable only in higher invertebrates; vitamin D only in vertebrates).
- *Minerals and trace elements:* vital inorganic substances that are not metabolized. Trace elements = minerals with a daily requirement

of <100 mg (chromium, iron, fluorine, germanium, iodine, cobalt, copper, manganese, molybdenum, nickel, selenium, silicon, vanadium, zinc, tin; total weight in the body is 8–9 g, of which iron comprises 4–5 g). Minerals (macroelements) = minerals of which the daily requirement is >100 mg (calcium, magnesium, phosphorus, sodium, potassium, chlorine, sulfur). Calcium is present in the largest proportion in the body at 1.5 kg (99% in the skeleton).

- *Antioxidants (free radical scavengers):* vitamins A (β-carotene), E, and C as well as the trace elements selenium, manganese, zinc, and molybdenum inactivate free radicals (highly reactive unstable molecules with unpaired electrons) that are metabolic by-products. Radicals are formed in the body during all reactions involving oxygen, but are reinforced by noxious substances and UV and radioactive radiation. The consequences might include malformed cells (cancer), arteriosclerosis, premature aging.

- *Active substances in plants:* chemical compounds that protect plants and humans from damaging environmental influences. Every plant contains several thousand active substances, most of which have not yet been studied and which might be active only in combination with each other.

- *Fiber:* indigestible vegetable carbohydrates that stimulate intestinal activity and increase the sensation of satiety.

■ The Digestive Organs

Divided into those of the head (oral cavity with salivary glands, oropharynx, and hypopharynx) and those of the trunk (esophagus; stomach; small bowel = duodenum + jejunum + ileum; large bowel = caecum + appendix + ascending, transverse, descending, and sigmoid colon + rectum; liver; pancreas).

The Oral Cavity

Ends posteriorly in the oropharyngeal isthmus (palatal arches with uvula). Function: to take up food and divide it into smaller pieces, and add saliva.

- *The tongue:* muscular transporting organ; assists in chewing and sucking. The dorsum of the tongue carries sensory organs (papillae) for touch, pressure, temperature, and pain sensation, and taste papillae for sour, salty, bitter, and sweet.

- *The teeth:* second dentition of 32 permanent teeth—8 incisors (cutters), 4 canines (tear and retain), 8 premolars (chew and grind), 12 molars (chew and grind). Dental formula for each half of each jaw: $I^2/2 \; C^1/1 \; P^2/2 \; M^3/3$. Milk teeth (first dentition) has 20 teeth—8 incisors, 4 canines, 8 milk molars. Structure of tooth: crown (above the gum; coated with enamel), root (in the alveolus; coated with cementum), and neck (transition from enamel to cementum). Cementum and enamel cover the dentine. The dental cavity with the dental pulp lies inside the tooth. Vessels and nerves reach the dental cavity through the root canal. The junction of dentine and pulp is lined with odontoblasts.
- *Salivary glands:* exocrine glands; they produce 1–1.5 liters of saliva/day. Function: increase lubrication of food after chewing, initiate splitting of carbohydrates (amylase). They are divided into bilateral small (in the mucosa of the lips, cheeks, tongue, and palate) and large salivary glands (parotid, submandibular, and sublingual glands), with ducts draining into the oral cavity.

The Pharynx

Part common to the digestive and respiratory tracts: nasopharynx (junction with the nasal cavity), oropharynx (junction with the oral cavity; crossing of the respiratory and digestive pathways), and hypopharynx (junction of the laryngeal opening and esophagus). At the junction of the nasal and oral cavities: tonsils of Waldeyer's tonsillar ring (midline pharyngeal tonsils [adenoids], palatine tonsils, midline lingual tonsils, lymphatic tissue of the lateral pharyngeal wall). During swallowing, the larynx is closed by the epiglottis (producing a momentary respiratory pause), so that no food can reach the larynx. The initiation of the act of swallowing (contraction of the floor of the mouth) is voluntary. This triggers the swallowing reflex (involuntary, coordinated by the swallowing center of the medulla).

The Esophagus

Function: moves the food from pharynx to stomach by peristalsis; length: 25–30 cm. Cervical and thoracic parts run behind the trachea. After piercing the diaphragm (esophageal hiatus), it enters the abdomen and opens into the stomach. Large boluses can become wedged in the esophageal constrictions (cricoid cartilage, aortic arch, esophageal hiatus) and cause pain.

The Stomach

Lies directly under the diaphragm; volume about 1200–1600 ml. It is divided into inlet (cardia: esophagus → stomach), fundus, body, pyloric antrum, and pylorus (circular sphincter muscle: stomach → duodenum). Function: chemical maceration and liquefaction of the food by gastric juice (pH 1.5; 2–3 l/day; water, mucus, pepsin, hydrochloric acid). Its secretion is triggered by sensory input (vagus nerve) and by entry of food into the stomach stimulating secretion of tissue hormones from the gastric mucosa (gastrin). Tissue hormones from the duodenal mucosa also inhibit (secretin) or stimulate (gastrin) secretion of gastric juice as needed. The gastric mucosa forms longitudinal folds. Several gastric glands drain into punctiform pits in the folds, where their cells secrete hydrochloric acid (parietal cells) and pepsinogen (chief cells). The necks of the glands contain neck cells that produce mucus (protection against autodigestion). In contrast to the rest of the gastrointestinal tract (circular and longitudinal muscle layers), the wall of the stomach is made up of three muscle layers (additional inner oblique muscle layer for kneading movements).

The Small Intestine

Total length 3–5 m; divided into duodenum (25–30 cm, begins distal to the pylorus), jejunum, and ileum. Function: degradation by pancreatic enzymes of food into compounds that can be absorbed (e. g., glucose, amino acids, fatty acids), and absorption of nutrients. Food is moved by peristalsis (alternating contraction and relaxation of longitudinal and circular muscle). To facilitate absorption, the mucosa of the small bowel (especially the jejunum) includes folds (Kerckring's folds), villi (projections on the folds), and crypts (crypts of Lieberkühn = depressions between the villi). The villi are lined by simple columnar absorbing epithelial cells with microvilli (total absorbent surface formed by all the surface extensions: 120 m^2) and mucus-forming goblet cells. Each villus contains a network of capillaries by which the nutrients reach the bloodstream, a central lymph vessel (removal of chylomicrons), and the arteriole and venule supplying the villus. The mucosa also contains collections of lymphoid follicles (especially dense in the mucosa of the appendix and the ileum = Peyer's patches): part of specific immunity.

The Large Intestine

Total length 1.5–1.8 m; ileocecal valve at junction of ileum and large bowel. Large bowel is divided into caecum (outpouching below the ileocecal valve), vermiform appendix (specific immunity), colon (four segments: ascending, transverse, descending, and sigmoid colon), and rectum (15 cm with ampulla, anal canal, and anus = distal end of gastrointestinal tract). Function: reabsorption of salt and water (the mucosa therefore consists mainly of mucus-forming goblet cells; surface extension only by crypts) and decomposition of indigestible food remnants by bacteria. External appearance of the large bowel: longitudinal muscle (taeniae) as well as constrictions and sacculations (by contraction of the circular muscle). The intestinal content is mixed and moved toward the rectum by alternating contraction and relaxation of the longitudinal and circular muscle. Closure of the anal canal: internal smooth muscle (= involuntary) and external striated (= voluntary) sphincter and the puborectalis muscle (most important muscle for closure, part of the musculature of the pelvic floor).

The Pancreas

Consists of head, body, and tail of the pancreas. The head is surrounded by the duodenum, into which drains the pancreatic duct (usually together with the common bile duct). The pancreas lies behind the stomach and is an exocrine gland secreting ca. 2 liters of alkaline (high bicarbonate content) pancreatic juice a day. The juice contains the most important digestive enzymes: lipases (fat), proteases (proteins), amylases (carbohydrates). Secretion is regulated by sensory input (vagus nerve) and the food itself (tissue hormones secretin and pancreozymin/cholecystokinin). The endocrine activity of the islet apparatus secretes insulin and glucagon (regulation of blood sugar).

The Liver

Lies directly under the diaphragm, to which it is partially adherent. Divided into left and right lobes (division on the surface by the falciform ligament) and two smaller lobes, the quadrate and caudate, both on the visceral side. In the visceral area of the right hepatic lobe the vessels and nerves enter and exit (porta hepatis): portal vein, hepatic artery proper (enter); bile duct (exits); lymph vessels and nerves (enter and exit). Weight: 1500–2000 g. Function: exocrine gland (secretes bile: bile salts for the emulsification of fats); the largest metabolic and detoxifying organ (nutrients absorbed in the intestines reach the liver through the portal vein). The liver is subdivided into hexagonal liver lobules (diameter 1–2 mm) (structure: hepatic epithelial cells, central vein, hepatic sinusoids, cholangioles), between which lie the portal canals, each with a branch of the portal vein and the hepatic artery as well as a biliary ductule. Blood flows through the portal vein into the central veins of the hepatic lobules, leaves the liver through the hepatic veins, and eventually drains into the inferior vena cava. The secreted bile flows through the biliary ductules to the common hepatic duct and the cystic duct into the gallbladder.

The Gallbladder

The reservoir for the bile (30–50 ml). When needed, the concentrated gallbladder bile is transported back through the cystic duct and the common bile duct (choledochous duct) to the duodenum at the head of the pancreas (usually together with the pancreatic duct). During digestive quiescence, bile flow into the duodenum is prevented (sphincter at the distal end of the common bile duct).

■ Digestive Processes
Fat Digestion

Splitting of fats begins in the stomach (10–30%) by lipase from the palatine part of the tongue, followed by emulsification (bile acids) and enzymatic splitting by pancreatic lipase and phospholipase A_2 in the duodenum. Fatty acids, monoglycerides, cholesterol, and phospholipids are absorbed in the form of fat droplets (micelles) by the mucosa of the small intestine, where the individual components together with proteins are immediately transformed in part into chylomicrons (mode of transportation of alimentary fats to the cells of the body). These bypass the liver and reach the blood by lymphatic pathways. Only short-chain fatty acids reach the bloodstream directly and are carried by the portal vein to the liver and thence to the cells of the body.

Carbohydrate Digestion

The splitting of carbohydrates begins in the mouth with salivary amylase (starch → oligosaccharides, disaccharides). In the small intestine there is further splitting by pancreatic amylase, as well as by glycosidases and disaccharidases from the mucosa of the small intestine, into monsaccharides (e. g., glucose, fructose). Absorption is by the mucosa of the small intestine and from there into the bloodstream, through the portal vein into the liver, and eventually into the cells of the body.

Protein Digestion

Begins only in the stomach. Proteins are denatured by acid gastric juice and split by pepsin (pepsinogen from the chief cells of the gastric glands → pepsin by the action of hydrochloric acid from the parietal cells) into polypeptides and peptides. In the duodenum (neutral milieu) there is further cleavage by trypsin and chymotrypsin (pancreas) into tripeptides and dipeptides, part of which are absorbed. Carboxypeptidases and aminopeptidases (pancreas, mucosa of the small intestine) continue cleavage into amino acids, which are also absorbed (active transport systems), enter the bloodstream, and reach the cells of the body through the portal vein and the liver.

10

The Kidneys and Urinary Tract

Contents

The ducts of the urinary and genital organs (urogenital organs) are closely associated during development. By its embryology, the *urogenital system* can therefore be divided into two parts:

- **The kidneys and urinary tract (urinary system)**
- **The genital system**

Both systems develop from the middle germ layer, the mesoderm (p. 518), and during embryonic development both systems drain initially into a common cavity, the cloaca.

■ Role of the Kidneys

The kidneys have the task of preparing urine, in which toxic metabolic products (waste products) and water are eliminated. This mechanism regulates the internal milieu of the tissues, balances fluid metabolism, and keeps the hydrogen ion concentration constant (maintaining blood pH). Specifically, the kidney has the following roles:

- Elimination of metabolic products and toxic substances (e. g., the products of protein breakdown such as urea and uric acid, or medications)
- Maintenance of electrolyte concentration (e. g., sodium and potassium salts), regulation of acid–base balance, water balance, and the osmotic pressure of body fluids
- Playing a part in regulating the circulation and forming blood by producing hormone-like substances (e. g., renin, erythropoietin)

■ Overview of Structure and Function of the Kidneys

With a 20% share of the cardiac output (CO) (corresponding to a blood flow of about 1.2 liters a minute when CO is 5–6 l/min; see Chapter 5: Cardiac Output), the daily perfusion of the kidneys amounts to about 1700 liters of blood. Each kidney consists essentially of about 1.2 million microscopic structural elements, the *nephrons*, each of which can produce urine. The nephron is therefore the functional unit of the kidney and mirrors the activity of the whole kidney. Each nephron consists of a *renal corpuscle* (*malpighian corpuscle*) and its *renal tubule* (see Fig. 10.**6**). The renal corpuscle consists of capillary tufts (glomerulus), surrounded by the proximal portion of the renal tubule (see Fig. 10.**5a**). This forms a double-walled cup (*Bowman's capsule*) with a capsular space into which the *glomerular filtrate* is secreted. Glomerular filtrate is an ultrafiltrate of the blood plasma and, except for proteins, contains dissolved substances in about the same concentration as that of the plasma. Subsequently, certain substances (e. g., inorganic and organic ions, glucose, amino acids, small protein molecules, vitamins) are reabsorbed from the glomerular filtrate (about 170 liters a day) together with water. Essentially this happens while the glomerular filtrate flows through the various segments of the renal tubules. Several hundred renal tubules drain into a common *collecting duct*. Here, after concentration to about 1 % of the original urinary volume, the definitive *urine* (about 1.5 liters a day) is formed. The collecting ducts channel the urine through the renal papillae into the renal pelvis, from where it is voided through the urinary tract (ureter, urinary bladder, urethra).

■ The Kidney (Ren, Nephros)

Shape and Position

The kidneys are shaped like beans and are about 10 cm long, 5 cm wide, and 4 cm thick. They have an upper and a lower *pole* and a medial and a lateral margin. They weigh between 120 and 300 g and lie in the lumbar region in a connective tissue space behind the abdominal cavity (retroperitoneal space, see also Chapter 9: Relations of the Peritoneum and Mesenteries of the Organs, and Fig. 9.**25b**) on each side of the vertebral column (Fig. 10.**2a**, **b**). The right kidney lies below the liver, the left below the spleen. In most people the upper pole of the right kidney lies about half a vertebra lower than that of the left. The side facing the vertebral column is notched and contains the hilus, through which the blood vessels, nerves, and renal pelvis enter and leave (Fig. 10.**1**).

Each kidney is surrounded by a fatty capsule (adipose capsule) and is sheathed in a connective tissue sac (renal fascia). Both make it possible for the kidney to move in its site. If the fatty tissue (storage fat) shrinks

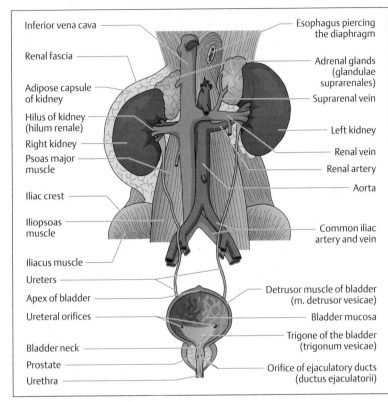

Inferior vena cava

Renal fascia

Adipose capsule
of kidney

Hilus of kidney
(hilum renale)

Right kidney

Psoas major
muscle

Iliac crest

Iliopsoas
muscle

Iliacus muscle

Ureters

Apex of bladder

Ureteral orifices

Bladder neck

Prostate

Urethra

Esophagus piercing
the diaphragm

Adrenal glands
(glandulae
suprarenales)

Suprarenal vein

Left kidney

Renal vein

Renal artery

Aorta

Common iliac
artery and vein

Detrusor muscle of bladder
(m. detrusor vesicae)

Bladder mucosa

Trigone of the bladder
(trigonum vesicae)

Orifice of ejaculatory ducts
(ductus ejaculatorii)

Fig. 10.**1** **The male urinary organs**

during starvation, the mobility of the kidney increases. The upper pole of
each kidney is capped by an adrenal gland, which is also enclosed in the
fatty capsule (Fig. 10.**1**).

Fig. 10.**2 a, b** **Position of the kidneys** ▷
a Projection of the kidneys on the posterior abdominal wall
b Horizontal section at the level of the kidneys (plane of section shown in **a**). The axes of
the two kidneys meet in a right angle (R) in front of the spinal column. The black arrows mark the inferior lumbar triangle (trigonum lumbale). (After Frick, Leonhardt,
and Stark)

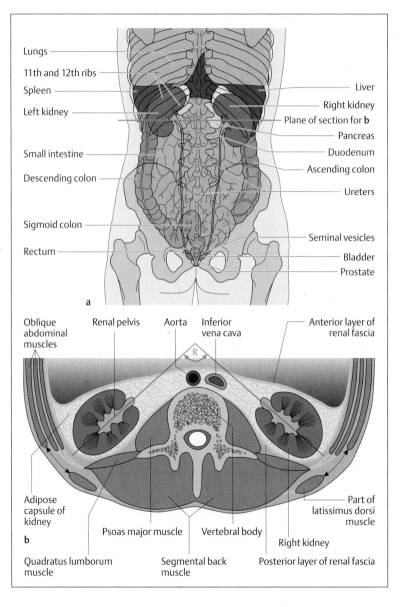

a

Lungs
11th and 12th ribs
Spleen
Left kidney
Small intestine
Descending colon
Sigmoid colon
Rectum

Liver
Right kidney
Plane of section for **b**
Pancreas
Duodenum
Ascending colon
Ureters
Seminal vesicles
Bladder
Prostate

b

Oblique abdominal muscles
Renal pelvis
Aorta
Inferior vena cava
Anterior layer of renal fascia

Adipose capsule of kidney
Psoas major muscle
Vertebral body
Part of latissimus dorsi muscle
Right kidney

Quadratus lumborum muscle
Segmental back muscle
Posterior layer of renal fascia

Renal Cortex and Renal Medulla

A longitudinal section through the kidney reveals the division of the kidney tissue into renal cortex and renal medulla, which can be seen with the naked eye. The cortex is a dark red stripe, about 8 mm wide, lying directly under the capsule of the organ (Fig. 10.**3**). The color of the cortex can be seen with a lens to be due to the numerous small renal corpuscles, each containing a *capillary tuft* (*glomerulus*). The proximal and distal ends of the renal tubules, parts of the nephron not visible to the naked eye, lie in the cortex, while their long descending and ascending segments reach in part deep into the medulla (Fig. 10.**4**).

The renal cortex borders on the renal medulla, which is formed by 10–12 *renal pyramids*. The broad base of a pyramid is directed toward the cortex and they run from there in medullary rays (bundles of collecting ducts). Between the renal pyramids, columns of cortex penetrate deep

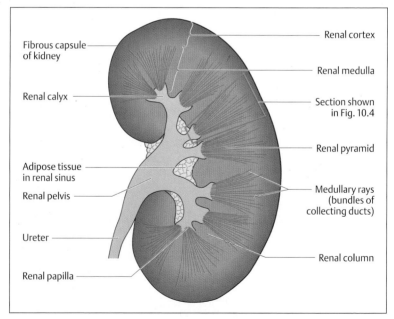

Fibrous capsule of kidney

Renal calyx

Adipose tissue in renal sinus

Renal pelvis

Ureter

Renal papilla

Renal cortex

Renal medulla

Section shown in Fig. 10.4

Renal pyramid

Medullary rays (bundles of collecting ducts)

Renal column

Fig. 10.**3**   **Simplified median section through a kidney**

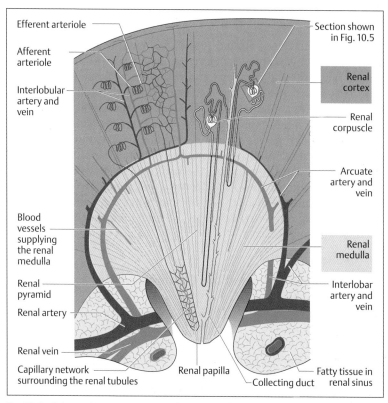

Efferent arteriole

Afferent arteriole

Interlobular artery and vein

Blood vessels supplying the renal medulla

Renal pyramid

Renal artery

Renal vein

Capillary network surrounding the renal tubules

Section shown in Fig. 10.5

Renal cortex

Renal corpuscle

Arcuate artery and vein

Renal medulla

Interlobar artery and vein

Fatty tissue in renal sinus

Collecting duct

Renal papilla

Fig. 10.**4** **Schematic representation of a prepared section of the blood vessels of the kidney.** (After Leonhardt.) Section from Fig. 10.**3**

into the medulla (Fig. 10.**3**). The apices of the pyramids form the renal papillae, into which drain the collecting ducts. The renal papillae drain into the renal calices, which together form a large part of the renal pelvis. Between the calyces lies loose areolar and fatty tissue (*renal sinus*), which contains the renal vessels.

The Renal Vessels

About 20% of the blood ejected by the heart into the aorta is channeled to the kidneys by the two *renal arteries* (*aa. renales*). At the hilus of the kidney (Fig. 10.**1**) the renal artery divides into 5–6 interlobar arteries (Fig. 10.**4**), which give rise to the *arcuate arteries* that run in an arc between the cortex and the medulla. The arcuate arteries give off branches (interlobular arteries) that enter the cortex and at regular intervals give rise to arterioles (*afferent arterioles*), which bring blood to the capillary tufts of the glomeruli. Other arterioles (*efferent arterioles*) lead blood away from the capillary tufts into a second capillary network that in part runs toward the renal medulla and forms a web around the renal tubules (Fig. 10.**4**). Finally, the blood collects in small veins that drain through the *arcuate veins* into the *interlobar veins* and from there into the *renal veins* and the inferior vena cava.

The Renal Corpuscles and the Glomerular Filter

Apart from its blood vessels, the kidney possesses a system of tubules that consists of nephrons and collecting ducts. *Nephrons form the structural and functional units of the kidney* and consist of a *renal corpuscle* (*malpighian body*) and its associated *renal tubule* (Figs. 10.**4** and 10.**6**). The ca. 2.4 million renal corpuscles of the two kidneys lie in the renal cortex (Fig. 10.**4**) and contain the glomerular filter, which filters the glomerular filtrate from the blood. Urine is formed in the renal tubules by about 90% reabsorption of the glomerular filtrate. The definitive concentration takes place in the collecting ducts that channel the urine into the renal pelvis.

Each renal corpuscle has a *vascular pole* and a *urinary pole* (Fig. 10.**5a**). At the vascular pole the proximal end of the renal tubule forms a blind sac that is invaginated by about 30 capillary loops (glomerulus), resulting in a double-walled cup (*Bowman's capsule*). The space between the two walls receives the glomerular filtrate and channels it into the efferent renal tubule at the urinary pole (Fig. 10.**5a**). The glomerular filtration barrier measures about 1 m^2 in total and is essentially composed of three layers:

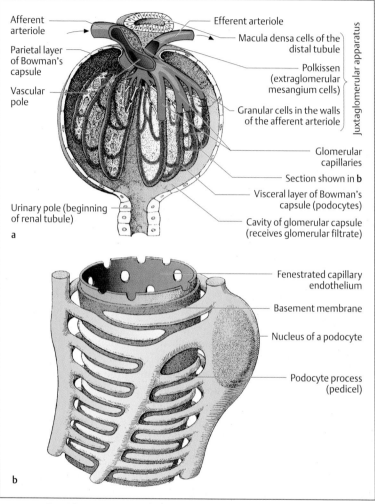

Afferent arteriole

Parietal layer of Bowman's capsule

Vascular pole

Urinary pole (beginning of renal tubule)

a

Efferent arteriole

Macula densa cells of the distal tubule

Polkissen (extraglomerular mesangium cells)

Granular cells in the walls of the afferent arteriole

Juxtaglomerular apparatus

Glomerular capillaries

Section shown in b

Visceral layer of Bowman's capsule (podocytes)

Cavity of glomerular capsule (receives glomerular filtrate)

Fenestrated capillary endothelium

Basement membrane

Nucleus of a podocyte

Podocyte process (pedicel)

b

Fig. 10.**5 a, b**   **Schematic representation of a renal corpuscle and structure of the glomerular filter**
a   Renal corpuscle; the section indicated by the blue box is magnified in **b**
b   Glomerular filter. (After Leonhardt.). Section from **a**

- The capillary endothelium
- The cells forming the visceral (inner) wall of Bowman's capsule (podocytes)
- The basement membrane common to the endothelial cells and the podocytes

Of these three layers, the *basement membrane* and the *podocytes* are especially important (Fig. 10.**5b**). While the basement membrane resembles a thick felt of collagen and glycoproteins, the podocytes with their multiple interdigitating processes (pedicels) form the so-called *slit-pores*, which allow particles only up to a certain size to pass. The glomerular filter is cleaned by the podocytes and the mesangium cells (lacis cells) (Fig. 10.**5a**), which lie between the capillaries and remove (phagocytose) the used-up basement membrane, for example. It is likely that the podocytes and endothelial cells continually renew the substance of the basement membrane.

Properties of the Glomerular Filter

Filtration through the glomerular filter is a passive process and therefore depends essentially on the arterial blood pressure, the properties of the filter, and the properties of the filtered molecules. The glomerular filter acts like a sieve, and the size of its pores determines its permeability to molecules of different sizes (mechanical filter). Hence, water and substances with small molecules (e. g., urea, glucose, salts, amino acids, sodium chloride) can pass through the filter unhindered, while large protein molecules (albumins and globulins) as well as blood cells (e. g., red blood cells) do not normally penetrate. Since the glomerular filtration barrier, especially the basement membrane, carries many negative charges (glycoproteins), it provides an *electrical* as well as a *mechanical filter*. This retains negatively charged molecules more effectively than those that are positively charged.

Glomerular Filtration

Glomerular Filtration Rate

The glomerular filtration rate (GFR) is the volume of fluid filtered per unit time by all the glomeruli. *It is a measure of the ability of the kidney to excrete* and amounts to about 120 ml per minute. From the renal plasma flow (RPF), i.e., the volume of plasma perfusing the kidney each minute (about 600 ml at a hematocrit of 50), it can be calculated that the glomerular filtrate (about 180 l/day) is about 20% of the plasma volume (GFR/RPF = 0.2).

Since the extracellular, i.e., exchangeable, fluid volume of a 70 kg person amounts to about 14–15 liters (see Chapter 1: Exchange of Materials between the Cell and Its Environment), the extracellular fluid passes through the glomerular filter 10 times a day, the plasma volume (about 3 liters) as much as 60 times(!) a day.

Effective Filtration Pressure

The glomerular filtration rate depends on an effective filtration pressure and the *glomerular filtration surface*. The driving force for the process of filtration is the *blood pressure in the capillary tufts* of the glomerulus, which is about 48 mmHg. However, the effectiveness of this blood pressure is reduced because it is opposed by the protein pressure (colloid osmotic pressure) of about 20 mmHg and the hydrostatic pressure in Bowman's capsule of about 13 mmHg. The effective filtration pressure can be calculated as follows:

- **Effective filtration pressure = 48 – 20 – 13 = 15 mmHg**

The blood pressure does not diminish materially toward the end of the glomerular capillary, but the colloid osmotic pressure rises considerably during passage through the glomerulus, since the concentration of plasma proteins increases as the ultrafiltrate leaves the plasma. It is therefore assumed that the colloid pressure rises to 35 mmHg even before the end of the capillary, so that the effective filtration pressure is reduced to zero (48 – 35 – 13 = 0). This is the *point of filtration balance.*

With an increase in renal blood flow, the site of this filtration balance shifts toward the distal end of the capillary, and this shift increases the filtration surface. Hence, with increased blood flow the amount of fluid filtered and with it the filtration rate also increases.

Autoregulation of Renal Blood Flow

Certain mechanisms allow the kidney to maintain a constant glomerular filtration rate, even with considerable swings in blood pressure. This regulation usually functions very well between blood pressures of 80–200 mmHg. On the other hand, if blood pressure falls below 80 mmHg, renal perfusion falls rapidly and filtration fails (acute renal failure).

Renal Tubules and Collecting Ducts

The renal tubule is a small tube, a few centimeters long, unbranched and consisting of a single epithelial coat, beginning at the urinary pole of the renal corpuscle (Figs. 10.**5a** and 10.**6**). It consists of convoluted and straight segments, and the whole tubule is surrounded by a network of blood vessels in its entire course:

- A proximal tubule, initially convoluted, then straight
- A thin transition (Henle's loop)
- A distal tubule, initially straight, then convoluted
- A short initial collecting tubule (junctional tubule)

While the convoluted tubules are found mainly in the cortex, the straight segments of the tubules as well as Henle's loop run into the medulla. The collecting tubules join the tubule to the system of collecting ducts. The collecting ducts drain into the renal pelvis in tiny openings at the apex of the renal papillae (see Renal Cortex and Renal Medulla above, and Fig. 10.**4**).

Transport Processes in the Renal Tubules

The walls of the renal tubules and the collecting ducts consist of epithelial cells that allow transport through the cells (transcellular) and between the cells (paracellular). Since the epithelial cells in the various segments have different functions, the glomerular filtrate is altered fundamentally during its passage through the several segments of the tubules. During this process the major portion of the dissolved components (e. g., inorganic and organic ions, glucose, amino acids) and 99 %

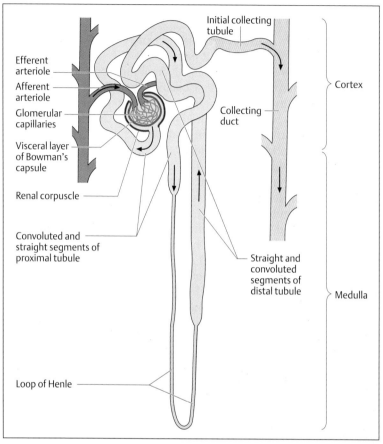

Fig. 10.**6**   **Nephron (functional unit of the kidney)**

of the water are reabsorbed, partly actively, partly passively; i.e., these substances are passed into the capillaries surrounding the tubules and so returned to the circulation. On the other hand, numerous substances (H^+ ions, uric acid, urea, creatinine, certain drugs such as penicillin, etc.) are secreted actively from the extracellular space into the lumen of the tubule.

The Na⁺−K⁺ pump (Na⁺,K⁺-ATPase)

Active and passive transport processes are often closely connected; for example, in the regulation of salt balance. For instance, the Na^+ ions of sodium chloride are reabsorbed actively from the tubule in exchange for H^+ ions (regulation of the acid–base balance by the kidney). To maintain electrical neutrality, Cl^- ions follow passively, together with water to maintain osmotic balance and additional sodium chloride dissolved in water. The necessary concentration gradient for sodium is maintained by what is called the Na^+−K^+ pump, located in the basement membrane of the tubule's epithelial cells, that transports Na^+ ions continuously from the cell back into the bloodstream with the aid of ATP. This mechanism creates a Na^+ gradient, which forms the basis for diffusion of Na^+ from the lumen of the tubule into the cell. The surface in the proximal tubule is greatly increased (presence of microvilli on the cell membrane of the lumen), and this location allows the reabsorption of large quantities of salt and water. *The active transport of NaCl is therefore the driving mechanism for the concentrating ability of the kidney.*

Of the 1.3 kg of sodium chloride normally contained in 180 liters of glomerular filtrate, only as much must ultimately be excreted as we ingest daily with our food, i.e., about 8–15 g, no more, no less. The kidney balances the Na^+ excretion with the daily salt intake. By this means, the Na^+ concentration and with it the extracellular fluid volume are kept relatively constant. This requires that about 99 % of common salt must be reabsorbed from the glomerular filtrate, more for a salt-restricted diet.

The kidney accomplishes this in what may be considered a two-step process: 90 % of sodium chloride and about 60–70 % of the filtered water are reabsorbed in the proximal convoluted tubule and the loop of Henle. The fine-tuning of sodium reabsorption is accomplished in the distal tubule, with the aid of the enzyme renin, which is formed in the kidney, and the adrenal cortical hormone aldosterone, which promotes the reabsorption of Na^+ and the excretion of K^+ by activating Na⁺,K⁺-ATPase. In this way, aldosterone can also prevent a rise in the plasma K^+ concentration. This is of major significance, since a rise in plasma potassium concentration can have serious consequences and is not compatible with life (e. g., a rise in plasma potassium concentration leads to cardiac arrhythmias, and a doubling can lead to life-threatening ventricular fibrillation).

How much urine will eventually be excreted, however, is determined by the influence of the antidiuretic hormone (ADH, vasopressin) released by the neurohypophysis (see Concentration of Urine in the Collecting Ducts, below).

Renin–Angiotensin–Aldosterone Mechanism

As previously mentioned in Chapter 1, extracellular fluid volume, and with it blood volume, is determined by its Na^+ content. Hence the excretion of Na^+ is of great importance. It is the result of a hormonal regulatory cycle, the renin–angiotensin–aldosterone mechanism, which fulfills an important function in the regulation of blood pressure. A decisive role in this is played by the "*juxtaglomerular apparatus*" (Fig. 10.**5a**), which involves:

- Specialized renin-producing cells in the vascular wall of the afferent arteriole, which contain secretory granules
- Macula densa cells in the wall of the distal tubule and in immediate proximity to the afferent arteriole running to its glomerulus
- Numerous connective tissue cells at the vascular end of the glomerulus, called the extraglomerular mesangium cells (lacis cells, polkissen)

The juxtaglomerular apparatus responds at a systemic (circulatory) and a local (glomerular) level. If, for instance, the blood pressure falls owing to a reduction in plasma volume (e. g., due to shock), the enzyme renin is secreted from the specialized cells of the afferent arteriole into the blood. There renin cleaves the protein molecule angiotensinogen, which is formed in the liver, into angiotensin I, which another enzyme (angiotensin-converting enzyme, ACE) converts into angiotensin II. Angiotensin II is one of the most potent vasoconstrictor substances and is effective in raising the peripheral resistance, and with it the blood pressure. Angiotensin II also causes aldosterone to be released from the adrenal cortex, increasing the absorption of Na^+ in the distal tubule. This leads to a reduction in water excretion in the kidney, increasing the blood volume and so increasing blood pressure. Finally, angiotensin II produces a sensation of thirst.

An equally effective stimulus for renin secretion and so for triggering the renin–angiotensin–aldosterone mechanism is an excess of sodium chloride in the distal tubule. For this reason the macula densa cells in the wall of the distal tubule are conceived as a "*chemosensitive area*" that measures the sodium chloride content of the urine, and in case of an excessive concentration liberates renin (through the polkissen). The increased aldosterone level in the blood then leads to an increase in the absorption of sodium ions in the distal tubule. Moreover, the vasoconstrictor activity of angiotensin II leads to vasoconstriction of the accompanying afferent arteriole, which reduces the glomerular filtration rate and reduces the sodium chloride concentration in the tubule. By this means the juxtaglomerular apparatus makes it possible for the glomerular filtration rate to be adapted to the sodium chloride content of the urine in the distal tubule. This is called a *tubulo-glomerular feedback mechanism*.

Concentration and Dilution of the Urine

The kidney can excrete a concentrated or a dilute urine as needed to regulate the water balance. For instance, maximally concentrated urine contains four time as many dissolved particles as extracellular fluid. Such urine is called *hypertonic*. If, on the other had, the organism must get rid of excess fluid intake, e. g., after drinking too much, it can excrete urine that is diluted to a concentration one-sixth of that of the extracellular fluid (*hypotonic urine*).

Concentration of Urine in the Collecting Ducts

Besides the active sodium resorption in the various tubular segments, renal water excretion is regulated by *antidiuretic hormone* (*ADH, vasopressin*), which is secreted in the hypothalamus and stored in the neurohypophysis. Vasopressin acts primarily on the collecting ducts, in that it raises the permeability of their walls to water. Consequently, water diffuses passively from the collecting ducts and moves along an osmotic gradient into the hypertonic interstitial fluid and eventually the blood. Hence the hormone opposes diuresis (hence *antidiuretic hormone*).

Vasopressin acts on the water balance by a hormonal regulatory cycle that depends on a center in the hypothalamic region of the diencephalon (see Chapter 13: The Brain, Diencephalon). The osmotic concentration of the plasma is monitored by sensors in the hypothalamus, the *osmoreceptors.* If the concentration of osmotically active particles (e. g., Na^+ ion concentration) in the plasma rises, ADH is liberated from the neighboring posterior lobe of the pituitary gland and transported by the blood .to the kidneys. As a result, more water flows out of the collecting ducts, leading to greater urine concentration. About 15–20 liters of water are resorbed daily in this way under the influence of vasopressin. A deficiency of ADH leads to the condition known as *diabetes insipidus*, in which up to 20 liters urine may be excreted daily.

Diuretics

Diuretics are medications that promote diuresis (substances promoting urinary flow). They are mostly used therapeutically to reduce the extracellular fluid volume in elevated blood pressure or water accumulation in the tissues (edema). The activity of these drugs rests mostly on inhibition of tubular Na^+ resorption.

Composition of Urine

In 24 hours an adult excretes about 0.5–2 liters of urine, which is composed of about 95% water. The light to dark yellow color is due to urochromes, which are related to bile pigments produced during the breakdown of hemoglobin. Urine is usually slightly acid, though slightly alkaline on a vegetarian diet. Apart from organic substances (especially urea, uric acid, and creatinine) it contains a number of inorganic components (e. g., sodium, potassium, calcium, chlorine. sulfate, phosphate, and ammonium ions) that can crystallize out in the urinary sediment. In disease, large amounts of red and white blood corpuscles and plasma proteins (especially albumin) and glucose (type II diabetes) can appear in the urine.

■ Urinary Tract

Urine travels from the renal papillae through the renal calyces into the renal pelvis and is then transported in small volumes by peristalsis along the ureter into the urinary bladder. From there it is voided to the outside through the urethra. The walls of the urinary tract are made of smooth muscle and are lined inside by a mucous membrane that is mainly composed of transitional epithelium (see Chapter 3: Surface Epithelia, and Fig. 3.**2**).

Renal Pelvis

The renal pelvis is a funnel-shaped tube with tubular extensions (*calyces*), into which project the *renal papillae* (Fig. 10.**3**). The renal pelvis is found in two basic forms, called dendritic or ampullar (Figs. 10.**7a**, **b**). In the ampullar type the calyces are short and rounded, while in the dendritic type the pelvis is branched like a tree and the calyces are long and narrow. The renal pelvis has a capacity of about 3–8 ml and can be visualized in radiographic contrast studies after administration of a contrast medium designed to be concentrated in the urine (intravenous urography, excretory urography) (Fig. 10.**8**).

Ureter

The ureter transports urine from the renal pelvis to the bladder. It is shaped like a flattened tube with a diameter of about 5 mm and a length of about 25 cm (Figs. 10.**1** and 10.**8**). The two ureters begin at the renal pelvis and run downward along the posterior abdominal wall, each crossing the psoas major muscle and, at the entrance to the true pelvis, the great pelvic vessels (common iliac artery and vein). They then run to the floor of the urinary bladder from both sides, pierce the bladder wall at an oblique angle about 5 cm apart, and enter the bladder by a slitlike opening (Figs. 10.**1** and 10.**9**).

Along the ureter there are three *physiological constrictions* where urinary stones (calculi) are most likely to become lodged. They are located at the ureteropelvic junction, at the point where the ureter crosses the common iliac vessels, and in its course through the bladder wall (Fig. 10.**1**).

The wall of the ureter consists of an inner mucous membrane lined with transitional epithelium, a smooth muscle layer, and an adventitia composed of connective tissue. The smooth muscle layer in the upper portion of the ureter is made up of a thinner inner layer of longitudinal

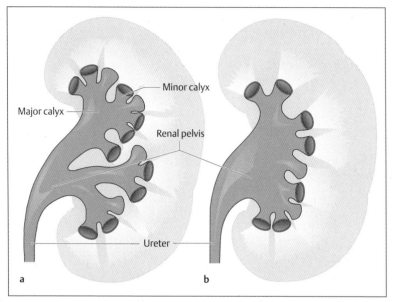

Fig. 10.**7 a, b Basic forms of the renal pelvis.** (After Faller)
a Dendritic form; **b** ampullar form

fibers and a thicker outer layer of annular fibers. The muscle cells of differing orientations form a spiral arrangement of fiber bundles. The structure of the wall allows the ureter to dilate substantially. Peristaltic waves advance the urine toward the bladder in batches (1–4 times a minute).

Urinary Bladder (Vesica Urinaria)

The urinary bladder in the adult lies in the true pelvis directly under the peritoneum (extraperitoneal, see Chapter 9: Relations of the Peritoneum and Mesenteries of the Abdominal Organs), immediately behind the symphysis on the pelvic floor. Laterally and anteriorly the bladder is covered by loose areolar tissue that contains blood vessels and nerves. The body of the bladder forms its roof. It runs forward and upward into

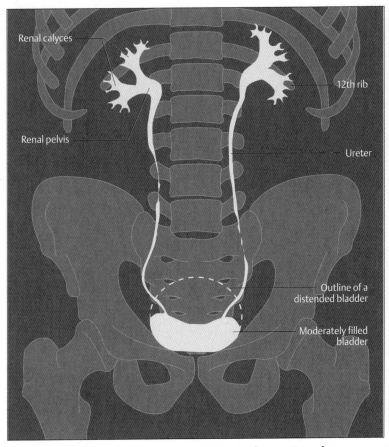

Fig. 10.**8**   **Simplified tracing of a radiographic image after injection of contrast medium (intravenous urogram)**
The contrast medium is filtered in the renal corpuscles and appears in the urine. The renal pelves, the ureters, and the bladder are outlined

the apex, which is fastened to the anterior abdominal wall in a mobile fashion. The part of the bladder directed toward the pelvic floor is called the base of the bladder. It narrows downward to a funnel, which forms the transition to the urethra (Fig. 10.**1**). The size of the bladder depends on the degree of its filling. The urge to urinate begins at a content of

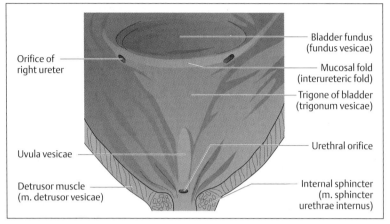

Fig. 10.**9** **Trigone of the bladder (trigonum vesicae).** (After Faller)

about 350 ml, but more than twice that amount can be retained voluntarily.

Bladder Muscle and Internal Surface

Like all hollow organs, the bladder possesses a muscle layer composed of a network of smooth muscle fibers (*detrusor of the bladder, detrusor vesicae muscle*) (Figs. 10.**1** and 10.**9**). The mucosa is lined with transitional epithelium that can adapt rapidly to changes in volume and that is protected against the urine by a special *differentiation of its surface*. The mucosa of the floor of the bladder has a smooth surface and is firmly attached to the muscle in the area between the ureteric orifices and the orifice of the urethra. This area is called the trigone of the bladder (Figs. 10.**1** and 10.**9**). Between the two ureteral orifices there is a fold in the mucous membrane (*interureteric fold, plica interureterica*). The *uvula of the bladder* (*uvula vesicae*), a longitudinal elevation, projects over the apex of the trigone. Depending on the state of contraction of the bladder, the mucosa forms more or less marked folds that project into the interior of the bladder over its remaining segments.

The muscular layer of the trigone is *structured in such a way that it can close or open* the ureteral and internal urethral orifices.

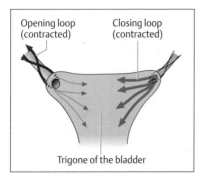

Opening loop (contracted)

Closing loop (contracted)

Trigone of the bladder

Fig. 10.**10**   **Opening and closure of the ureteric orifices.** The ureter is opened by contraction of the opening loop (red) and closed by contraction of the closing loop (blue). The arrows indicate the direction of contraction of the muscle fibers. (After Leonhardt)

Muscles of the Ureteral Orifices

External muscular bundles from the ureter loop around the ureteral orifices (Fig. 10.**10**). When the muscle fascicles contract, the orifice is lifted and opened (*opening loop*). Muscular loops that run between the two ureteral orifices pull the orifices downward and close them (*closing loop*).

Muscles of the Urethral Orifice

The internal involuntary smooth muscle sphincter of the bladder neck (*m. sphincter urethrae internus*) is formed by longitudinal muscle fascicles of the bladder and circular muscle bundles. The voluntary striated sphincter muscle consists of muscle fibers that split from muscles of the pelvic floor (*m. transversus perinei profundus*) and loop around the urethra spirally (*m. sphincter urethrae externus*) (Fig. 10.**11**).

The smooth muscle of the bladder and the urethral orifice is innervated by the sympathetic nervous system. When stimulated by the sympathetic, the bladder muscle (detrusor) relaxes and the involuntary internal urethral sphincter contracts. The bladder fills. When the parasympathetic is stimulated, the detrusor contracts and the smooth internal sphincter muscle relaxes. The bladder empties.

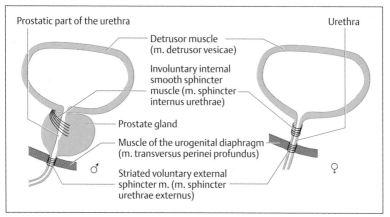

Fig. 10.**11**   **Urethral sphincters in the male and the female** (diagrammatic)

Urethra

From the bladder, urine reaches the outside through the urethra. The male and female urethras differ mainly in their length, and by the use of the urethra in the male as the duct for the sexual substances.

The Male Urethra

The male urethra is 20–25 cm long and becomes a combined urinary and spermatic tube by the entrance of the vas deferens and the sex glands. Its course is divided into three parts (Fig. 10.**12**):

- A portion about 3 cm long that begins at the internal urethral orifice and runs through the prostate (prostatic part)
- A very short but narrow portion that pierces the pelvic floor (membranous part)
- Finally, a long part that runs though the corpus spongiosum of the penis (pars spongiosa, spongy part) and ends at the external urethral orifice (urinary meatus)

The two *ejaculatory ducts*, the common duct of the spermatic ducts and the seminal vesicles (vesicula seminales) as well as the ducts of the pros-

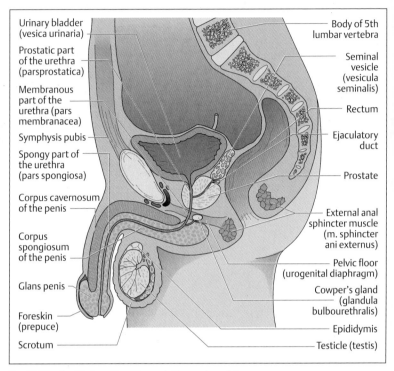

Urinary bladder (vesica urinaria)

Prostatic part of the urethra (parsprostatica)

Membranous part of the urethra (pars membranacea)

Symphysis pubis

Spongy part of the urethra (pars spongiosa)

Corpus cavernosum of the penis

Corpus spongiosum of the penis

Glans penis

Foreskin (prepuce)

Scrotum

Body of 5th lumbar vertebra

Seminal vesicle (vesicula seminalis)

Rectum

Ejaculatory duct

Prostate

External anal sphincter muscle (m. sphincter ani externus)

Pelvic floor (urogenital diaphragm)

Cowper's gland (glandula bulbourethralis)

Epididymis

Testicle (testis)

Fig. 10.**12** **Sagittal section through the male pelvis**

tate gland drain into the prostatic part. Muscle fibers from the pelvic dia-phragm form the voluntary sphincter of the urethra around the mem-branous part (see above). The pea-sized *Cowper's glands* (bulbourethral glands) have openings into the beginning of the pars spongiosa, which receives the ducts of numerous small urethral glands in its further course (Fig. 10.**12**).

The mucosa of the urethra is marked by longitudinal folds, which provide reserve and act as an additional closing mechanism. In the pros-tatic part the transitional epithelium of the mucosa changes to the stratified columnar epithelium of the urethra, and this in turn is replaced by stratified squamous epithelium in the glans penis.

The Female Urethra

The female urethra is 3–4 cm long and so markedly shorter than the male. It begins directly above the pelvic floor and runs forward between the symphysis and the anterior vaginal wall (see Chapter 11: Female Reproductive Organs, and Fig. 11.**8**). The urethra ends at the external urethral orifice in the vestibule just behind the clitoris.

The mucosa of the female urethra is marked by longitudinal folds that reduce its lumen. In addition, the connective tissue of the mucosa contains a network of elastic fibers and an extensive venous plexus that form a sort of *occluding cushion* that takes part in the closure of the urethra.

Summary **The Kidneys and Urinary Tract**

■ The Kidneys
The essential tasks of the kidneys are:

- The excretion of metabolic products and waste products
- Maintenance of electrolyte concentrations (acid–base balance), water content, and the osmotic pressure of body fluids
- A role in the regulation of the circulation and the production of red blood cells (renin, erythropoietin).

Shape and Position
The kidneys are shaped like beans (120–300 g), lie on each side of the vertebral column in the retroperitoneal space (left kidney below the spleen, right kidney below the liver), and are surrounded by a fatty capsule and a fascial sheath. The renal pelvis lies in the hilus, where vessels and nerves enter and exit. An adrenal gland sits on the upper pole of each kidney.

Renal cortex and Renal Medulla
Renal tissue includes a renal cortex and a renal medulla. The blood vessels, nephrons (functional units of the kidney) and the collecting ducts run in the renal cortex and medulla. A nephron is composed of a renal corpuscle (Bowman's capsule and glomerulus) and its renal tubule. The tubules drain into the collecting ducts, which begin in the

cortex (cortical collecting ducts) and run through the medulla (medullary collecting ducts) toward the renal papillae.

- *Renal cortex:* consists of a band about 8 mm wide directly under the capsule; it contains the renal corpuscles (about 1.2×10^6 in each kidney), the proximal and distal convoluted tubules, and the cortical collecting ducts that form the medullary rays (bundles of collecting ducts).
- *Renal medulla:* consists of 10–12 renal or medullary pyramids, the broad base of which forms its boundary with the cortex, and the apices form the renal papillae. Medullary rays run from the pyramids to the cortex. Between the medullary rays, the cortex extends deep into the medulla in the form of columns. The medulla contains the straight segments of the renal tubules, the junctional tubules, and the medullary collecting ducts.

The Renal Vessels

The kidneys receive about 20% of the cardiac minute volume from the aorta through the two renal arteries: At the hilus they divide into 5–6 interlobar arteries, which run toward the cortex between the renal pyramids and then arch as arcuate arteries between the cortex and the medulla. Interlobular arteries branch from the arcuate arteries toward the cortex, and these in turn give rise to afferent arterioles that supply the glomeruli of the renal corpuscles. Efferent arterioles take the blood into further capillary networks that supply both the cortex and the medulla. Finally, small and large veins collect the blood, which then flows through the renal veins into the inferior vena cava.

Renal Corpuscles and the Glomerular Filter

The renal corpuscles form the beginning of the nephron and filter the glomerular filtrate from the blood. They consist of a double-walled cup (Bowman's capsule) and a capillary tuft (glomerulus). Between the glomerular capillaries lie the mesangium cells (support cells that phagocytose and so clean the glomerular filter). They have a urinary pole and a vascular pole: the afferent arterioles enter and the efferent arterioles leave at the vascular pole, while the proximal tubule begins at the urinary pole. The glomerular filter (about 1 m²) forms the *glomerular filtration barrier.* It has three layers:

- Fenestrated capillary epithelium
- The visceral wall of Bowman's capsule (podocytes with slit-pores)
- The common basement membrane of endothelial cells and podocytes

Glomerular Filtration

A passive process, dependent on the arterial blood pressure level (autoregulation between 80 and 200 mmHg), the properties of the filter (mechanical and electrical filter), and the properties of the filtered molecule (size and charge).

Glomerular Filtration Rate

The volume of fluid filtered by all the glomeruli per unit time (120 ml/min = 180 l/day).

Effective Filtration Pressure

Depends on the arterial blood pressure in the glomerular capillaries (48 mmHg), colloid osmotic pressure (20 mmHg), and the hydrostatic pressure in Bowman's capsule (13 mmHg): effective filtration pressure = 48 – 20 – 13 = 15 mmHg.

Renal Tubules and Collecting Ducts

The renal tubule is a small tube a few centimeters long consisting of simple epithelium, and can be divided into several segments:

- A proximal tubule, initially convoluted, then straight
- A thin transitional limb (Henle's loop)
- A distal tubule, initially straight, then convoluted
- A short junctional tubule

The junctional tubule connects the nephron to the collecting duct, which drains into the renal pelvis through a fine orifice at the apex of the renal papilla.

Transport Processes in the Renal Tubule

After being filtered in the renal corpuscle, the glomerular filtrate (ultrafiltrate of plasma) is concentrated in the course of its passage through the various segments of the renal tubules and the collecting ducts (urine), i.e., mainly water, together with certain substances (e.g., inorganic and organic ions, glucose, amino acids, small protein molecules, vitamins) is reabsorbed (urine = 1% of the glomerular filtrate) and returned to the circulation. On the other hand, other substances, e. g., urea, uric acid, and creatinine, are excreted actively into the tubular lumen, especially in the proximal tubule.

Na^+-K^+ pump (Na^+,K^+-ATPase)

The concentration of the glomerular filtrate is closely linked to the reabsorption of the Na^+ ions of sodium chloride (Na^+Cl^-). Na^+ ions are actively (i.e., utilizing ATP) reabsorbed from the lumen of the tubules by means of Na^+,K^+-ATPase (Cl^- ions and water follow passively); that is, the active transport of NaCl is the driving force of the concentrating mechanism of the kidney.

Reabsorption of Water

A two-step process: 60–70% of water is reabsorbed in the proximal tubule and the loop of Henle, the rest in the distal tubule (renin–angiotensin–aldosterone mechanism) and the collecting duct (vasopressin, ADH).

Renin–Angiotensin–Aldosterone Mechanism

Extracellular fluid volume, and with it blood volume, is determined by the Na^+ content. The regulation of Na^+ excretion is accomplished by the renin–angiotensin–aldosterone mechanism by means of the *juxtaglomerular apparatus*, which includes the following structures:

- Renin-producing cells in the wall of the afferent arteriole
- Macula densa cells with chemoreceptors in the wall of the neighboring distal tubule belonging to its glomerulus
- Extraglomerular mesangium cells (polkissen) at the vascular pole

The juxtaglomerular apparatus has a local and a systemic response:

- *Systemic response:* a fall in blood pressure (e. g., reduction in blood volume) leads to liberation of renin into the blood; renin cleaves angiotensin into angiotensin I, which in turn is transformed by a "converting enzyme" into angiotensin II. Angiotensin II has two major effects: (1) direct vasoconstriction of blood vessels with a consequent rise in blood pressure and (2) liberation of aldosterone from the adrenal cortex. This triggers Na^+, K^+-ATPase, especially in the distal tubules, and so increases the reabsorption of water (consequence: increase in blood volume, and therefore rise in blood pressure).

- *Local response (tubuloglomerular feedback mechanism):* a high NaCl concentration in the distal tubule is sensed by the macula densa cells, and renin is liberated through the intermediary action of the extraglumerular mesangium cells. (1) Just as in the systemic response, the blood vessels (including the afferent arterioles) constrict and the blood pressure rises, with consequent reduction in the glomerular filtration rate (consequence: reduction in NaCl concentration in the distal tubule) and (2) aldosterone is liberated, followed by increased reabsorption of Na^+ in the distal tubule.

Concentration of Urine in the Collecting Ducts

The definitive regulation of water excretion occurs in the collecting ducts by antidiuretic hormone (ADH, vasopressin). Regulatory cycle: osmoreceptors in the hypothalamus monitor the osmotic concentration (especially NaCl concentration) of the plasma. If the concentration of osmotically active particles rises, ADH is formed in the hypothalamus and released into the bloodstream through the neurohypophysis. ADH raises the permeability to water of the walls of the collecting ducts (consequence: passive diffusion of water from the collecting ducts into the intercellular space and from there into the bloodstream) with consequent urine concentration (15–20 liters of water are reabsorbed daily by this route).

■ The Urinary Tract

The urinary tract includes the renal pelvis, ureter, bladder, and urethra. With the exception of the urethra, the mucosa of the urinary tract is lined by transitional epithelium.

The Renal Pelvis

A short, funnel-shaped tube with renal calyces into which project the renal papillae (capacity: 3–8 ml).

Ureter

Transports urine from the renal pelvis to the bladder (length about 25 cm, diameter about 5 mm). The smooth muscle is arranged spirally and permits marked dilatation (transport to the urinary bladder occurs in batches: 1–4 ml/min). There are three physiological constrictions (ureteral constrictions), where ureteral calculi become wedged by preference: (1) junction with the renal pelvis, (2) crossing over the common iliac vessels, and (3) course through the bladder wall.

Urinary Bladder

An extraperitoneal hollow organ situated in the true pelvis, with body (roof) of the bladder, apex (attached to the anterior abdominal wall), base (next to the pelvic floor), and bladder neck (transition to the urethra). The bladder muscle (detrusor) forms a network and is lined internally by mucosa (transitional epithelium with a surface differentiated to protect against the urine). The muscular layer of the trigone (triangle between the openings of the ureters and the urethra) forms mechanisms for the closing and opening the ureteral orifices (opening and closing loops) and for the internal urethral orifice at the bladder neck (internal sphincter of the urethra = involuntary smooth sphincter muscle; external urethral sphincter = voluntary striated sphincter. muscle).

Male Urethra

The 20–25 cm long urethra can be divided into three parts:

- *Prostatic part:* segment within the prostate, with entrance of the two ejaculatory ducts and the ducts of the prostatic glands.
- *Membranous part:* pierces the pelvic floor and contains the voluntary urethral sphincter; entrance of the ducts of the bulbourethral glands.
- *Spongy part:* longest segment; runs within the corpus spongiosum and ends at the external urethral orifice (urinary meatus).

Female Urethra

Has a total length of 3–4 cm and so is markedly shorter than the male urethra. Ends in the vaginal vestibule; surrounded by a venous plexus serving as an occluding cushion.

11

The Reproductive Organs

Contents

■ Function and Structure of the Reproductive Organs

The reproductive organs have the function of forming germ cells, promoting their union, and giving the fertilized ovum an environment in which it can develop from an embryo to a fetus mature enough to be born. In addition, the reproductive organs take part in developing the body shape specific to each sex by the hormones they form.

The male and female reproductive organs include:

- **The gonads,** which produce germ cells and sex hormones
- **The reproductive passages,** which serve the transport of reproductive products
- **The reproductive glands,** the secretions of which promote the union of ovum and sperm
- **The external sex organs,** which allow sexual union to occur

■ Male Reproductive Organs

Overview

The male reproductive organs are divided according to their development into internal and external organs. The internal male reproductive organs include the testes, the epididymis, the vas deferens, the seminal vesicles, and the prostate. The external male reproductive organs include the penis and the scrotum (Fig. 11.**1a**, **b**).

From the testes, which produce the germ cells and the male reproductive hormones, the sperm cells (spermatozoa) pass through a system of small tubules into the epididymis, which stores them. Through the vas deferens, which runs through the inguinal canal, the spermatozoa reach the urethra at the level of the prostate. Shortly before they open into the urethra, they receive the ducts of the seminal vesicles. The ducts of the prostate and Cowper's glands open directly into the urethra. The spermatozoa achieve mobility under the influence of secretions from these glands. The further transport of the spermatic fluid (semen) is taken over by the urethra, the corpora cavernosa of which generate the erection of the penis and so allow it to penetrate the vagina.

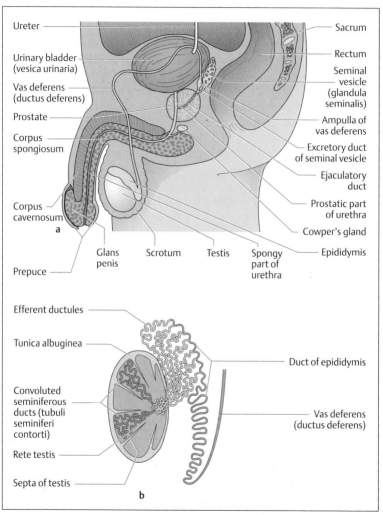

Fig. 11.**1 a, b   Internal and external male reproductive organs**
a   Overview
b   Ductules of the testis and epididymis

Testis (Orchis)

The two testes, each about the size of a plum, are the male gonads. They lie in a skin pocket, the *scrotum* (Fig. 11.**1a**). They develop on the posterior abdominal wall, and at the end of fetal development they leave a peritoneal pocket and descend along the posterior wall of the abdominal cavity through the inguinal canal into the scrotum (descensus testis). This mechanism withdraws them from experiencing the internal body temperature, which would impede maturation of the sperm. When the testes remain in the abdominal cavity or in the inguinal canal, the condition is called *cryptorchidism*.

Each testis is surrounded by a dense white *connective tissue capsule* (*tunica albuginea*), from which *connective tissue septa* (*septula testis*) run inward (Fig. 11.**1b**). In this way the tissue of the testis is subdivided incompletely into more than 200 compartments (*lobuli testis*). Each lobule is made up of two to four extensively convoluted *seminiferous tubules* (*tubuli seminiferi contorti*) that measure 350 m in total and the epithelium of which *forms the spermatozoa* (*spermatogenesis*) (Fig. 11.**1b**).

Testosterone Production

The connective tissue between the seminiferous tubules contains the *endocrine interstitial cells of Leydig* (*Leydig cells*) (Fig. 11.**2**) that produce the *male sex hormones* (chiefly *testosterone*) and secrete them into the bloodstream. Testosterone promotes the formation of spermatozoa, promotes the growth of the external reproductive organs, and determines sex-specific behavior. Additionally, the *secondary sexual characteristics* (e. g., hair distribution) develop under the influence of the male sex hormone. It also has an anabolic effect on metabolism. The production of testosterone in Leydig cells and spermatogenesis are controlled from the hypothalamus by releasing hormones that trigger the liberation of *luteinizing hormone* (*lutropin, LH*) and *follicle-stimulating hormone* (*follitropin, FSH*). FSH directly promotes spermatogenesis in the seminiferous tubules and LH stimulates Leydig cells to secrete testosterone. The blood testosterone level in its turn influences the *hypothalamopituitary system* through a feedback mechanism (see Chapter 7: Hypothalamic–Hypophyseal Axis).

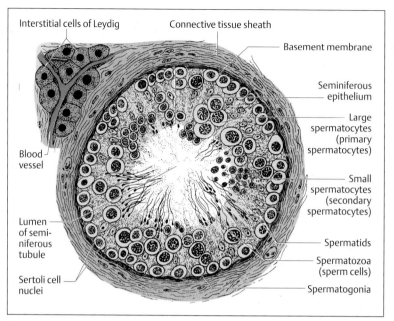

Fig. 11.**2**   **Cross-section of a seminiferous tubule of the testis (tubulus seminiferus contortus)**

Development of Sperm Cells (Spermatogenesis)

The wall of the seminiferous tubules is lined with *seminiferous epithe-lium* (Fig. 11.**2**) on a basement membrane. Within the seminiferous epithelium, the Sertoli cells form a support in which the germ cells are embedded. The formation of spermatozoa begins with puberty and con-tinues into old age. It develops in several steps as the cells migrate from the periphery into the center of the seminiferous tubule:

1. **Period of multiplication**
2. **Period of maturation**
3. **Period of differentiation**

During the period of multiplication, the diploid primitive germ cells (spermatogonia) divide by mitosis to form more spermatogonia. During the maturation period, large spermatocytes (primary spermatocytes) are formed, again by mitosis (Fig. 11.**2**). These then enter the first meiotic division (separation of the homologous chromosomes) (see Chapter 1: Reduction or Maturation Division [Meiosis] and Chapter 12: Germ Cells) and develop into the small spermatocytes (secondary spermatocytes) with only half a set of chromosomes. The secondary spermatocytes develop into smaller spermatids during the second meiotic maturation division (separation of the chromatids). In this way, at the end of the maturation period, which lasts about 72 hours, eight spermatids are generated from one spermatogonium. Of these, four contain an X and four a Y chromosome (see also Chapter 12: Germ Cells).

In the course of the period of differentiation, the spermatids are transformed into the motile form of germ cells, the spermatozoa, the tails of which protrude into the lumen of the seminiferous tubules. Every hour about 3–4 million spermatozoa pass from the testes into the epididymis—i.e., about 1000 spermatozoa are generated every second.

Spermatozoa

The spermatozoa are motile cells with tails, about 50–60 µm in length (1/20 mm). The head contains the haploid cell nucleus and possesses a caplike structure (acrosome) (Fig. 11.**3**) that allows the spermatozoon to penetrate the ovum (see Chapter 12: Fertilization). Below the head there follows a short neck, a relatively thick middle piece, a tail, and an end piece. The neck contains the centriole, which will form the cleavage spindle after the spermatozoon has united with the ovum. In the middle piece, the beginning of the flagellum (tail) is surrounded by numerous spirally arranged mitochondria that provide energy for the cell's motion. The flagellum continues into the tail.

By wriggling their tail, spermatozoa can advance at a speed of about 3–4 mm a minute. In order to reach the ovum for fertilization, spermatozoa must migrate through the uterine cavity and along to the end of the fallopian tube, a passage that takes about 1–3 hours. Once they reach the ampulla of the fallopian tube, the spermatozoa remain fertile for up to 4 days.

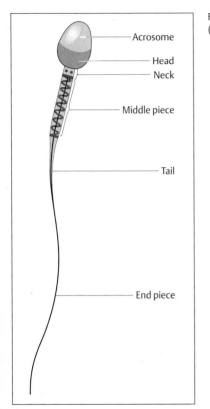

Fig. 11.**3** **Structure of a sperm cell** (magnified about 1650×)

- Acrosome
- Head
- Neck
- Middle piece
- Tail
- End piece

Epididymis

By way of the *rete testis*, a wide-meshed, dilated system of channels, the spermatozoa, swim in a fluid stream to reach the epididymis. This structure, which serves as a *store for sperm* (Fig. 11.**4**), sits on the testis like a horse's tail. The epididymis is divided into a head, a body, and a tail. It includes the *efferent ductules* of the testis and the *duct of the epididymis*, which is about 5 m in length (Fig. 11.**1b**). The ducts are markedly convoluted and are packed tightly into a single mass by connective tissue. In the tail of the epididymis the duct of the epididymis continues into the *vas deferens* (*ductus deferens*) (Fig. 11.**1b**).

The epithelium of the duct of the epididymis reabsorbs much of the fluid and secretes substances that promote the *definitive maturation* of the spermatozoa and their protection against the acid medium of the duct. This acid medium depresses the spermatozoa's motility, so that they do not use up their energy.

The transport of spermatozoa through the epididymis takes about 12 days. It takes several ejaculations in the course of 24 hours to empty the epididymis completely. In the absence of ejaculation for a prolonged period, the spermatozoa are broken down and the epithelium or macrophages take up the breakdown products.

Vas Deferens

The vas deferens is 50–60 cm long. It transports the spermatozoa during ejaculation (Fig. 11.**4**). It is sheathed in connective tissue together with the testicular vessels and nerves, forming the *spermatic cord* (*funiculus spermaticus*), which runs through the inguinal canal and on into the pelvis. Toward its end, the vas deferens widens into a *spindle-shaped ampulla* (*ampulla ductus deferens*), is joined by the duct of the seminal vesicle to form the *ejaculatory* duct, pierces the prostate, and opens into the prostatic part of the urethra (Fig. 11.**1a**).

The vas deferens has a smooth muscle coat, about 1.5 mm thick, with three layers. These are arranged in a spiral fashion, so that when they contract (during ejaculation) they widen and simultaneously shorten the vas. This mechanism actually sucks the spermatozoa out of the epididymis. Because of its firm consistency, the vas deferens can easily be palpated in the spermatic cord.

Seminal Vesicles (Vesiculae Seminales) or Seminal Glands (Glandulae Seminales)

The two seminal vesicles (seminal glands) are large thin-walled glands, about 10 cm long, that lie on the posterior wall of the urinary bladder, abutting on the rectum (Figs. 11.**1a** and 11.**5**). The *excretory duct* of the seminal vesicle runs at an acute angle into the vas deferens below the ampulla. The common ejaculatory duct so formed then pierces the pros-

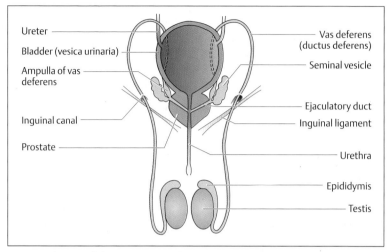

Fig. 11.**4** **Course of the spermatic pathways**

tate from behind and laterally and drains into the prostatic part of the urethra.

Contrary to their name, the seminal vesicles do not contain spermatozoa, but produce a slightly alkaline, protein-rich secretion that mobilizes the sperm in the acid environment of the vagina. The secretion also contains fructose, a simple sugar, which provides energy for the motion of the spermatozoa.

Prostate Gland

The prostate has the shape and size of a large chestnut and lies between the pelvic floor (urogenital diaphragm) and the base of the bladder (Figs. 11.**1a** and 11.**5**). Its posterior aspect abuts directly on the rectum, through which it can be palpated with a finger (*rectal examination of the prostate*). It consists of 30–50 individual glands surrounded by a dense white connective tissue capsule. Their secretory ducts drain into the urethra, which runs vertically through the prostate. The prostatic stroma is largely composed of smooth muscle fibers.

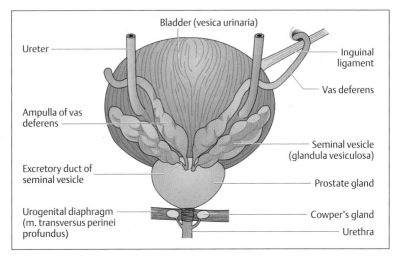

Fig. 11.**5** **Urinary bladder and prostate seen from behind**

The prostate forms a slightly acid, thinly fluid, opalescent secretion with an odor of chestnuts. It contains numerous enzymes (e. g., acid phosphatase), immunoglobulins, and prostaglandins to stimulate the uterus. Spermine, a protein found in prostatic secretion, promotes the motility and fertility of the spermatozoa. In dried semen it forms crystals, which, when demonstrated in the vagina, can document a rape in legal medicine.

Three poorly delineated zones can be made out in the glandular tissue of the prostate (Fig. 11.**6**): an *outer zone*, an *inner zone*, and a *periurethral zone* that lies in direct contact with the urethra. The outer zone lies under the connective tissue capsule and includes the major part of the glandular tissue. This zone is often a site for the development of *malignant tumors* (*prostatic carcinoma*). Prostatic cancer is one of the commonest tumors in elderly men. The periurethral zone is very often the site for the development of *benign tumors* (*prostatic adenoma*), which affect more than half of men over 60 years of age. Prostatic adenoma leads to a narrowing of the urethra, with consequent difficulty in emptying the bladder.

Cowper's Glands (Bulbourethral Glands)

The two pea-sized Cowper's glands lie in the musculature of the pelvic floor (urogenital diaphragm) and their ducts drain into the first part of the spongy portion of the urethra (Figs. 11.**1a** and 11.**5**). Their weakly alkaline secretion precedes ejaculation and neutralizes the acid environment of the urethra.

Composition of the Ejaculate

The major portion of the fluid part of the ejaculate derives from the prostate (25%) and the seminal vesicles (75%). The semen as a whole is weakly alkaline and so protects against the acid environment of the vagina. After three days of sexual continence, one emission contains about 3–6 ml semen with at least 20 million spermatozoa per milliliter (*normospermic*). Among the spermatozoa of one ejaculate, as a rule 10–20% are not fully developed or are malformed. A sperm count of less than 20 million per milliliter is termed *oligospermia*. The condition in which there are no spermatozoa in the semen is *azoospermia*.

Castration and Sterilization

In castration, both testes are removed surgically, e. g., as treatment for a malignant testicular tumor. Castration leads not only to infertility but to profound hormonal disturbances. In sterilization, the vas deferens on each sides is merely divided; since the hormonal system remains intact, *libido* (*sexual desire*) and *potency* (*ability to have an erection*) remain intact.

External Male Sex Organs

The external male reproductive organs, the penis and scrotum, are developed from the abdominal wall.

Scrotal Sac (Scrotum)

The testes lie outside the abdominal cavity in the scrotal sac. Here the ambient temperature is about 3 °C lower than the body temperature in the abdominal cavity. This temperature difference is a prerequisite for optimal development of the sperm. The skin of the scrotum is provided with numerous smooth muscle cells (tunica dartos, dartos), that can wrinkle or smooth the skin surface and so play a role in temperature regulation (reduced surface).

Penis (Male Member)

The penis consists of a *root*, which is firmly anchored to the pelvic floor and the two pubic rami, and a freely movable *body (shaft)* ending in the *glans penis*. The skin is freely movable over the penis and is folded back over the glans as the prepuce (Fig. 11.**1a**). Constriction of the prepuce is called phimosis.

To facilitate copulation the penis has three *cavernous bodies of erectile tissue* that enable the penis to become erect (Figs. 11.**1a** and 11.**7**):

- Two paired cavernous bodies (corpora cavernosa)
- A single urethral cavernous body (corpus spongiosum)

The corpus spongiosum runs along the underside of the penis and surrounds the urethra. Posteriorly it widens into a bulb (*bulb of the penis*), while anteriorly it ends in the glans penis (Fig. 11.**1a**). The bulb of the penis is covered by the two bulbospongiosus muscles, which are joined in the midline. They help to express the content of the urethra. The dorsum of the penis is formed by the two corpora cavernosa, which are separated by a connective tissue septum. Two crura (legs) attach the corpora cavernosa to the pubic rami. All three cavernous bodies are surrounded by a dense white connective tissue sheath that is about 1–3 mm thick (*tunica albuginea*) (Fig. 11.**7**).

Structure of the Penis

The structure of the penis is determined principally by the blood-filled spaces of the cavernous bodies (Fig. 11.**7**). The paired cavernous body of the penis is a spongy network of collagen and elastic fibers lined with

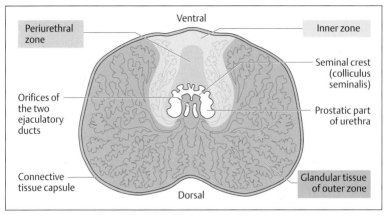

Fig. 11.**6** **Horizontal section through the prostate.** (After Leonhardt)

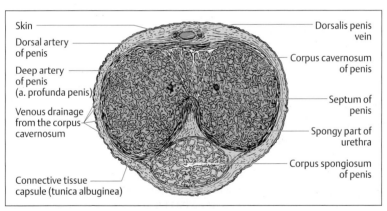

Fig. 11.**7** **Transverse section through the penis**

endothelium. When empty, the spaces are slits; when they are filled with blood, they attain a diameter of several millimeters. The corpus spongiosum, on the other hand, is mainly filled with a dense network of veins.

In the middle of each cavernous body runs an artery (*deep artery of the penis, arteria profunda penis*), of which the branches run a helical course (helicine arteries). They run into the spaces of the corpora cavernosa and their ends can be occluded. From the spaces, veins that can be occluded run through the tunica albuginea and drain into the *dorsal vein of the penis*.

Erection

During erection, the helicine arteries open and blood pours in, distending the tunica albuginea. At the same time, the veins running through the tunica albuginea become compressed, so that blood enters while drainage is occluded. The body of the penis therefore swells and becomes very hard. When the penis relaxes, the helicine arteries close, and as the tunica albuginea becomes less distended more blood can flow out through the vein.

During erection the venous network of the corpus spongiosum is repeatedly filled with blood, which, however, can flow out at any time. Hence the swelling remains relatively soft, allowing semen to flow through the urethra.

Ejaculation

Erection and ejaculation are complex processes that are regulated by the autonomic nervous system. While erection is a process influenced by the parasympathetic system, ejaculation is triggered by the sympathetic system. Ejaculation begins with contraction of the smooth musculature of the prostate, the seminal vesicles, and the vas deferens, as well as closure of the bladder neck. Once the semen has been positioned in the prostatic part of the posterior portion of the urethra, the pelvic floor contracts spasmodically. This movement drives the ejaculate in rhythmic thrusts out of the external urethral orifice.

■ Female Reproductive Organs

Overview

The female reproductive organs, similarly to the male, are divided into internal and external organs. The internal reproductive organs lie in the true pelvis and include the two ovaries, the two fallopian tubes, the uterus, and the vagina. The external organs include the major and minor labia, the clitoris, the vestibule, the vestibular glands, and the mammary glands (Fig. 11.**8**).

In the ovary of a woman, ova grow in response to the female sexual cycle (menstrual cycle), undergo ovulation, and reach the fallopian tube. After fertilization occurs in the ampullae of the tube, the fertilized ovum

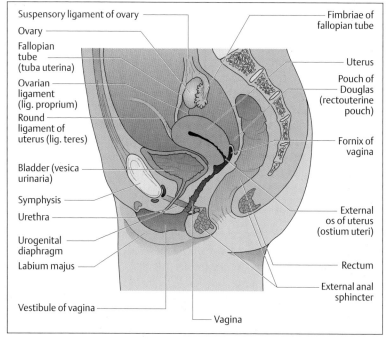

Fig. 11.**8**   **Median section through a female pelvis**

migrates in a fluid stream into the uterus, where nidation (nesting) into a mucosa prepared by hormones follows. After just a few days the fertilized ovum signals the beginning pregnancy to the pituitary gland, which influences the ovary to secrete hormones that secure the maintenance of the pregnancy during the months that follow. The uterine muscle adapts to the size of the growing embryo by undergoing hypertrophy. As the pregnancy progresses a combination of embryonic and maternal tissue forms the placenta, by which the fertilized ovum receives nutrition and oxygen. During labor, repeated contractions of the uterine muculature push the infant out of the birth canal and the placenta becomes detached from the uterine mucosa as the afterbirth.

Ovaries

The ovaries, like the testes, originate on the posterior abdominal wall and in the course of development migrate downward (*decensus*) toward the true pelvis. They come to rest at the junction of the true and false pelves, about the level of the division of the common iliac artery. They are attached by ligaments to the pelvic wall (*suspensory ligament of the ovary*) and the uterus (*ovarian ligament*) (Figs. 11.**8** and 11.**13**). Anteriorly they are loosely attached to the *broad ligament of the uterus* (*ligamentum latum uteri*) by a suspending ligament (*mesovarium*) (Fig. 11.**13**). In size and shape the ovaries resemble two almonds, each weighing about 14 g.

After maturation and preparation of the ovum, the ovary secretes hormones into the bloodstream that coordinate the processes in the uterus and vagina (estrogen, progesterone).

Structure of the Ovary

The ovary consists of a *cortex* and a *medulla*. The medulla contains blood vessels that enter the ovary through the mesovarium (Fig. 11.**9**). The cortex of an ovary in a woman during her reproductive years lies directly under the surface. It contains ovarian follicles in various stages of maturation (*primary, secondary*, and *tertiary or graafian follicles*), involuted follicles (atretic follicles), usually no more than one yellow body (corpus luteum), and the scarred remains of old corpora lutea (corpora albicantia) (Figs. 11.**9** and 11.**10**).

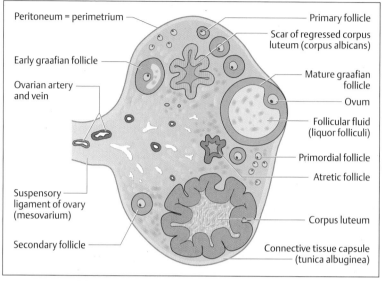

Fig. 11.**9** **Prepared section of an ovary** (longitudinal section, schematically represented)

Development of the Ovum (Oogenesis) and Follicle Maturation

Like spermatogenesis, the development of the ovum can be divided into a period of multiplication and a period of maturation. There is no period of differentiation. In contrast to the development of sperm in the male, which can continue into old age, the period of multiplication is already completed at birth. The germ cells (oogonia) develop into primary oocytes toward the end of the fetal period. These enter the prophase of the first maturation division (see Chapter 1: Reduction or Maturation Division [Meiosis]). They remain in this phase (dictyotene phase of the prophase) until the beginning of puberty or their atrophy. If an ovum matures after puberty (follicle maturation) (Fig. 11.**10**), the primary oocyte ends the first meiotic maturation division shortly before ovulation. It then forms two ova of different sizes, (a secondary oocyte and a first polar body, see also Chapter 12: Germ Cells), each with a haploid set of chromosomes. The second meiotic maturation division is initiated during ovulation, but is only completed if the egg is fertilized. During the

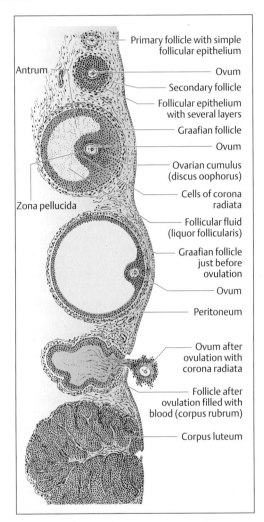

Fig. 11.**10** **Maturation of a follicle, ovulation and corpus luteum.** (After Leonhardt)

second maturation division, the chromatids separate to form a mature ovum and another (second) polar body (see Chapter 12): Germ Cells.

The ovarian follicles develop during maturation of the ovum. Follicular epithelial cells surround the primary oocytes and provide them with nutrients. According to the type of follicular epithelium surrounding the oocyte, follicles are divided into primordial, primary, secondary, and graafian. At birth, both ovaries contain about one million primary follicles, of which a large number perish up to the time of puberty (follicle atresia). With puberty, some of the remaining follicles develop into secondary follicles, of which a small number continue to develop into graafian (tertiary) follicles during each menstrual cycle.

Ovulation

In the course of development from primary to secondary follicle and eventually to graafian follicle, the follicular epithelium divides and, under the influence of the *follicle-stimulating hormone* (*FSH, follitropin*) of the hypophysis, forms several layers (Figs. 11.**10** and 11.**11**). The cells surrounding the follicle are hormonally active and secrete female sex hormones (e. g., estradiol), which reach the uterus by way of the bloodstream and cause the mucosal cells to proliferate (*proliferative phase*).

The cavity (antrum) of a tertiary follicle (Fig. 11.**10**) is filled with fluid rich in hyaluronic acid and proteoglycans (follicular fluid, liquor follicularis), and is enclosed by a multilayered follicular epithelium consisting of granulosa cells. The oocyte lies within a clump of granulosa cells called the cumulus oophorus. The granulosa cells surrounding the oocyte are called the corona radiata; they supply nutrients to the oocyte and are connected to it by gap junctions. The oocyte is closely enveloped by a layer of glycoproteins that it largely produces, the zona pellucida. This structure plays a major role in fertilization (Chapter 12: Fertilization) and in the early development of the embryo (segmentation; Chapter 12: Transport through the Uterine Tube and Segmentation).

In the middle of the menstrual cycle, one of the mature tertiary (graafian) follicles moves toward the surface of the ovary. The pressure of the fluid in the follicle, together with enzymes, initiates ovulation. The fluid pouring out of the follicle floats the ovum surrounded by a several surrounding follicular cells (corona radiata, Fig. 11.**10**) from the follicle into the distal end of the fallopian tube, which grasps the ovary with its fimbria at the time of ovulation. Suction in the fallopian tube brings the ovum into the ampulla (ampulla tubae), where fertilization takes place (Fig. 11.**13**). If the ovum is not fertilized within 12 hours, it perishes.

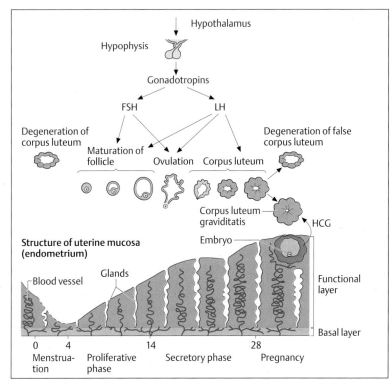

Fig. 11.**11** **Schematic representation of the ovarian cycle and the changes in the endometrium.** The anterior pituitary hormones FSH (follicle-stimulating hormone) and LH (luteinizing hormone) induce growth of the follicle in the ovary, ovulation, and formation of the corpus luteum. Ovarian hormones (estradiol and progesterone) reach and act on the endometrium through the bloodstream. During pregnancy, the implanted fertilized ovum forms HCG (human chorionic gonadotropin), which stimulates the corpus luteum to secrete more progesterone (corpus luteum of pregnancy). (After Langman)

Corpus Luteum

Under the influence of *pituitary luteinizing hormone* (*LH, lutropin*) the follicular epithelium left in the ovary is transformed within a few days into a corpus luteum and begins to secrete luteal hormones (e. g., progesterone) (Figs. 11.**10** and 11.**11**). This acts on the uterine mucosa to prepare it for nidation (nesting) of the fertilized ovum (*secretory phase*). If

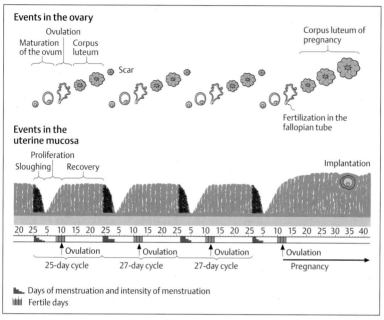

Events in the ovary

Ovulation

Maturation | Corpus
of the ovum | luteum

Scar

Corpus luteum of
pregnancy

Fertilization in the
fallopian tube

**Events in the
uterine mucosa**

Proliferation

Sloughing | Recovery

Implantation

20 25 5 10 15 20 25 5 10 15 20 25 5 10 15 20 25 5 10 15 20 25 30 35 40

↑Ovulation   ↑Ovulation   ↑Ovulation   ↑Ovulation

25-day cycle   27-day cycle   27-day cycle   Pregnancy

Days of menstruation and intensity of menstruation
Fertile days

Fig. 11.**12** **Simplified representation of the regular cyclic changes in the ovary and
the endometrium**

fertilization occurs, the germ cell takes over the secretion of *chorionic
gonadotropins* (*human chorionic gonadotropin, HCG*), which in turn
stimulates the corpus luteum to secrete more progesterone. The corpus
luteum becomes a *corpus luteum of pregnancy* (*corpus luteum gravidi-
tatis*) and fulfills its task up to about the 4th month of pregnancy. After
that it degenerates and the placenta takes over the functions of the corpus luteum.

If the ovum is not fertilized, the corpus luteum stops functioning
after about 2 weeks (*false corpus luteum, corpus luteum of menstruation =
corpus luteum menstruationis*). As the progesterone level declines, the
uterine mucosa undergoes menstrual bleeding and the mucosa is
sloughed off (Fig. 11.**12**).

The Menstrual Cycle

During the period of sexual maturity, the ovarian cycle causes cyclic changes in the uterine mucosa that lead to periodic sloughing of the mucosa (menstrual bleeding). The menstrual cycles begin (*menarche*) between the 10th and 15th years of life; they end (*menopause*) about the 50th year of life, beginning the "change" (climacteric). During this phase of life, the secretion of ovarian hormones gradually declines, follicular growth and ovulation no longer take place, and the uterine mucosa becomes increasingly thinner. The menstrual cycle is divided into three phases and lasts on an average 28 days (Fig. 11.**12**). Longer or shorter cycles are common. The day when menstrual bleeding begins is designated as the first day of the cycle. The phases are:

1. **Phase of desquamation and regeneration (day 1–day 4)**
2. **Follicular (proliferative) phase (day 5–day 14)**
3. **Luteal (secretory) phase (days 15–28)**

The proliferative phase shifts into the secretory phase on the day of ovulation (day 14 of a 28-day cycle). The secretory phase always lasts about 14 days, regardless of the duration of the cycle. Therefore, the day of ovulation shifts correspondingly.

If pregnancy does not occur, the corpus luteum involutes after 13–14 days. The interruption in progesterone secretion then causes menstrual sloughing of the uterine mucosa. At the same time, there is a transient diminution in the number of thrombocytes and blood clotting is reduced. Immediately afterward, the mucosa begins to regenerate from the basal layer (Fig. 11.**11**).

In the following proliferative phase, the endometrium grows and the mucosal glands enlarge. These processes are controlled by estrogens that are formed in the growing follicle and reach the uterine mucosa through the bloodstream. The proliferative phase ends on the day of ovulation (usually on or around the14th day).

The secretory phase that follows is controlled by the corpus luteum. It prepares the mucosa for the *nidation* (*implantation*) of the germ cell. In this phase the mucosal glands reach their greatest length and produce a mucous secretion. After ovulation, progesterone effects a rise in body temperature of 0.5–1 °C.

Fallopian Tube (Uterine Tube, Salpinx)

The fallopian tubes are about 10–15 cm long and are incorporated into the broad ligament of the uterus by a ligament (mesosalpinx) (Figs. 11.**13** and 11.**14**). It begins at the level of the ovary at the abdominal ostium (opening) as a funnel lined with fringes (*infundibulum, fimbriated end*) and runs into the uterus at an angle. It is usually divided into the narrow uterine end (*isthmus, isthmus tubae uterinae*) and the wider outer part (*ampulla, ampulla tubae uterinae*) in which fertilization takes place (Fig. 11.**13**).

The mucosal surface of the fallopian tube is greatly magnified by several longitudinal folds. It is lined with a simple columnar ciliated epithelium with numerous glandular cells that secrete mucus at certain stages of the cycle. The kinocilia of the epithelium direct the fluid stream toward the uterus, against which the spermatozoa must swim but which helps to transport the fertilized ovum toward the uterus. The migration of the germ cell through the tube, which lasts 4–6 days, is aided by *peristalsis of the tubal musculature directed toward the uterus.*

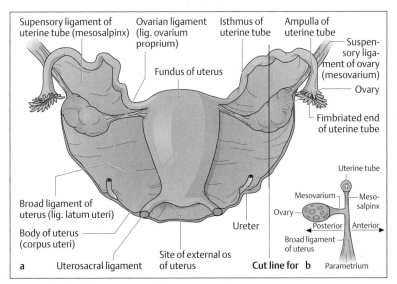

Fig. 11.**13 a**, **b**   **Uterus, fallopian tubes and ovaries**
a   Dorsal view
b   Section through **a** along the indicated cut line

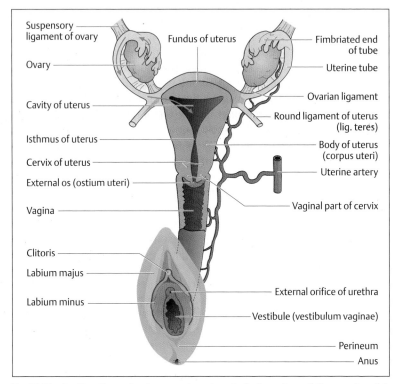

Fig. 11.**14** **Section through uterus and vagina, including view of the ovaries, fallopian tubes, and external sex organs** (blue arrows indicate the path of the ovum from ovary to uterus)

Uterus

During pregnancy, the uterus supports the fertilized ovum. In shape and size it resembles a pear, and it lies between the urinary bladder and the rectum (Figs. 11.**8**, 11.**13**, and 11.**14**). It is divided into a *body* (*corpus uteri*), a *fundus* situated between the tubal ostia, and a *narrow portion* (*isthmus uteri*), situated at the transition from the uterine body to the *uterine neck* (*cervix uteri*). The cervix is conical and below is directed backward into the vaginal vault. There is an external opening in the part projecting into

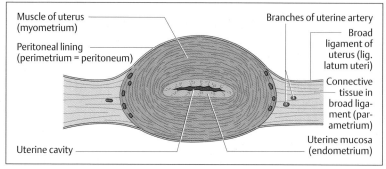

Muscle of uterus (myometrium)

Peritoneal lining (perimetrium = peritoneum)

Uterine cavity

Branches of uterine artery

Broad ligament of uterus (lig. latum uteri)

Connective tissue in broad ligament (parametrium)

Uterine mucosa (endometrium)

Fig. 11.**15** **Cross-section through a human uterus**

the vagina (*portio vaginalis*), the *external os* (*ostium uteri externum*) (Fig. 11.**14**).

The *uterine cavity* is a narrow slit lined with mucous membrane (*endometrium*). The rest of the wall consists of a muscular layer (*myometrium*) up to 2 cm thick and a peritoneal covering over the corpus and fundus (*perimetrium*). The connective tissue space on each side of the uterus is called the parametrium. It contains important structures including the ureter and vessels running toward the uterus (e. g., the uterine artery) (Figs.11.**13** and 11.**14**).

Depending on the phase of the cycle, the uterine mucosa is 2–8 mm thick and is lined by a simple epithelium. The mucosal connective tissue contains numerous tubular glands with ducts opening into the uterine cavity. The mucosa is made up of two layers, one immediately adjacent to the muscular layer, the basal layer (stratum basale) and the functional layer (stratum functionale), which overlies it (Fig. 11.**11**). The cyclic changes of the uterine mucosa affect chiefly the functional layer.

Vagina

The vagina is a thin-walled tube, about 10 cm long, with a weakly developed muscle layer (Figs. 11.**8** and 11.**14**). Its blind end surrounds the vaginal portion of the uterus, forming the *vaginal vault* (*fornix of the vagina, fundus of the vagina*). Its anterior end opens into the *vaginal vesti-*

bule. It is lined with a stratified squamous epithelium that shows changes with the menstrual cycle: during the second phase of the cycle, the superficial epithelial cells, which in this phase have an especially high glycogen content, are increasingly desquamated. The mucus of the cervical glands and the desquamated epithelial cells together form the acid vaginal secretion. The acidity (pH 4–4.5) of the vaginal milieu is due to a physiological lactobacillus (*Lactobacillus acidophilus* = Döderlein's bacillus), that transforms the desquamated epithelial cells into lactic acid. This physiological vaginal flora is an effective barrier against invasion of the vagina by bacteria or other pathogens.

External Female Sex Organs (Vulva)

The external female sex organs as a whole are called the *vulva*.

Vestibule (Vestibulum Vaginae), Labia Majora and Minora, and Clitoris

The urethra, the vagina, and the various vestibular glands all terminate in the vestibule (Fig. 11.**14**). It is bounded laterally and posteriorly by skin folds, the labia majora and minora, anteriorly by the clitoris, and posteriorly by a small skin fold, the *frenulum* (*posterior commissure, fourchette, frenulum labiorum pudendi*). The two bulbospongiosus muscles are not fused as in the male, but lie on either side of the labia minora and join at the level of the *perineum*. The two muscles cover the *vestibular bulbs*, two dense erectile venous networks that correspond to the corpus spongiosum in the male.

The labia majora contain adipose tissue and sebaceous, sweat, and scent glands. The clitoris arises by two crura from the inferior pubic rami and ends in the *glans* (*glans clitoridis*), an erectile body comparable to the male glans. The vaginal orifice can be partly occluded by a membrane (*hymen*) until the first sexual intercourse. The ducts of the large *glands of the vestibule* (*Bartholin glands*), about 1–2 cm long, end on each side of the vaginal opening and moisten it.

The Female Breast (Mamma) and Mammary Gland

The female breast and mammary gland are structures derived from skin and are functionally related to the female sex organs. They develop during puberty under hormonal influence and are composed of glandular, adipose, and connective tissues (Figs. 11.**16** and 11.**17**).

The sexually mature breast has the shape of a pliable hemisphere and is freely movable over the pectoralis major muscle at the level of the 3rd

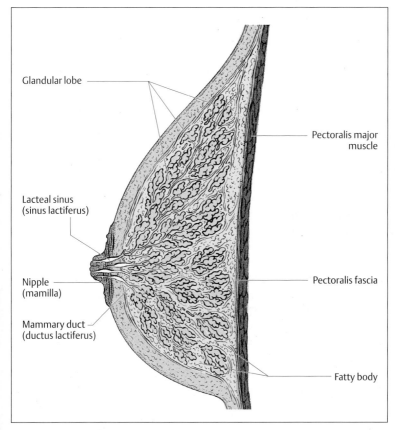

Glandular lobe

Pectoralis major muscle

Lacteal sinus (sinus lactiferus)

Nipple (mamilla)

Pectoralis fascia

Mammary duct (ductus lactiferus)

Fatty body

Fig. 11.**16**   **Longitudinal section through a female breast.** (After Leonhardt)

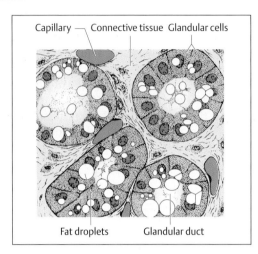

Capillary — Connective tissue Glandular cells

Fat droplets   Glandular duct

Fig. 11.**17** **Section through a lactating milk gland** (the glandular cells form the fatty droplets of milk)

to 7th ribs. From about the middle of the breast projects the *nipple* (*mamilla, mammary papilla*), on which open the 15–20 lacteal sinuses (*sinus lactiferi*), the ends of the *lactiferous ducts* (*mammary ducts*), which are the ducts from the lobes of the gland.

During pregnancy, the duct system and the glands proliferate under the influence of estrogens and progesterone, the breast increasing considerably in size. At the same time, the nipple becomes more prominent and the areola darkens. During the last month of pregnancy, the breast at first secretes a precursor to the milk, the colostrum, which consists of droplets of fat and sloughed cells. Compared to milk, colostrum contains less fat and more protein, as well as maternal antibodies that help protect the newborn against exogenous pathogens. After delivery, prolactin— a pituitary hormone (see Chapter 7: Adenohypophysis [Anterior Lobe of the Pituitary Gland])—leads to milk secretion. Later, a posterior pituitary hormone, oxytocin, promotes lactation by stimulating specialized cells in the gland, the *myoepithelial* cells, to contract.

Summary **The Reproductive Organs**

The role of the reproductive organs is to form haploid germ cells, to enable their union, and to ensure the development of the fertilized ovum through the embryonic and fetal stages until birth. The reproductive organs also secrete hormones to regulate the development of the germ cells and the cyclic changes in the endometrium. Finally, they take part in the expression of the specific sexual characteristics of the human body.

■ Structure and Function of the Reproductive Organs

- *Gonads:* produce germ cells and sex hormones
- *Reproductive passages:* transport the reproductive substances
- *Reproductive glands:* produce secretions that promote the union of ovum and sperm
- *External sex organs:* allow sexual union to occur

■ Male Reproductive Organs

- *Internal male reproductive organs:* testes, epididymis, vas deferens, seminal vesicles, and prostate
- *External sex organs:* penis and scrotum

Testes: paired organ, about the size of a plum with a dense connective tissue capsule (tunica albuginea); testicular tissue is divided into about 200 lobules each with 2–4 convoluted seminiferous tubules (tubuli seminiferi contorti), the walls of which form the germinal epithelium from Sertoli and germ cells.

- *Spermatogenesis* is divided into periods of multiplication (mitotic division of spermatogonia throughout life), maturation (by mitosis the spermatogonia develop into primary spermatocytes that enter the first maturation division and form haploid secondary spermatocytes; the second maturation division creates spermatids), and differentiation (spermatids are transformed into the mobile form: sperm cells). It is regulated by the anterior pituitary (FSH); duration: about 72 days.
- *Testosterone production:* interstitial cells of Leydig outside the seminiferous tubules; regulated by the anterior pituitary (LH).

Epididymis: through the rete testis, spermatozoa reach the epididymis, in which the spermatozoa mature and in which their motility is reduced; duration: 10–12 days.

Vas deferens: runs in the spermatic cord (funiculus spermaticus) is accompanied by vessels and nerves; about 50–60 cm in length; transports the spermatozoa from the epididymis to the urethra. It is wider at the end (ampulla of the vas deferens), is joined by the duct of the seminal vesicle, and opens as the ejaculatory duct into the prostatic urethra.

Seminal vesicles: also called seminal glands; secrete the major part of the ejaculate (about 75%), of which most important component is the sugar fructose (delivers energy for spermatic motility).

Prostate: chestnut-sized gland between base of bladder and urogenital diaphragm; posteriorly abuts on rectum (rectal examination of the prostate). The glandular tissue is divided into an outer zone (most likely site for the development of malignant tumors), an inner zone, and a periurethral zone surrounding the urethra (commonest site for benign prostatic adenomata). The prostate secretes one-quarter of the spermatic fluid (major components: acid phosphatase, immunoglobulins, prostaglandins, spermine). The ducts of the prostatic glands open into the prostatic part of the urethra.

Semen (ejaculate): comprises 3–6 ml fluid (chiefly from the seminal vesicles and the prostate), with about 20 million spermatozoa/ml (normospermia) after three days of sexual continence (oligospermia corresponds to less than 20 million sperm cells; azoospermia is the absence of sperm cells in the ejaculate).

Cowper's glands: pea-sized paired glands at the level of the urogenital diaphragm; open into the proximal portion of the spongy part of the urethra and with their alkaline secretion neutralize the urethral environment.

Scrotum: contains the two testes and makes possible an optimal ambient temperature (3 °C lower than body temperature) for spermatogenesis.

Penis: consists of a root, a body, and a glans, as well as the freely movable penile skin. Three erectile bodies (corpora cavernosa penis, paired erectile bodies; corpus spongiosum, unpaired urethral erectile body) permit the erection of the penis and are surrounded by a dense connective tissue sheath (tunica albuginea). The corpus spongiosum protects the urethra and allows the sperm to be transported during an erection.

Erection (regulated by the parasympathetic system): blood flows from the deep arteries of the penis (aa. profundae penis) into the cavities of the erectile bodies and the tunica albuginea becomes tense. This compresses the penile veins and blood flows in while drainage is impeded.

Ejaculation (regulated by the sympathetic nervous system): contraction of the smooth muscle of the prostate, the seminal vesicles and the vas deferens, while semen is made available to the prostatic urethra (emission). Closure of the bladder neck and contraction of the urogenital diaphragm leads to rhythmic expulsion of the ejaculate from the urethral opening.

▪ Female Reproductive Organs

- *Internal female reproductive organs:* ovaries, fallopian tubes, uterus, and vagina
- *External female reproductive organs:* labia majora and minora, vestibule, vestibular glands, and clitoris
- *Breast and mammary glands*

Ovaries: paired almond-sized intraperitoneal organs, attached to the pelvic wall by the suspensory ligament of the ovary, to the uterus by the ovarian ligament, and to the broad ligament of the uterus by the mesovarium (entry of blood vessels). It is divided into a cortex (contains various stages of ovarian follicles) and a medulla (contains blood vessels).

- *Oogenesis, maturation of the follicle, and ovulation:* oogenesis includes a multiplication period and a maturation period. The multiplication period is completed before birth, after which the primary oocytes are surrounded by a flattened simple follicular epithelium (about 1 million primordial or primary follicles at birth) and enter the first maturation division, which, however, is not completed until puberty (resting stage = dictyotene stage). After puberty, ovarian follicles mature in the cortex with the cycle (maturation sequence: primary, secondary, and graafian follicles). Shortly before ovulation in the middle of the cycle, the primary oocyte completes the first maturation division (separation of homologous chromosomes) with two resulting haploid cells: a secondary oocyte and a first polar body. The second maturation division follows during ovulation (result: the mature ovum and another polar body), but it is not completed until successful fertilization has occurred.

- *Hormonal regulation of follicular maturation:* The pituitary gonadotropic hormones (FSH = follicle-stimulating hormone and LH = luteinizing hormone) generate the cycle of follicle maturation (FSH) and trigger ovulation (LH). The follicular epithelium remaining after ovulation is transformed into a corpus luteum under the influence of LH). The female hormones secreted into the bloodstream by the follicular epithelium (estradiol) and the corpus luteum (progesterone) reach the uterine mucosa (endometrium), which undergoes cyclic changes under hormonal influence (menstrual cycle).

Fallopian tubes: paired tubes 10–15 cm in length with a funnel-shaped opening near the ovary and an opening into the uterus at the fundus; by their ciliated epithelium they transport the ovum, after fertilization in the ampulla, into the uterine cavity over 4–6 days.

Uterus: The uterus is a pear-shaped organ lying between the bladder and the rectum. It consists of a uterine body, a fundus (ostia of the fallopian tubes), uterine cavity, isthmus, and neck, as well as a cervix, the vaginal part that projects into vagina. It has an opening, the external os. Layers of the uterine wall: endometrium, myometrium, and perimetrium. The endometrium is composed of a basal layer and a functional layer.

- *Menstrual cycle:* menstruation begins (menarche) between the 10th and 15th years of life; it ends around the 50th year of life, followed by the menopause ("change", climacteric). Average duration of one menstrual cycle is 28 ± 3 days. There are three phases, beginning with the first day of menstrual bleeding:
  - Phase of desquamation and regeneration: days 1–4
  - Follicular phase (proliferative phase): days 5–14
  - Luteal phase (secretory phase): days 15–28
- *Mucosal (endometrial) changes during the cycle:* if ovulation is not followed by fertilization, the corpus luteum stops secreting progesterone after 2 weeks (= corpus luteum of menstruation), lead-

ing to menstrual bleeding and sloughing of the endometrium (phase of desquamation). Regeneration begins at the basal layer. During the ensuing proliferative phase the endometrium is regenerated (triggered by estradiol), and the secretory phase (the mucosa is prepared for implantation) begins at ovulation (formation of the corpus luteum). Should pregnancy occur, the trophoblast, after nidation (days 20–23 of the cycle), secretes human chorionic gonadotropin (HCG), which stimulates the corpus luteum to continue secretion of progesterone (corpus luteum of pregnancy). Desquamation does not occur and pregnancy can begin.

Vagina: thin-walled tube with little muscle between the vestibule and the vaginal portion of the uterus. The stratified squamous epithelium shows changes with the menstrual cycle. During the second half of the cycle desquamation of superficial epithelial cells containing glycogen increases. These are transformed into lactic acid by a lactobacillus (*Lactobacillus acidophilus* = Döderlein's bacillus). This permanent physiological vaginal flora (pH 4–4.5) protects against bacteria and pathogens, and is especially effective in the second half of the cycle (protecting nidation in case of a fertilized ovum).

External female reproductive organs (vulva): include the vestibule, the labia majora and minora, the vestibular glands, and the clitoris. The vestibule receives the openings of the urethra, the vagina, and the vestibular glands.

The female breast and mammary gland: Derivatives of skin that develop during puberty under hormonal influence and are made up of glandular, adipose, and connective tissue. The lacteal ducts (mammary ducts) open as 15–20 lacteal sinuses (sinus lactiferi) on the nipple (mamilla). During pregnancy, hormones (estradiol, progesterone) cause the glands and ducts to grow. The secretion of milk begins after birth, triggered by prolactin (anterior pituitary hormone). Lactation is facilitated by oxytocin (posterior pituitary hormone).

12

Reproduction, Development, and Birth

Contents

Human sexual reproduction is characterized by the union of a male sperm cell with a female ovum (fertilization), the ensuing transport of the germ cell through the uterine tube, its nidation (implantation) into the uterine mucosa, and the subsequent development into a viable newborn infant (embryonic and fetal development). At the end of the 8th week of gestation, *embryonic development* (*embryogenesis*), during which the primordial organs are laid down, becomes *fetal development* (*fetation*), characterized by the growth and differentiation of the organ systems.

■ Germ Cells

The development of germ cells (*oogenesis* and *spermatogenesis*) begins when diploid primitive germ cells (oogonia and spermatogonia) first form more diploid primary oocytes and spermatocytes (primary oocytes and primary spermatocytes) by mitosis. These develop into haploid cells (spermatozoa and ova) during the first and second maturation division (see Chapter 1). During fertilization, the sperm cell and the ovum fuse and form a zygote (see below).

A female diploid germ cell (primary oocyte) with 44 autosomes and 2 sex chromosomes (44, XX) eventually forms four haploid daughter cells, each with 22 autosomes and one X chromosome (22, X) (Fig. 12.**1a**). Only one, however, develops into an ovum, the other three form polar bodies that contain hardly any cytoplasm and degenerate during further development.. The male diploid germ cell (primary spermatocyte) with 44 autosomes and 2 sex chromosomes (44, XY) also forms four daughter cells (spermatids), of which two each possess 22 autosomes and either an X or a Y chromosome (22, X and 22, Y) (Fig. 12.**1b**). In contrast to oogenesis, however, all develop into mature sperm cells.

■ Fertilization

The spermatozoa must seek the ovum actively to fertilize it. The arduous passage through the uterus to the ampulla of the uterine tube at a migrating speed of 3 mm per minute requires about 1–3 hours. Of the 200–300 million spermatozoa deposited in the posterior vaginal fornix

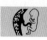

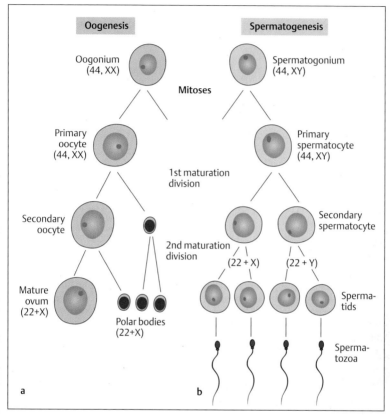

Fig. 12.**1 a, b   Formation of ovum and spermatozoa.** (After Sadler.) **a** Oogenesis: the oogonia first form primary oocytes with a diploid set of chromosomes (44, XX) by mitosis. The primary oocytes then pass through the first and second maturation divisions, which lead to four haploid cells (one mature ovum and three polar bodies). **b** Spermatogenesis: diploid spermatogonia divide by mitosis and form primary spermatocytes (44, XY). These divide by meiosis and form four haploid spermatids, each with one X (22, X) or one Y (22, Y) chromosome. The spermatids develop into the motile spermatozoa

during intercourse only about 300 reach the ovum. In contrast to the sperm cells, which can survive up to 4 days in the female genital apparatus, the ova must be fertilized within 6–12 hours after ovulation, otherwise they perish.

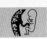

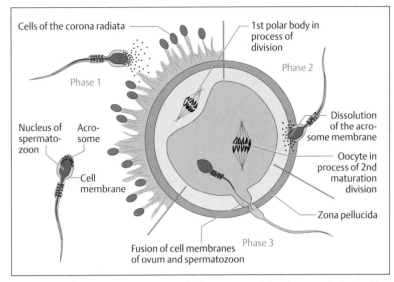

Fig. 12.**2** **Schematic representation of the process of fertilization.** (After Sadler.) During the first stage, the spermatozoon penetrates the cells of the corona radiata; during the second stage, the acrosome dissolves and the zona pellucida is digested by enzymes. In the third stage, the cell membranes of ovum and spermatozoon fuse and the sperm cell enters the ovum

During fertilization, the spermatozoon penetrates the attached follicular epithelial cells (corona radiata) and the zona pellucida by the action of the enzymes in the acrosome. This process of fertilization can be divided into three phases (Fig. 12.**2**):

- **Phase 1:** Penetration of the corona radiata
- **Phase 2:** Dissolution of the zona pellucida
- **Phase 3:** Fusion of the cell membranes of ovum and sperm

As a spermatozoon passes through the corona radiata and the zona pellucida, the so-called acrosome reaction takes place. Initially this involves the liberation of acrosomal enzymes (hyaluronidase and proteases) to disperse the follicular epithelial cells. Once the sperm cell has made contact with the glycoproteins of the zona pellucida, which have specific binding sites for spermatozoa, the acrosomal membrane dissolves and the enzymes so released facilitate the passage of the spermatozoon to the ovum. The cell membranes of the ovum and sperm cell then fuse and the spermatozoon penetrates the ovum. When the sperm cell touches the ovum, it elicits the so-called cortical reaction. Specific membrane receptors on the surface of the ovum are activated, triggering an action potential throughout the cell membrane. This leads to a sort of chain reaction that leads to exocytosis (outpouring) of intracytoplasmic vesicles from the ovum (cortical granules), the content of which empties into the space (perivitelline space) between the cell membrane of the ovum and the zona pellucida. This reaction (known as polyspermy block) prevents more than one sperm cell from entering the ovum. The head of the spermatozoon that has penetrated the ovum swells and forms the male pronucleus (Fig. 12.**3a–f**). Almost simultaneously, the ovum completes its second maturation division and forms the female pronucleus and the third polar body (Fig. 12.**3**). The first polar body also completes the second maturation division. Thus, at the end of oogenesis, a female pronucleus and three polar bodies have been formed, each with a haploid set of chromosomes. The two haploid pronuclei with 23 maternal or paternal chromosomes fuse into one diploid cell, called a *zygote*. The first mitotic division, in which two daughter cells, each with 46 chromosomes, is formed follows after about 30 hours. The number of cells then continues to be doubled by mitotic cell divisions.

Sex Determination

The genetic sex is determined during fusion by the *sex chromosome* (X or Y) of the male pronucleus. While all haploid ova always contain an X chromosome, sperm cells possess either an X or a Y chromosome (Fig. 12.**4**). Depending on whether the sperm cell meeting an ovum contains an X or a Y chromosome, the zygote that is formed will have XX (female) or XY (male) sex chromosomes.

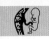

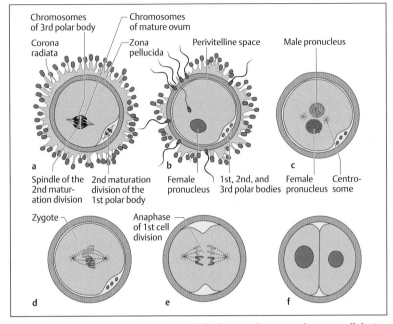

Fig. 12.**3 a–f** **Simplified representation of the fusion of ovum and sperm cell during fertilization.** (After Sadler)
a Secondary oocyte with the surrounding corona radiata cells immediately after ovulation during the second maturation division (anaphase). Under the zona pellucida, the first polar body is also dividing. **b** After the spermatozoon has penetrated the ovum, the second maturation division is completed with the formation of the female pronucleus (red) and a third polar body. **c** The head of the sperm cell develops into the male pronucleus (blue). **d** Formation of the zygote and beginning of the first mitotic cell division. **e** Anaphase of the first mitotic cell division. The three polar bodies have degenerated. **f** Two-cell stage, each with a complete set of chromosomes

Fig. 12.**4** **Sex determination**

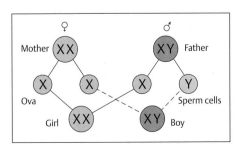

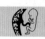

■ Transport through the Uterine Tube and Segmentation

After fertilization in the ampulla, the ovum divides in the course of its 4–5-day migration through the fallopian tube to the uterus (Figs. 12.**5** and 12.**6**) and arrives in the uterine lumen at approximately the 16-cell stage. The fertilized ovum is transported in the direction of the uterus by a fluid stream and by the cilia of the epithelial cells beating toward the uterus. Should this tubal transport be impeded, the germ cell can become implanted in the tubal mucosa, leading to a *tubal pregnancy*. In such a case, the growth of the embryo can lead to rupture of the tube after a short time (6–9 weeks), followed by massive, mostly life-threatening hemor-

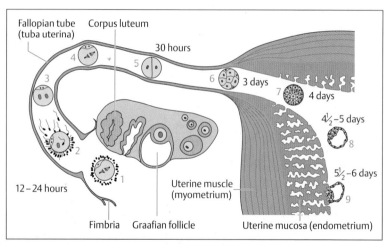

Fig. 12.5 Schematic representation of human developmental processes during the first week. (After Sadler)
1 Ovum immediately after ovulation
2 Fertilization within 12 hours
3 Stage of male and female pronucleus
4 First cleavage division
5 2-cell stage
6 Morula stage
7 Entry into the uterine cavity
8 Blastocyst
9 Early nidation (implantation) stage

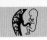

rhage. A fertilized ovum reaching the abdominal cavity leads to an *abdominal pregnancy*. In this case the ovum usually implants in the pouch of Douglas (see Chapter 11, Figs. 11.**8** and 11.**14**).

The segmented cells (blastomeres) formed during continued cell divisions form a *morula*, which is hardly larger than the fertilized ovum (Fig. 12.**6**). The morula enters the lumen of the uterus, where it develops, over the ensuing two days, into a *blastocyst* consisting of an *outer cellular envelope* (*trophoblast*) and an *inner cell mass* (*embryoblast*). Development up to the morula stage takes place within the zona pellucida; the blastocyst usually exits from the zona pellucida on the fifth day. At this point, the blastocyst becomes embedded in the endometrium with the aid of enzymes, a process called *nidation* or *implantation*. (Premature implan-

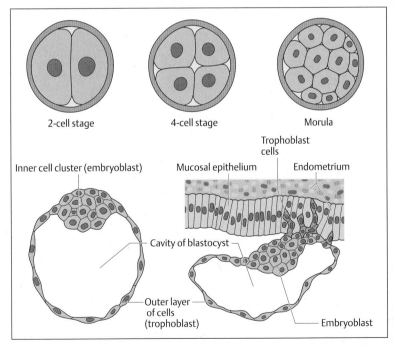

Fig. 12.**6**   **Schematic representation of the development of a zygote (zygote = fertilized ovum) from the two-cell stage to implantation of the blastocyst in the endometrium on day 5–6** (After Sadler)

tation into the wall of the fallopian tube is prevented by the zona pellucida.) While the embryoblast goes on to develop into the embryo, the trophoblast forms the fetal part of the placenta.

■ Implantation and Development of the Placenta (Afterbirth)

Normally, the germ cell is implanted into the part of the uterine cavity near the fundus (fundus uteri, see Fig. 11.**14**). At this time, about 5–6 days after ovulation, the endometrium is at the height of its secretory phase. For the rest of the period of gestation it is called *decidua* (*membrane that falls off*), because after delivery it is expelled as part of the afterbirth.

When it is implanted into the uterine mucosa, the trophoblast forms villi (chorionic villi or chorion) (Figs. 12.**7** and 12.**9**) that first contain a connective tissue core and later fetal blood vessels (*fetal part of the placenta*). These, together with parts of the uterine mucosa (*maternal*

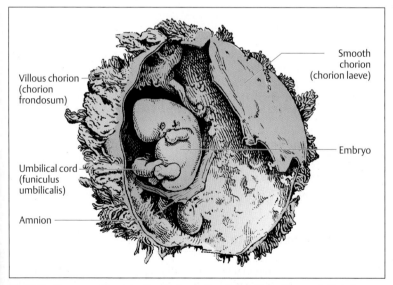

Fig. 12.**7** **Human embryo in the 2nd month of gestation. The gestational membranes have been opened**

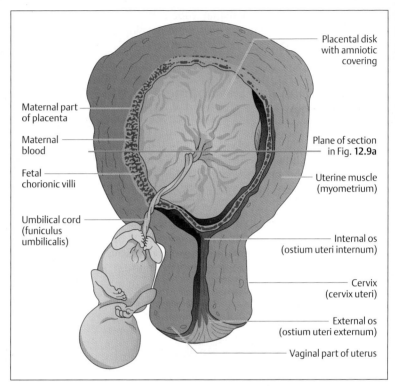

Placental disk
with amniotic
covering

Maternal part
of placenta

Maternal
blood

Fetal
chorionic villi

Umbilical cord
(funiculus
umbilicalis)

Plane of section
in Fig. 12.9a

Uterine muscle
(myometrium)

Internal os
(ostium uteri internum)

Cervix
(cervix uteri)

External os
(ostium uteri externum)

Vaginal part of uterus

Fig 12.**8** **Uterus, fetus, afterbirth (placenta), umbilical cord, and fetal membranes in the 6th month of gestation** (plane of cross-section shown in Fig. 12.**9a**)

part of the placenta), form the discoid placenta (afterbirth). The umbilical cord connects the embryo to this organ, which nourishes the growing germ and takes over the gas and substance exchange between the maternal and fetal bloodstreams.

Structure of the Placenta

The mature, fully formed placenta has a discoid shape with a diameter of about 18 cm (Figs. 12.**8**, 12.**9a**, **b**, and 12.**10a**, **b**). It weighs between 450 and 500 g and has the shape of a flat pot. The bottom of the pot is formed

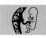

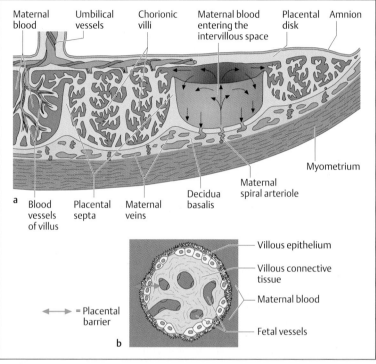

Fig. 12.**9 a, b** **Cross-section of a placenta (a) and a placental (chorionic) villus (b)**
a See Fig. 12.**8** for the plane of cross section
b The chorionic villi are bathed in maternal blood and contain fetal vessels. The placental barrier (arrow) consists of the villous epithelium, the villous connective tissue, and the wall of the fetal vessels

by the uterine mucosa (*decidua basalis*), the lid by parts of the fetal trophoblast (*chorionic disk*). From the chorionic disk project about 15–20 cotyledons, distinct structures formed by villi branching like trees from that part of the placenta that is filled with maternal blood. The maternal blood flows through spiral arterioles into the intervillous spaces, that are divided incompletely by placental septa. The intervillous spaces of a mature placenta contain about 150 ml of blood, which is exchanged about 3 to 4 times a minute. The placental villus is lined by an epithelium, and carries fetal vessels in the villous connective tissue inside it (Fig. 12.**9**). The total surface of the villi of a mature placenta is between 8 and 14 m². The gas and substance transport between maternal and fetal blood must pass through the epithelium and connective tissue of the villi and the wall of the fetal vessels (*placental barrier*) (Fig. 12.**9b**). As a rule, maternal and fetal blood do not mix. The placenta becomes detached from the uterine wall after the birth of the infant and is itself "born" (afterbirth). On examination of the maternal side of the placenta, 15–20 slightly elevated areas can be seen, the cotyledons, covered by a thin layer of decidua basalis. The grooves between the cotyledons are created by the placental septa (Fig. 12.**10a** and **b**).

The placenta has numerous tasks beside gas and substance transport. It ensures the stability of the pregnancy by taking over the tasks of the hypophysis and the ovary, forming important hormones such as estrogens, progesterone, and chorionic gonadotropins (placental hormones).

Umbilical Cord (Funiculus Umbilicalis)

After being oxygenated in the placenta, fetal blood reaches the fetus through a single umbilical vein. Deoxygenated blood returns to the placenta through two umbilical arteries (see Chapter 5: The Fetal Circulation). The umbilical arteries and vein run in a gelatinous connective tissue envelope, the umbilical cord, about 1.5 cm thick and up to 1 m long (Figs. 12.**8**, 12.**9**, and 12.**10**).

■ Development of the Embryo

After completed implantation, the cells of the embryoblast form a two-layered embryonic disk, consisting of an inner (*endoderm*) and an outer (*ectoderm*) germ layer, from which the embryo develops. The endoderm and ectoderm are each covered by a fluid-filled sac, the endoderm by the yolk sac and the ectoderm by the amnion, which forms the amniotic sac (Fig. 12.**11**). While the yolk sac regresses slowly, the embryo grows into the *amniotic cavity* that forms in the amnion. By the end of pregnancy, the latter contains about 1 liter of amniotic fluid ("waters"), the function of which is to protect and nourish.

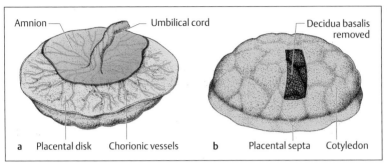

Fig. 12.**10 a, b   Placenta after birth. a** View from the fetal side (the amniotic epithelium has been partially removed). **b** View from the maternal side (the decidua basalis has been partly removed. The cotyledons bulge out and are separated from each other by the placental septa

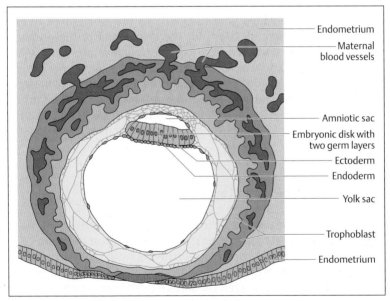

Fig. 12.**11   Diagrammatic representation of a 12-day-old human blastocyst.** (After Sadler)

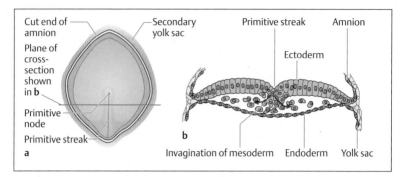

Fig. 12.**12 a, b**   **Diagrammatic representation of a 16-day-old human embryonic disk**
(After Sadler)
a   View of the embryonic disk from above
b   Cross-section of the embryonic disk; in the region of the primitive streak cells migrate
inward and form the middle germ layer, the mesoderm, between ectoderm and endoderm

The *primitive streak* (Fig. 12.**12a**, **b**), a narrow groove that deepens
and becomes the *primitive groove*, appears on the ectoderm of an embryo when it is about 16 days old. The cranial end of the primitive
streak (primitive node) develops into the *primitive pit*, from which
later the rudimentary *notochord* (*chorda dorsalis*) slides under the ectoderm in the direction of the eventual head. In this area occur extensive cell migrations and shifts (gastrulation). In the area of the primitive streak cells migrate inward and form the middle germ layer, the
mesoderm between the endoderm and the ectoderm (forming the
three germ layers).

Derivatives of the Germ Layers

The rudimentary organs develop from the three germ layers laid down at
the beginning of embryonic development (3rd week of gestation). The
outermost germ layer (*ectoderm*) essentially forms the rudiments of the
central nervous system (brain and spinal cord, as well as the otic vesicle,
nasal pit, and optic lenses) and the surface epithelium (epidermis). The
skeleton, the skeletal musculature, the circulatory organs, and the genitourinary organs develop from the *middle germ layer* (*mesoderm*). Finally

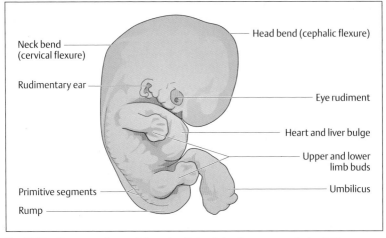

Neck bend (cervical flexure)

Rudimentary ear

Primitive segments

Rump

Head bend (cephalic flexure)

Eye rudiment

Heart and liver bulge

Upper and lower limb buds

Umbilicus

Fig. 12.**13**   **Human embryo at 6 weeks.** Natural size (crown–rump) about 13 mm

the *endoderm* (*innermost germ layer*), as it develops, forms chiefly the epithelial rudiments of the digestive and respiratory organs.

Evolution of the Body

The embryo is at first flat and shaped like a shield; it then begins to constrict at the anterior and posterior ends. At the end of the 4th week, the basic form of the trunk has been elaborated. The head grows very rapidly and occupies about one third of the total length of the embryo. Its shape is determined by the three primary brain vesicles and the ocular vesicles. At the beginning of the 5th week, the upper and lower limbs (limb buds) appear as plump buds on the lateral walls of the trunk. The trunk bulges owing to the rudiments of the cardiac tube and the liver. Caudad, it tapers to the rump (Fig. 12.**13**).

In the course of the 2nd month, the embryo bends markedly, with emphasis on bends in the neck and head (cervical and cephalic flexures). The head by this time takes up about half of the total length; the rudimentary forebrain is especially prominent. The eyelids are laid down as folds, and nose, lips, and chin can be identified. The pinnae of the external ear can be seen where the neck begins. Fingers and toes are seen as rays in the limb buds.

■ Development of the Fetus

The germ is called a fetus from the beginning of the 3rd month of gestation. Fetal development involves growth and the differentiation of the organ systems. Growth occurs in spurts. While the rate of growth is small up to the 26th week of gestation, the rate of physical growth then accelerates until the 27th week. This is followed by a period of maximal growth that continues until the 37th week. During this time the amniotic cavity (Fig 12.**14a**, **b**) also reaches its final size.

At the beginning of the 3rd month, the head takes up about one-half the size of the whole body, in the 5th month one-third, and at birth one-quarter (see Fig. 12.**17**).

The relationship between total length of the embryo and its age is given by Haase's rule, which can indicate the age of a fetus from the measurement of its length. According to this rule the total length (*crown–heel length*) of the fetus in centimeters (Arey's rule gives an equivalent calculation in inches) in the 4th and 5th months of gestation equals the square of the age in months, while from the 6th month on it equals 5 times the number of months. Table 12.**1** additionally lists the body weights in grams. The data for length in the 1st, 2nd, and 3rd months of gestation deviate from Haase's rule and refer to the crown–rump length, since the lower extremity is at first present only as a short bud.

Body length increases about 50-fold from the first month of gestation to birth, while weight increases about a thousandfold. After birth, until growth is complete, body length increases only about 3.5 times, while body weight increases 20 times.

Fetal growth can be monitored very precisely by the use of ultrasound. One measure used for this purpose is the distance between the two parietal bones (*biparietal diameter*), since the head is easily visualized by ultrasound. An approximate determination of fetal length can be obtained by the formula:

■ Biparietal diameter in cm × 5.5 = body length in cm

At birth, the biparietal diameter measures about 9 cm.

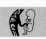

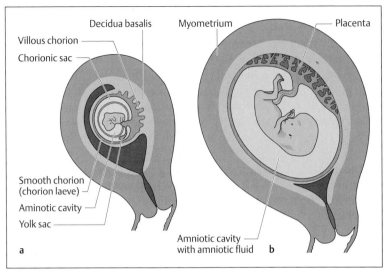

Fig. 12.**14 a, b** **Diagrammatic representation of the relation between fetal mem-branes and uterus.** (After Sadler)
a At the end of the 2nd month of gestation. Chorion frondosum (= villous chorion) be-comes the fetal part of the placenta; chorion laeve (= smooth chorion) does not take part in the formation of the placenta. The chorionic sac disappears at the end of the 2nd month. Decidua basalis = maternal part of the placenta
b End of the 3rd month. The placenta is fully developed

Table 12.**1** **Body length and weight of the human fetus**

Month of gestation		Body length (cm)	Body weight (g)
At the end of:	1st month	0.4	1
	2nd month	3	3
	3rd month	6	20
	4th month	16 (4 × 4)	130
	5th month	25 (5 × 5)	400
	6th month	30 (6 × 5)	700
	7th month	35 (7 × 5)	1100
	8th month	40 (8 × 5)	1800
	9th month	45 (9 × 5)	2750
	10th month	50 (10 × 5)	3300

Signs of Maturity

A full-term infant has a crown–heel length of about 49–51 cm with a sitting length (crown–rump length) of about 33 cm. Average weight is 3200 g for girls and 3400 g. for boys. (A neonate weighing less than 2500 g, regardless of gestational age, is said to be of *low birth weight*, by definition.) Lanugo hair is barely present and head hair is about 2 cm long. The fingernails and toenails project beyond the ends of the digits. In the male infant the testes have reached the scrotum and in the female infant the labia minora are just covered by the labia majora.

Other criteria used to determine the maturity of the newborn are the condition of the skin (color, turgidity, development of subcutaneous fat), stiffness of the nasal and auricular cartilages, the presence of certain neuromuscular reflexes, and the respiratory state, heart rate, and muscle tone. Radiologically, an epiphyseal center can be seen at the lower end of the femur.

Duration of Gestation and Calculation of the Date of Delivery

The date of reference for determining the duration of gestation is the date of last menstruation. Using the first day of the last menstrual period for this calculation, the average duration of pregnancy is 280 days, while the mean duration of gestation calculated from the time of ovulation is 266 days. For the sake of simplicity, the normal duration of pregnancy is given as 10 lunar months of 28 days = 280 days = 40 weeks.

■ **Naegele's rule is used to calculate the precise expected date of delivery on the basis of a 28-day menstrual cycle:**

- Subtract 3 calendar months from the first day of the last menstrual period, then add 7 days and 1 year = expected date of delivery.
- If the menstrual cycle is shorter (e. g., 25 days) or longer (e. g., 30 days) the difference above or below the normal must be subtracted (3 days) or added (2 days).

Example: first day of the last menstrual period: 22/10/1999. Calculated on the basis of a 28 day cycle:

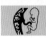

– Subtract 3 months from 22/10/1999 (= 22/07/1999)
– Add 7 days (= 29/07/1999)
– Add 1 year (expected date of delivery = 29/07/2000)
  For a 25-day cycle the expected date would be 26/07/2000; for a 30-day cycle it would be 31/07/2000.

■ Birth

At the end of the period of gestation, the infant lies in the uterus ready for delivery with its body bent and arms and legs crossed (Fig. 12.**15**); the head (*cephalic presentation*) or the breech (*breech presentation*) may be the *presenting part* that is directed toward the cervix. Labor is usually divided into three stages, of which the first is the stage of dilatation, the second the stage of expulsion, and the third the placental stage.

The *descent of the fetus,* i.e., the entry of the head of the fetus into the pelvic inlet, occurs toward the end of pregnancy in a woman who is giving

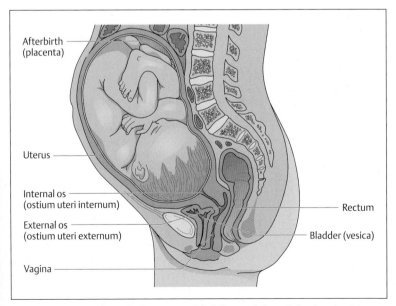

Fig. 12.**15**   **Section through the uterus with full-term infant.** (After Leonhardt)

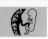

birth for the first time (*primipara*), or at the beginning of labor in one who has given birth before (*multipara*). During the first stage, the "waters," a sac filled with amniotic fluid, forms and precedes the head, widening the soft tissues of the birth canal. For this stage, the cervix, vagina, and perineum form a canal of constant diameter. The amnion usually ruptures ("breaking of the waters") toward the end of the first stage of labor, though it may do so earlier; indeed, amniotic rupture sometimes triggers the first stage. The amniotic fluid drains through the vagina.

The expulsion stage begins as soon as the external os of the cervix is fully dilated (fully dilated cervix). While the abdominal muscles bear down in support, rhythmic contractions of the uterus shorten the uterine musculature (Fig. 12.**16a**, **b**) and the child is pushed into, and through,

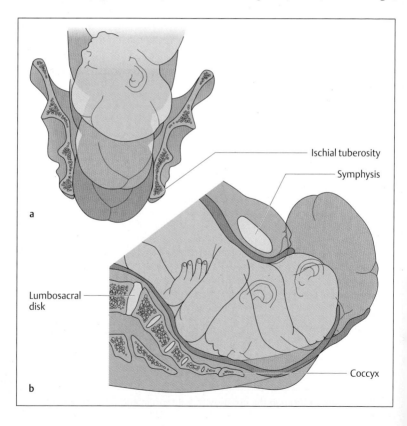

the birth canal. Because the pelvic inlet is oval with the longer diameter set transversely and the pelvic outlet is oval with the longer diameter set anteroposteriorly, the infant's head must rotate 90° during passage through the canal. Following the head, the shoulders align themselves first with the transverse diameter, then the anteroposterior diameter. The head, which has already been born, is forced into a renewed 90° rotation, which is assisted and supported by the obstetrician or midwife. The passage of the baby's head through the vulva is known in obstetrics as "crowning."

The third stage of labor begins with the completed expulsion of the child and ends with the expulsion of the placenta and fetal membranes. The cord is clamped and cut when delivery of the infant is complete. This procedure leads to carbon dioxide enrichment in the baby's blood and this helps to activate the respiratory center. The newborn begins to breathe with the "first cry." At the same time, the fetal circulation changes to the baby's own systemic and pulmonary circulation. After delivery, the uterus contracts, so that the placenta separates from the uterine wall. It is usually "born" about $1/4$–$1/2$ hour later (afterbirth) (Fig. 12.**10a, b**).

■ Postnatal Development

At birth, prenatal development ends and postnatal development begins. It is divided for practical purposes into various stages of development and age:

- Infancy: from birth to the end of the 1st year of life
- Early childhood: from the beginning of the 2nd year of life through the 6th year
- School years: from the 7th year of life to the beginning of puberty

◁ Fig. 12.**16a, b Childbirth (parturition).** (After Leonhardt)
a Bony pelvis and the baby's head seen from in front
b "Crowning" of the baby's head during childbirth, seen from the side. Because the pelvic inlet is oval with the longer diameter set transversely and the pelvic outlet is oval with the longer diameter set anteroposteriorly, the infant's head must rotate 90° during crowning

■ Puberty: the period from the appearance of the first secondary sexual characteristics up to complete sexual maturity
■ Youth or adolescence: continues to the completion of physical growth

The rate of growth differs among these various developmental stages. Normal physical development is best defined by correlating age with body length or height and body weight. As growth is followed from birth to its completion, it may be seen at different times to occur at slower or more rapid rates.

Body Length

The most rapid rate of growth is noted during the first year of life. For instance, growth during the first half-year is about 16 cm, while in the second half-year it is about half that (8 cm). About 50% of definitive body length is attained as early as the end of the 2nd year of life. To the beginning of puberty, annual growth is about 5–6 cm. After that, both sexes show a noticeable growth spurt (*pubertal growth spurt*), more marked in boys than in girls (9–10 cm as opposed to 8–9 cm). At 12 years of age, girls are in general taller than boys of the same age, as their pubertal growth spurt begins about two years earlier. Growth ends at different ages in different populations. In central Europe, for example, growth usually ends at age 17 or 18 years in women and at about age 19 in men The mean height of an adult woman is about 167 ± 11 cm, of an adult man 177 ± 13 cm.

Body Weight

Body weight, like body length, shows characteristic changes during the developmental stages. Thus birth weight (3200–3400 g) has about doubled by 5 months and has tripled by the end of the first year of life. It is fivefold by age 4–5 years. By the end of growth, body weight is about 20 times birth weight.

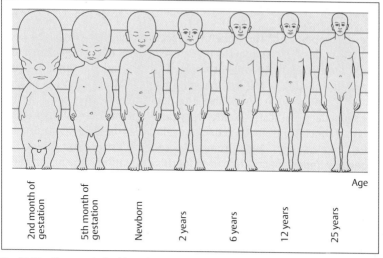

2nd month of gestation

5th month of gestation

Newborn

2 years

6 years

12 years

25 years

Age

Fig. 12.**17**   **Changes in bodily proportions during growth.** (After Rauber-Kopsch)

Physical Proportions

At each age the various regions, limbs, and organs of the body change in their relative size (proportions); i.e., their growth rates differ. Just as in the prenatal period, such changes in proportions are seen especially in infancy and early childhood. While the length of the head constitutes about one-half of the length of the embryo at the end of the 2nd month (Fig. 12.**17**), it measures about one-quarter of the total body length in the newborn, about one-sixth the body height in the 6-year-old child, and one-eighth in the adult. Acceleration of growth in the extremities brings with it an upward shift of the umbilicus, which is the middle of the body in the newborn. The middle of the body in the adult is the symphysis pubis.

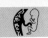

Growth of the Skeleton

The development of the skeleton, especially the part played by bone growth, is closely related to the total development of the organism and is considered when evaluating disorders of growth and in estimating eventual body height. In this estimation, radiological examination plays a major diagnostic role, for example, to determine at what point in time the secondary ossification centers appear. From these it is often possible to draw conclusions about general development by referring to the so-called "*skeletal age*." Apart from the secondary ossification centers, an especially important criterion used for this evaluation is the fusion of the epiphyseal and apophyseal disks (growth disks). For this, by convention, a radiograph is performed on the left hand of the infant or small child. The rate of development may be *retarded* or *accelerated*. Growth and development depend on many factors. For instance, body weight and especially growth in height depend on genetic influences, but external influences, such as the quality and quantity of the nutrients ingested with food, can also be demonstrated.

Summary **Reproduction, Development, and Birth**

Human sexual reproduction takes place in several stages:

- Union of a male sperm cell with a female ovum (fertilization)
- Subsequent transport of the germ cell through the uterine tube (tubal transport)
- Implantation (nidation) in the uterine mucosa (endometrium)
- Development into a viable infant (development of the embryo and fetus)

■ **Germ Cells**
- *Oogenesis:* oogonia (primitive germ cells, 44, XX)—primary oocytes (44, XX)—secondary oocytes (22, X)—ovum (mature egg cell, 22, X) plus 3 polar bodies (22, X).
- *Spermatogenesis:* spermatogonia (primitive germ cells, 44, XY)—primitive spermatocytes (44, XY)—secondary spermatocytes (22, X

or 22, Y)—spermatids (22, X or 22, Y)—sperm cells (spermatozoa, 22, X or 22, Y)

■ Fertilization

The spermatozoa must find the ovum after ovulation in the uterine tube (only 200–300 of 200–300 million reach the ovum, speed of migration: 3 mm/min). While spermatozoa can survive in the uterine tube up to 4 days, ova must be fertilized within 6–12 hours.

Process of fertilization (*3 phases*)*:* Acrosomal reaction (phase 1 and phase 2): penetration of the corona radiata and enzymatic dissolution of zona pellucida. Phase 3: fusion of the cell membranes of ovum and sperm cells, followed immediately by the cortical reaction (prevents penetration of the ovum by other spermatozoa = polyspermy block).

At the time of fertilization the ovum ends its second maturation division and forms the female pronucleus, which then fuses with the male pronucleus to form the diploid zygote. A female (XX) or male (XY) germ cell then forms, depending on the sex chromosome of the male pronucleus (X or Y).

■ Transport through the Uterine Tube and Cleavage

The zygote begins to divide (cleavage) during the 5 days of transport through the uterine tube into the uterus: zygote—2-cell stage—4-cell stage, etc. After the 16-cell stage, the germ is called a morula (mulberry), which is followed by a blastocyst with an outer shell of cells (trophoblast) and an inner cluster of cells (embryoblast).

When transport through the tube is impeded, a tubal pregnancy occurs.

■ Implantation and Placenta Formation

Implantation: Nidation of the blastocyst into the endometrium 5–6 days after ovulation or fertilization (endometrium at the peak of the secretory phase):

- *Trophoblast:* forms the fetal part of the placenta
- *Embryoblast:* forms the embryo, later fetus

Placenta:
- *Function:* provides the growing germ with nutrition, takes over substance and gas exchange, secures maintenance of pregnancy,

and secretes hormones (e. g., estrogens, progesteone, chorionic gonadotropins)

- *Structure:* consists of a fetal part with chorionic disk and chorionic villi, containing the fetal vessels, and a maternal part with decidua basalis (endometrium), spiral arterioles, and placental septa, between which the intervillous spaces are filled with maternal blood. Total surface of the villi: 8–14 m²; diameter of a mature placenta: ca. 18 cm; weight: 450–500 g.
- *Placental barrier:* separates maternal and fetal blood; formed by the villous epithelium, villous connective tissue, and the walls of the fetal vessels; selectively permeable to various substances.
- *Umbilical cord* (funiculus umbilicalis): connects the placenta with the fetal organism; contains an umbilical vein (v. umbilicalis; oxygenated blood flows from the placenta to the fetus) and two umbilical arteries (aa. umbilicales: deoxygenated blood flows from the fetus to the placenta).

■ Development of the Embryo

The period of embryonic development (formation of the embryonic disk, formation of the germ layers and organogenesis) begins following early development (transport through the uterine tube and implantation, 1st and 2nd week).

Formation of the embryonic disk: at first two germ layers (inner endoderm, outer ectoderm), later three germ layers including the middle germ layer (mesoderm). The mesoderm develops in the primitive streak on the ectodermal surface of the embryonic disk and migrates inward. The rudimentary head (notochord, chorda dorsalis) forms from its anterior end (primitive node).

Derivatives of the germ layers: ectoderm (central nervous system and surface epithelium); mesoderm (skeleton, skeletal muscle, circulatory organs, genitourinary apparatus), endoderm (epithelial lining of the digestive and respiratory passages).

Development of the body: folds form in the embryonic disk at the end of the 4th week; rudimentary extremities form at the beginning of the 5th week; embryonic curvature and appearance of the cephalic and cervical flexures between weeks 5 and 7. At the end of the embryonic period, the head makes up about 50 % of the total length.

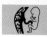

At the end of embryonic development, the embryo lies protected by amniotic fluid in the amniotic cavity, which continues to grow and contains about 1 liter of amniotic fluid at the end of gestation.

■ Development of the Fetus
At the beginning of the 9th week of gestation, the germ becomes a fetus. During the fetal period the organ systems grow and differentiate.

Growth in length (crown–heel length or crown–rump length depending on the month of gestation). Haase's rule: total length of the fetus in centimeters during the 4th and 5th month is the square of the number of months; from the 6th month onward it is 5 times the number of months.

- Monitoring of fetal growth by ultrasonography: biparietal diameter in cm × 5.5 = body length in cm.

Anatomical signs of maturity at term: crown–heel length (49–51 cm); crown–rump length (33 cm); weight (3200–3400 g); fingernails and toenails project beyond the ends of the digits. In boys the testes are in the scrotum; in girls the labia majora cover the labia minora.

Functional signs of maturity at term: evaluation of skin color, respiration, heart rate, muscle tone, and neuromuscular reflexes.

Duration of pregnancy: 280 days (= 10 lunar months of 28 days), calculated from the first day of the last menstrual period; 266 days, calculated form the time of ovulation or fertilization.

- *Naegele's rule* to calculate the expected date of delivery: subtract 3 calendar months from the first day of the last menstruation, add 7 days, add 1 year (valid for a 28 day cycle).

■ Labor
Divided into three stages. first stage (*stage of dilatation*), second stage (*stage of expulsion*), third stage (*placental stage*). During the phase of dilatation, the fetal head enters the pelvic inlet; the amnion, filled with amniotic fluid, dilates the soft tissues of the birth canal (soft tissue canal: cervix, vagina, and perineum) and the external os of the cervix dilates. The expulsion phase begins with rhythmic uterine contractions (supported by bearing down of abdominal muscles), rota-

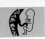

tion of the baby's head in the birth canal followed by the passage ("crowning") of the head through the vulva. When parturition is complete, the umbilical cord is divided. The placenta separates and appears as afterbirth about 30 minutes later.

■ Postnatal Development

- Divided into stages of development and age: *infancy* (1 year); *early childhood* (2nd to 6th years); *school age* (7th year to puberty); *puberty* (to full sexual maturity); *youth* or *adolescence* (to the completion of physical growth).
- *Physical development* is described by correlating rapidity of growth, body length or height, body weight, and physical proportions with age.
- *Skeletal age* (timely appearance of centers of ossification and epiphyseal fusion); used to evaluate disorders of growth and estimate eventual body height. Left hand is examined radiologically.

13

The Central and Peripheral Nervous Systems

Contents

■ Classification of the Nervous System

The nervous system connects the organism with its environment (*somatic nervous system*) and its internal organs (*autonomic or vegetative nervous system*). The characteristics of the somatic nervous system are conscious sensation, voluntary movement, and rapid processing of information. The vegetative nervous system, on the other hand, is responsible for maintaining a constant internal milieu (homeostasis) and for the autonomous regulation of organ functioning in response to environmental demands.

The somatic and the autonomic nervous systems include sensory (*afferent*) as well as motor (*efferent*) connections. Afferent conduction occurs when impulses are conducted from the periphery (e. g., sensations from skin or internal organs) to the center (brain and spinal cord). In efferent conduction, impulses are conducted from the center to the periphery (e. g., skeletal muscle, smooth muscle, gland cells) (Fig. 13.**1**).

By its spatial distribution the nervous system is divided into a *central nervous system* (*CNS*) and a *peripheral nervous system*. The CNS includes the brain and spinal cord. The peripheral nervous system includes all somatic and autonomic nerves, including the collections of nerve cells called ganglia.

■ Role of the Nervous System

The central and peripheral nervous systems coordinate the performance of organ systems directly (through nerves) or indirectly (through endocrine glands). They regulate the activities of the locomotor apparatus, the respiratory, circulatory, digestive, and urogenital systems, and the system of endocrine glands. Integration and evaluation of incoming impulses occur in the central nervous system, while the peripheral nervous system conducts impulses originating in the CNS to the periphery of the body and conducts impulses from the periphery to the CNS. (For a discussion of the generation, conduction, and transmission of nerve impulses, see Chapter 3: The Nerve Impulse [Action Potential], and Chapter 3: The Synapse.) Beyond these functions, the so-called "higher functions" of the nervous system (memory, ability to learn and think, judgment, language) are tied to the activity of the central nervous system.

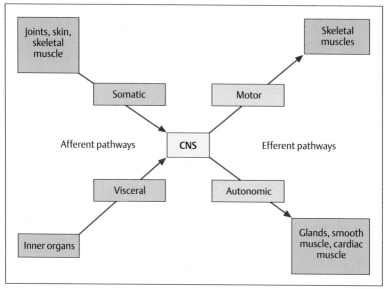

Fig. 13.**1**   **Diagram showing the connections between the central and peripheral nervous systems.** CNS = brain and spinal cord

■ Development of the Nervous System

The components of the central and peripheral nervous system develop from the outer germ layer, the *ectoderm*. The first rudiment appears about the 18th day of embryonic development as a platelike thickening of the ectoderm of the embryonic disk (*neural plate*) (Chapter 12: Derivatives of the Germ Layers). Within the neural plate, between two lateral folds (*neural folds*), develops a depression—the neural groove—which subsequently closes to form the *neural tube* and migrates inward. Parts of the neural folds that do not take part in the formation of the neural tube form the neural crests (Fig. 13.**2a–c**).

The neural tube becomes the central nervous system (brain and spinal cord), while the neural crests form the peripheral nervous system (peripheral nerves and ganglia).

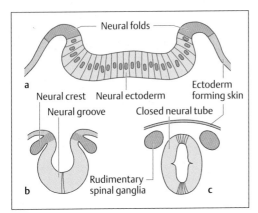

Fig. 13.**2a–c** Develop-
ment of the nervous sys-
tem. Schematic cross- section through the superior
portion of a 20-day-old
human embryonic disk.
(After Faller)

- Neural folds
- Neural crest Neural ectoderm
- Neural groove
- Ectoderm forming skin
- Neural groove Closed neural tube
- Rudimentary spinal ganglia

a Neuroderm (neural plate), laterally turning into skin at the neural folds
b Formation of the neural groove and extrusion of the neural crests
c The neural groove has closed to form the neural tube and now lies under the dermal
part of the ectoderm. The substance of the neural crests forms, among others, the spinal ganglia

■ Central Nervous System

The central nervous system is divided into the *brain* (*encephalon*) and the
spinal cord (*medulla spinalis*). Both parts are well protected against external influences by bony walls and the cushioning effect of the cerebrospinal fluid (CSF, liquor cerebrospinalis). The brain is enveloped in a bony
capsule, the cranial cavity, while the spinal cord lies in the vertebral
canal, surrounded by the bones of the vertebral column. *Cranial or spinal
membranes* enclose a space filled with cerebrospinal fluid around the
brain and spinal cord, respectively.

Development and Organization

The division of the brain into cerebrum, midbrain, pons, cerebellum, and
medulla oblongata (Fig. 13.**4a, b**) is based on its development from the
three *embryonic primary brain vesicles* (forebrain, midbrain, and hind-

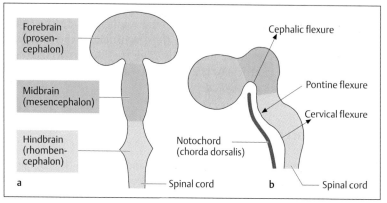

Fig. 13.**3 a, b   Development of the brain (stage of three primary brain vesicles).**
(After Faller)
a View from above
b Lateral view. The three primary embryonic brain vesicles form at the anterior end of
the neural tube; the posterior end becomes the spinal cord

brain) formed from the anterior end of the neural tube (Fig. 13.**3a, b**). The
posterior part of the neural tube becomes the spinal cord. The wall of the
neural tube develops into the gray and white matter of brain and spinal
cord, while its lumen develops into a system of cavities in the brain (ventricles) and a narrow canal (central canal) in the spinal cord.
   The derivatives of the primary brain vesicles are as follows:

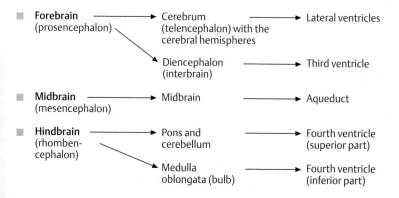

The ventricular system (see Cerebrospinal Fluid [CSF] and the Ventricular System below) consists of four cavities inside the brain, namely, the two lateral ventricles, the third ventricle of the midbrain, and the fourth ventricle of the hindbrain. They are interconnected (e. g., the third and fourth ventricle by the aqueduct = aqueduct of Sylvius) and are filled with *cerebrospinal fluid.*

The Brain (Encephalon)

The brain of a newborn weighs about 400 g and grows in the course of the first 9 months of life to about 800 g. It reaches close to its final weight of about 1310 g at about 5–7 years of age and is fully formed at 10 years. Data concerning brain weight vary remarkably (1100–1600 g). The brain of a man weighs on average 1375 g, that of a woman about 1245 g. The lesser weight in the woman is ascribed to the weaker development of her locomotor system and its consequently reduced representation in the CNS. However, when the actual brain weight is compared to body weight (brain/body weight ratio), women show on an average 22 g of brain weight per kg of body weight, while in men the figure is 20 g.

The striking example of the blue whale shows that the absolute weight of the brain is of no significance. A whale weighing about 74000 kg has a brain weight of 7 kg. If, now, we again compare brain weight to body weight, 1 kg body weight corresponds to 0.1 g brain weight. If a similar body/brain weight ratio were applied to a human brain, it would weigh on average 7 g.

Cerebrum or Forebrain (Telencephalon)

Cerebral Hemispheres

The cerebrum is the *highest integration center of the CNS* and for this reason is the most markedly differentiated segment of the human brain. Essentially it is composed of two structures: the two cerebral hemispheres and several bilateral gray nuclei (basal ganglia). The latter have a partial role in motor activity, especially the initiation and performance of slow movements. They lie deep inside the hemispheres and cannot be seen

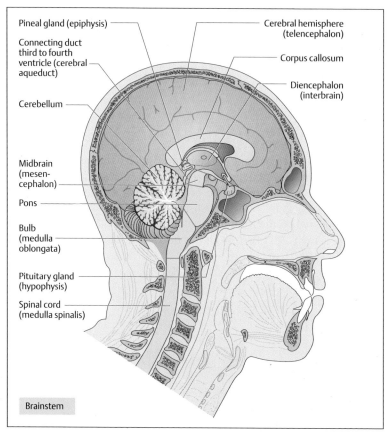

Pineal gland (epiphysis)

Connecting duct third to fourth ventricle (cerebral aqueduct)

Cerebellum

Midbrain (mesencephalon)

Pons

Bulb (medulla oblongata)

Pituitary gland (hypophysis)

Spinal cord (medulla spinalis)

Cerebral hemisphere (telencephalon)

Corpus callosum

Diencephalon (interbrain)

Brainstem

Fig. 13.**4 Organization of the brain.** Sagittal section through the head of an adult man; view of the left half from the medial side. The midbrain, pons, and medulla oblongata together form the brainstem

until the brain is cut. The two voluminous cerebral hemispheres are separated by a deep division, the *longitudinal fissure* (Fig. 13.**7**) and comprise the major part of the visible substance of the brain.

Lobes of the Brain (Cerebral Lobes)

The surface of the brain is formed by convolutions (gyri) separated by fissures (sulci). The two lateral sulci and the central sulcus may be considered to divide each hemisphere into four lobes (Fig. 13.**5**):

- **Frontal lobe**
- **Parietal lobe**
- **Temporal lobe**
- **Occipital lobe**

The frontal lobe lies in front of the central sulcus, the parietal lobe behind it. The temporal lobe lies below the lateral sulcus, and an imaginary line drawn down from the parieto-occipital sulcus separates the parietal lobe from the occipital lobe. Deep inside the lateral sulcus lies the insula (island), covered by the frontal, parietal, and temporal lobes. The insula is often regarded as a fifth lobe. It has no known function in the human brain.

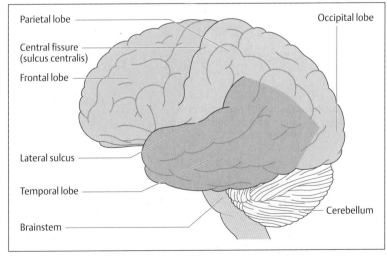

Fig. 13.**5**   **Lobes of the cerebrum.** Seen from the left side. (After Frick et al)

Each lobe in turn has its specific convolutions and fissures. For instance, the frontal lobe comprises the *precentral gyrus*, which lies immediately in front of the central fissure. It is the motor center that sends impulses to the voluntary muscles. The point situated closest to the forehead, the frontal pole, is the seat of personality.

Gray and White Matter

In a brain cut in the horizontal or coronal plane, the cerebral hemisphere can be seen to consist of an outer gray cortical layer; the cerebral cortex, about 2–5 mm thick, mainly composed of cell bodies; and an inner white core composed mainly of nerve fibers (myelinated axons) (Figs. 13.**6a**, **b** and 13.**7a**, **b**). The cerebral cortex has a total surface of about 2,200 cm², with about 10000–20000 nerve cells per mm³. This may be contrasted with the white matter, which houses about 300000–400000 km of nerve fibers.

Medullary Tracts and Internal Capsule

Fibers interconnecting the hemispheres are called *commissural fibers*. One example is the vast *corpus callosum* (Figs. 13.**4** and 13.**6a**), a fiber system containing about 200 million nerve fibers. Nerve fibers confined to one hemisphere are called *association fibers*. These run within the same hemisphere from lobe to lobe or fissure to fissure. Finally, there are fibers that run from the cerebral cortex to other parts of the CNS, called *projection fibers*. The majority of these form the *internal capsule* (Figs. 13.**6a**, **b** and 13.**7a**, **b**). This structure consists of an *anterior limb* (*crus anterius*), a *posterior limb* (*crus posterius*), and a segment between them, the *genu* (*knee*).

Basal Ganglia

Several basal ganglia are located next to the genu of the internal capsule (Figs. 13.**6a**, 13.**7a**, and 13.**8**), e. g., the *globus pallidus* and the *putamen*. The globus pallidus and the putamen together are also known as the *lentiform nucleus*. The anterior limb of the internal capsule is bounded by the *caudate nucleus* and the *lentiform nucleus*, which together form the *corpus striatum* (*striate body*). The posterior limb of the

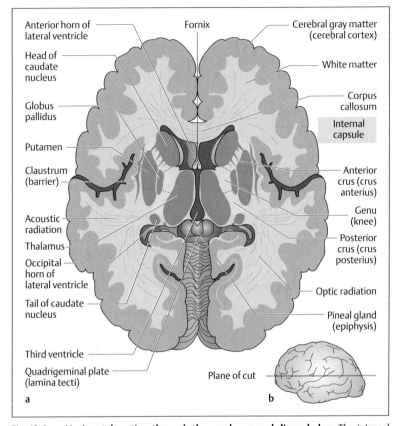

Anterior horn of lateral ventricle

Head of caudate nucleus

Globus pallidus

Putamen

Claustrum (barrier)

Acoustic radiation

Thalamus

Occipital horn of lateral ventricle

Tail of caudate nucleus

Third ventricle

Quadrigeminal plate (lamina tecti)

Fornix

Plane of cut

Cerebral gray matter (cerebral cortex)

White matter

Corpus callosum

Internal capsule

Anterior crus (crus anterius)

Genu (knee)

Posterior crus (crus posterius)

Optic radiation

Pineal gland (epiphysis)

a   b

Fig. 13.**6** **a Horizontal section through the cerebrum and diecephalon.** The internal capsule is shown in yellow. **b** Plane of the horizontal section

internal capsule is bounded medially by the *thalamus*. This is an important nuclear area of the diencephalon and is not considered part of the basal ganglia.

The basal ganglia have an important function in the so-called *extrapyramidal motor system* (see later in this chapter). The current view is that their function is to regulate the extent and direction of voluntary movements. The symptoms of lesions of the basal ganglia include disturbances of muscle tone and involuntary movements.

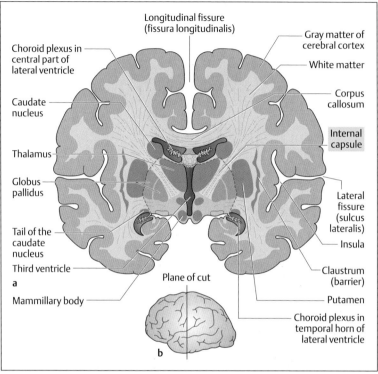

Fig. 13.7 a Coronal section through the cerebrum and diencephalon. The broken blue line shows the junction of the diencephalon and the telencephalon. The internal capsule is highlighted in yellow. **b** Plane of the coronal cut

Lateral Ventricles

The lateral ventricles are situated in the two cerebral hemispheres. They are a part of a system of cavities (ventricles) that contain the cerebrospinal fluid (CSF). The CSF is formed by an arterial plexus (choroid plexus) that extends into both lateral ventricles. The lateral ventricles possess a frontal horn, a body, an occipital horn, and a temporal horn (see Cerebrospinal Fluid [CSF] and the Ventricular System below and Fig. 13.**25a**, **b**). Each

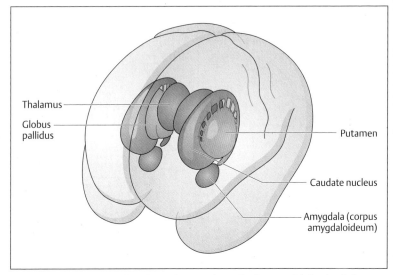

Fig. 13.**8**   **Location of the basal ganglia seen from the front and left.** The thalamus is shown for orientation, as it is not one of the basal ganglia. Putamen and globus pallidus = lentiform body. Caudate nucleus and lentiform body = corpus striatum. (After Duus)

lateral ventricle is connected with the third ventricle of the diencephalon by an opening, the interventricular foramen.

Limbic System

The term "limbic system" derives from the anatomical relation to the corpus callosum, which it surrounds like a hem (limbus) (Fig. 13.**9**). In the course of evolution, the limbic system was formed from an old part of the cerebrum that consisted mainly of the *paleocortex* and the *archicortex* (*archipallium*). The paleocortex and archicortex are often lumped together under the term *allocortex*, which takes up the major part of the cortex in lower mammals, for example. In humans these older parts of the brain are overgrown by the newer, strongly developed *neocortex* (*isocortex*).

The paleocortex consists essentially of the olfactory brain. The archicortex includes among other structures the amygdala (almonds) the

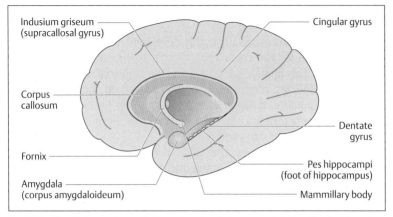

Fig. 13.**9** **The limbic system.** Right cerebral hemisphere, medial view. The limbic system is highlighted in yellow

hippocampus, the dentate gyrus, the cingulate gyrus, and the indusium griseum (supracallosal gyrus). From the hippocampus, a fiber tract (fornix) arches to areas of the hypothlamus, especially the mammillary bodies. From the mammillary bodies, in turn, pathways run to the reticular formation in the brainstem (see p. 555). The hippocampus and the cingulate gyrus are the central structures of the limbic system. The hippocampus plays an important role in aggression and in behavioral motivation, as well as in learning processes, particularly the formation of explicit memories, i.e., those that are accessible to deliberate, conscious recall. Short-term and long-term memory are components of explicit memory.

The limbic system evaluates experience affectively and triggers emotional reactions. Stimulation of these regions triggers rage, for example, but also pleasurable reactions. Thus, it is hardly surprising that many of their pathways end in the hypothalamus (see Diencephalon), which is the major coordinating and reflex center for many sensations such as smell and taste. Since the hypothalamus also regulates the autonomic nervous system (see p. 605), it makes sense that emotional reactions lead to autonomic disturbances (rise in blood pressure, blushing, becoming pale, etc.), while autonomic disturbances express themselves in emotions and psychosomatic illnesses.

Functional Cortical Areas

The cerebral cortex is especially highly developed in humans (Fig. 13.**10**). It is responsible for the characteristics that distinguish human beings from animals. This includes, for instance, the ability to use the hand for skillful and difficult movements, highly developed language, logical thinking, personality, and conscience. All this has become known because these characteristics are lost or are severely diminished when certain cortical areas are damaged.

Of the two hemispheres, the left is dominant in 80–90% of cases, mostly demonstrated by right-handedness (projection of the left hemisphere on the right half of the body by crossing of the nerve fibers). The two cerebral hemispheres are also known to differ in their intellectual abilities. For instance, the ability to read, speak, and write is especially marked in the left hemisphere. On the other hand, aptitudes such as memory, language comprehension, visualization of spatial relationships, and musical comprehension dominate in the right hemisphere.

The cerebral cortex in lower animals is small and almost exclusively responsible for the processing of olfactory stimuli (archicortex and paleocortex), which are among the most important sensations for these animals. The thalamus processes all stimuli from the sensory nerves and special senses, while the basal ganglia are the motor centers.

In the course of evolution the cerebral cortex has increased in size (neocortex) and has taken over other functions. For instance, the *postcentral gyrus*, situated behind the central fissure, has become the most important center for conscious somatic perception (somatosensory area). Meanwhile, the phylogenetically older center, the thalamus, has become a transmission and relay station for all impulses from general and special senses flowing toward the cerebral cortex and into consciousness. From the development of the motor cortex (*precentral gyrus*) it follows that the human basal ganglia perform only gross motor activities (see p. 542).

As the neocortex increases in size and takes over more functions, the number of neurons also increases. They are arranged in six layers. In order to be able to greatly increase its surface without increasing its volume, the cerebral cortex develops folds, the characteristic gyri and sulci. In lower mammals, as for instance the rat, the cerebral surface remains smooth.

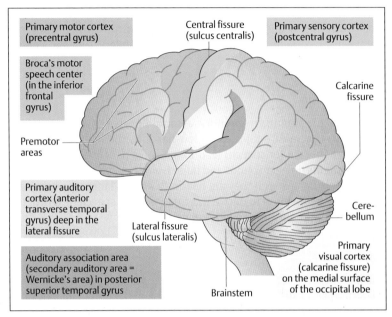

Fig. 13.**10**   **Functional cortical areas of the left cerebral hemisphere.** (After Frick et al)

As mentioned earlier, certain areas of the brain have specific functions. These can be divided into *primary* and *secondary (association) areas.* The primary areas contain the beginning or termination of specific projection pathways. For instance, large portions of the pyramidal tract originate in the precentral gyrus, and sensory tracts from the thalamus end in the postcentral gyrus. Some 80 % of the cerebral surface is taken up by association areas that surround isolated primary areas and process information.

The precentral gyrus (Fig. 13.**10**) is responsible for the execution of voluntary movements (*primary motor cortex*), while the postcentral gyrus is the somatosensory center for conscious sensations (*primary sensory cortex*). On the medial side of the two occipital lobes, a region on each side of the calcarine fissure (visual fissure) is the center for conscious vision (*primary visual cortex*) (Fig. 13.**10**). It is surrounded by visual association areas in which visual stimuli are recognized. The transverse gyri deep in the lateral sulcus of the temporal lobe form the acoustic cortex (*primary acoustic cortex*). They are framed by the auditory association area (secondary acoustic center) (Fig. 13.**10**).

Sensory Aphasia

Lesions of the dominant auditory association area (Wernicke's area) (Fig. 13.**10**) (for most people, even left-handers, the left hemisphere is the dominant side for speech) lead to receptive or sensory aphasia. Affected patients do hear sounds and noises, but they have no significance. The patients behave as if they are hearing a foreign language. Aphasia is defined as the inability to derive information from speech or writing or to understand it and subsequently pass it on.

Motor Aphasia

The *motor speech center* (*Broca's area*) can be found on the inferior frontal gyrus (Fig. 13.**10**). With lesions of this area on the dominant side of an adult, the patient cannot speak even though the laryngeal muscles are not paralyzed (motor aphasia). Patients know what they want to say, but all they can produce are distorted sounds or words that are repeated over and over. If the lesion occurs in childhood, the child relearns speech by using the nondominant side.

Diencephalon

The diencephalon is an area of the brain that lies between the cerebral hemispheres and surrounds the third ventricle (Figs. 13.**11**, 13.**6**, and 13.**7**). It consists of the *thalamus*, which is the central relay station of the sensory pathways (pain, temperature, pressure, touch, as well as vision and hearing) and the *hypothalamus* below it.

The thalamus is the major subcortical relay station for all incoming impulses except those dealing with smell (the olfactory pathway). In the thalamus, these impulses are synaptically transmitted to neurons that mostly project to the cerebral cortex. Thus, the thalamus is sometimes called "the gateway to the cortex," or even "the gateway to consciousness."

The hypothalamus is an area essential to life. It regulates body temperature, manages water balance, controls food intake, governs emotional life, and regulates the autonomic nervous system. Through the *hypophysial stalk* (*infundibulum*), the diencephalon becomes the most important connection to the chief organ of hormonal regulation, the *hypophysis* (Chapter 7).

The diencephalon also includes the *medial* and *lateral geniculate bodies*, important relay stations in the visual and auditory pathways subsumed under the term metathalamus, the *pineal body* (*pineal gland*), and the *habenular nuclei* forming the epithalamus.

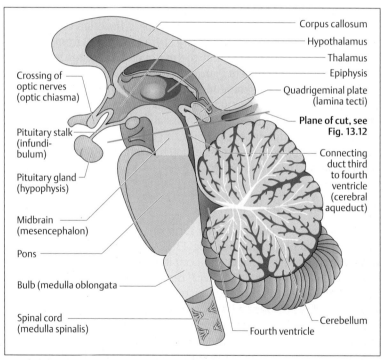

Fig. 13.**11** **Diagrammatic representation of a longitudinal section through the diencephalon, the brainstem, and the cerebellum.** The thalamus, hypothalamus, pineal gland, and pituitary gland are part of the diencephalon; the brainstem (in color) is formed by the midbrain, pons, and medulla. (After Duus)

Midbrain (Mesencephalon)

The midbrain is the smallest part of the brain, lying between the diencephalon and the pons (Figs. 13.**11** and 13.**12**). The area above the aqueduct is the *roof of the midbrain* (*tectum*), composed of four projections resembling hills, the *lamina tecti*. The two upper hills form the superior colliculi, the four lower hills the inferior colliculi. Together, the four colliculi are known as the corpora quadrigemina. They give rise to optic and acoustic reflex pathways to the spinal cord.

A number of bundles of fibers run to the *tegmentum* (*cover*), which lies under the tectum. This structure also includes the *red nucleus* (*nucleus ruber*) and the nuclei of the extrinsic eye muscle nerves, cranial nerves III (oculomotor nerve) and IV (trochlear nerve). At the base of the midbrain run a pair of massive bundles of fibers, the crura cerebri, made up of descending projection fibers (e. g., pyramidal tract) from the internal capsule. The last structure of the midbrain that needs to be mentioned is the *substantia nigra* (*black substance*), which, together with the crura cerebri and the tegmentum, forms the *cerebral peduncles* (*pedunculi cerebri*). The red nucleus and the substantia nigra form the basal ganglia of the midbrain. An expanding mass above the tentorium, such as a hematoma in or adjacent to the brain, can cause acute wedging (herniation) of the midbrain in the tentorial notch, leading rapidly to a decline of consciousness, coma, and death.

Pons (Bridge) and Cerebellum

The pons and cerebellum together form the metencephalon part of the hindbrain (rhombencephalon) (Fig. 13.**11**). The cerebellum lies in the posterior cranial fossa under the occipital lobe of the cerebrum, separated from it by the *tentorium (tent) cerebelli*. Its anterior surface forms the roof of the fourth ventricle. It is connected to the midbrain, the pons, and the medulla oblongata by the cerebellar peduncles. The function of the cerebellum is to maintain equilibrium and muscle tone and to coordinate the activity of voluntary muscles (coordination of antagonistic muscle groups, e. g., flexor/extensor). It works with the basal ganglia (p. 542) in the programming of movement.

The cerebellum weighs about 130–140 g and consists of a central *vermis* (worm) and bilateral *cerebellar hemispheres* (Fig. 13.**13a**, **b**). The cere-

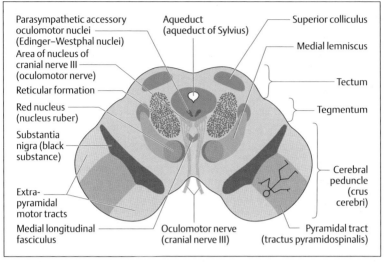

Parasympathetic accessory oculomotor nuclei (Edinger–Westphal nuclei)

Area of nucleus of cranial nerve III (oculomotor nerve)

Reticular formation

Red nucleus (nucleus ruber)

Substantia nigra (black substance)

Extra-pyramidal motor tracts

Medial longitudinal fasciculus

Aqueduct (aqueduct of Sylvius)

Oculomotor nerve (cranial nerve III)

Superior colliculus

Medial lemniscus

Tectum

Tegmentum

Cerebral peduncle (crus cerebri)

Pyramidal tract (tractus pyramidospinalis)

Fig. 13.**12   Transverse section through the midbrain at the level of the superior colliculus.** The individual nerve fibers are arranged in somatotopic order in the pyramidal tract. The periaqueductal gray substance (substantia grisea centralis) is distributed around the cerebral aqueduct. For plane of section, see Fig. 13.**11**

bellar surface shows a large number of narrow, almost parallel folia (gyri) and sulci (fissures), much more marked than in the cerebrum. If the total surface of the cerebrum is compared to that of the cerebellum, the cerebellar surface is about 75 % that of the cerebrum, though with only one-tenth of its weight.

The phylogenetically oldest part of the cerebellum (*archicerebellum*) consists of the nodulus of the vermis and the bilateral flocculus (Fig. 13.**13a, b**). Together they form the flocculonodular lobe, which is responsible for the maintenance of equilibrium. The *paleocerebellum* is the second oldest part of the cerebellum, composed of the anterior lobes of the cerebellar hemispheres and part of the vermis. Its primary function is to regulate muscle tone. The phylogenetically youngest and largest part of the cerebellum is the *neocerebellum*, composed of the posterior lobes of the cerebellar hemispheres and the major part of the vermis. It is responsible for the coordination of voluntary muscles.

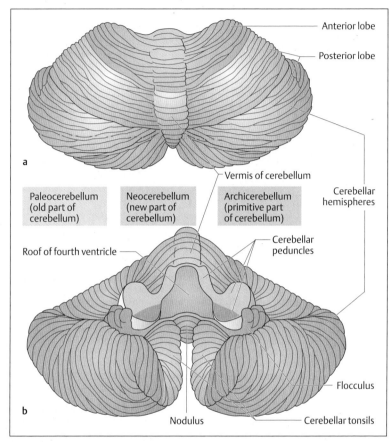

Fig. 13.**13 a**, **b**   **Cerebellum.** (After Duus.) **a** Seen from above; **b** seen from below. The cerebellar peduncles have been divided

The cerebellar surface is made up of a gray cortex, below which is a core of white matter containing four important gray nuclei (cerebellar nuclei). The most important of these is the *dentate nucleus*. A median section of the cerebellum shows a treelike structure on the cut surface, called the *arbor vitae* (tree of life) (Fig. 13.**11**).

The tracts entering and leaving the cerebellum form the three cerebellar peduncles: the superior, middle, and inferior peduncles (Figs. 13.**13** and 13.**15**). The pons lies between the midbrain and the medulla oblongata and is separated from the cerebellum above it by a cavity, the fourth ventricle. Several ascending and descending tracts run through the pons: it contains the nuclei of cranial nerves V, VI, and VII (trigeminal, abducens, and facial nerves) (Fig. 13.**14**).

Medulla Oblongata

The medulla oblongata (myencephalon, medulla, bulb), about 4 cm long, ends at the transition between the brain and the spinal cord (Figs. 13.**14** and 13.**15**) at the level of the foramen magnum of the skull. Anteriorly it has a median groove (median sulcus, fissura mediana anterior) (Fig. 13.**15**), interrupted by the *decussation of the pyramidal tracts* (p. 566) (Fig. 13.**14**). The pyramidal tract, the most important tract of the voluntary motor system (see Voluntary Motor Tracts [Pyramidal Tracts] below) runs on each side of the groove, thickening below the pons into the pyramids. The olive, a folded gray nucleus, bulges beside it (Fig. 13.**14**).

The posterior surface of the medulla is partly covered by the cerebellum. If the cerebellum is removed, the floor of the fourth ventricle can be seen, known as the rhomboid fossa because of its shape (Fig. 13.**15**). The anterior portion of the rhomboid fossa forms part of the pons; the posterior part is part of the medulla. The bulges in the rhomboid fossa are formed by the nuclei of certain cranial nerves. On each side of the groove the medulla has two raised areas (nucleus cuneatus and nucleus gracilis), relay station in the ascending sensory tracts of the posterior spinal funiculus (fasciculi cuneatus and gracilis).

The medulla, like the pons and the midbrain, contains ascending and descending fibers and nuclei of cranial nerves (VIII to XII). It is also the seat of the *respiratory* and *circulatory centers*. If the intracranial pressure rises (e. g., due to hemorrhages or tumors), the medulla becomes compressed and this may lead to coma or death.

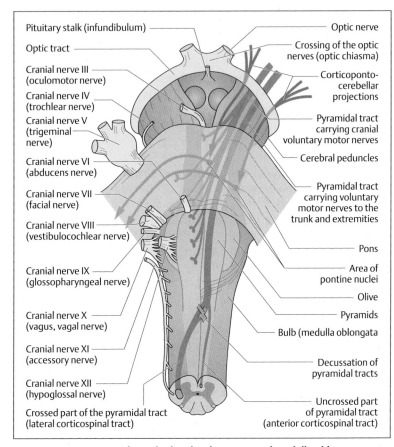

Pituitary stalk (infundibulum)

Optic tract

Cranial nerve III
(oculomotor nerve)

Cranial nerve IV
(trochlear nerve)

Cranial nerve V
(trigeminal
nerve)

Cranial nerve VI
(abducens nerve)

Cranial nerve VII
(facial nerve)

Cranial nerve VIII
(vestibulocochlear nerve)

Cranial nerve IX
(glossopharyngeal nerve)

Cranial nerve X
(vagus, vagal nerve)

Cranial nerve XI
(accessory nerve)

Cranial nerve XII
(hypoglossal nerve)

Crossed part of the pyramidal tract
(lateral corticospinal tract)

Optic nerve

Crossing of the optic
nerves (optic chiasma)

Corticoponto-
cerebellar
projections

Pyramidal tract
carrying cranial
voluntary motor nerves

Cerebral peduncles

Pyramidal tract
carrying voluntary
motor nerves to the
trunk and extremities

Pons

Area of
pontine nuclei

Olive

Pyramids

Bulb (medulla oblongata

Decussation of
pyramidal tracts

Uncrossed part
of pyramidal tract
(anterior corticospinal tract)

Fig. 13.**14   Brainstem with cerebral peduncles, pons, and medulla oblongata; anterior view.** The right side shows the cranial nerves, the left side the most important descending tracts. (After Faller)

Brainstem

The midbrain, pons, and medulla oblongata together form a wedge-
shaped structure, the brainstem (Figs. 13.**14** and 13.**15**), extending from
the base of the brain to the foramen magnum. The nuclei of the cranial
nerves lie in the brainstem, and their nerves leave the brainstem in 12

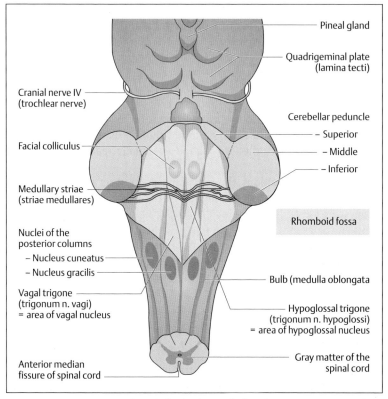

Pineal gland

Quadrigeminal plate
(lamina tecti)

Cranial nerve IV
(trochlear nerve)

Cerebellar peduncle

– Superior

Facial colliculus

– Middle

– Inferior

Medullary striae
(striae medullares)

Rhomboid fossa

Nuclei of the
posterior columns

– Nucleus cuneatus
– Nucleus gracilis

Vagal trigone
(trigonum n. vagi)
= area of vagal nucleus

Bulb (medulla oblongata

Hypoglossal trigone
(trigonum n. hypoglossi)
= area of hypoglossal nucleus

Anterior median
fissure of spinal cord

Gray matter of the
spinal cord

Fig. 13.**15 Brainstem seen from behind.** The cerebellum has been removed and the rhomboid fossa exposed. (After Faller)

pairs of cranial nerves. With the exception of the first two cranial nerves (olfactory and optic nerves), the rest are true peripheral nerves (see Peripheral Nervous System below).

Reticular Formation

The area called the reticular formation consists of a group of diffuse nuclei deep in the brainstem (Fig. 13.**12**). It extends from the medulla through the whole brainstem to the diencephalon. Its development is most marked in the tegmentum of the midbrain.

These nuclear areas receive impulses through the hypothalamic tracts and are also connected to the basal ganglia. Through descending tracts they connect with anterior horn cells and preganglionic neurons of the autonomic lateral horn (see p. 610). They also receive information from all important sensory and special sense organs (e.g., pain, temperature, pressure, touch, as well as vision and hearing), and pass this on to the thalamus, relay station of numerous sensory and motor tracts, and from there the information eventually reaches the cerebral cortex.

Among other functions, the reticular system plays an important role in the state of consciousness, that is, in alert wakefulness as well as the sleep–wake cycle. It is believed that wakefulness and/or sleep depend on the number of stimuli that reach the cerebral cortex via the reticular formation. If, for instance. the number of environmental stimuli decreases, attention flags and this leads to transition to a state of sleep. On the other hand, an increase in the number of stimuli reaching the cerebral cortex increases attention and this leads to transition to the waking state.

The Electroencephalogram (EEG)

Every stimulation of nerve cells in the brain elicits rhythmic potential oscillations of a few microvolts. Hence, as with the ECG, these oscillations can be conducted from the body surface (scalp) by metal electrodes and recorded as an electroencephalogram. The waves (α, β, δ, and θ waves) of the EEG vary from region to region, especially in their height (amplitude) and frequency. Hence it is possible to make relatively crude interpretations concerning normal and pathological activities of the brain.

Sleep and Wakefulness

As in almost all living forms, an internal (biological) clock regulates the normal human sleep–wakefulness cycle. Such sleep–wake cycles are called *circadian rhythms*, because they correspond to about (= Latin *circa*) the duration of one day (= Latin *dies*). In actual life, these circadian rhythms are adapted to the 24-hour rhythm of the day by external time divisions (work, leisure, and sleep phases, as well as light and dark periodicity).

While an awake organism is actively connected to the environment and reacts to external stimuli, contact with the surroundings is largely suspended during sleep. Nevertheless, the electroencephalogram demonstrates that sleep is not simply a state of cerebral rest, but simply an alternative state of consciousness. Depending on the depth of sleep, the EEG changes in characteristic ways. Several stages of sleep can be distinguished and these are repeated several times during the night, with a lightening of the depth of sleep toward morning.

REM Sleep

A special role is taken by the stage of sleep called REM (rapid eye movement) sleep, characterized by jerky eye movements and distinctly lower muscle tone. Such REM stages last on average 10–20 minutes and repeat about every 90 minutes. The experience of dreams frequently present during REM sleep mirrors the lively activity of the central nervous system during these stages. The percentage of REM sleep relative to total sleep is noticeably high in infants and small children (about 50%). It is believed that this high proportion of REM sleep accompanies increased neuronal activity and is important for maturation of the brain. With increasing age, the relative proportion of REM sleep declines and amounts to about 20% of total sleep in the adult.

Spinal Cord (Medulla Spinalis)

The spinal cord is a cylindrical cord, about the thickness of a finger and about 40–45 cm long, that runs in the vertebral canal from the foramen magnum to the level of the 1st to 2nd lumbar vertebra. In it run the *ascending* and *descending nerve tracts* that connect the peripheral nerves with the brain. The peripheral nerves leave the spinal cord in *31 pairs of spinal nerves* (Figs. 13.**16** and 13.**17**). The spinal cord is thickened above and below, where there is a special accumulation of nerve cells (*intumescentia cervicalis* and *lumbosacralis*) (Fig. 13.**16**).

These nerve cells, with their set of spinal nerves, supply the upper and lower limbs.

Spinal Nerves

Each pair of spinal nerves leaves the vertebral canal between two adjacent vertebrae through the *intervertebral foramen* (Fig. 3.**17**). The number of spinal nerve pairs corresponds to the number of vertebrae with one exception (in the cervical region eight pairs of spinal nerves, seven cervical vertebrae). There are eight spinal nerves from the cervical spine (C1–C8), 12 thoracic (T1–T12) from the thoracic spine, five lumbar (L1–L5) from the lumbar spine, five sacral (S1–S5) from the sacral spine, and 1 or 2 coccygeal from the coccyx (Co1–Co2). The first pair of spinal nerves (C1) leaves the vertebral canal between the base of the skull and the 1st cervical vertebra (atlas). Each part of the spinal cord giving rise to a pair of nerves is called a segment.

Spinal Nerve Roots

The spinal nerves are derived from *anterior* and *posterior roots* (*radix anterior* and *posterior*) (Fig. 13.**18a**) that arise from the spinal cord in the form of *root filaments of spinal nerves* (*fila radicularia nervi spinalis*) (Fig. 13.**16**) The posterior root is marked by a swelling (dorsal root ganglion) that contains the sensory nerve cells of the afferent nervous pathways from the periphery. The efferent nervous pathways from the spinal cord to the periphery run exclusively in the anterior roots (Fig. 13.**18**). Both roots come together just below the dorsal root ganglion and form a mixed spinal nerve (afferent and efferent nerve fibers), that, after a short course (1.5 cm), first divides into an *anterior* and a *posterior branch* (*r. dorsalis* and *r. ventralis*) (Figs. 13.**18a** and 13.**29**).

The roots of the upper spinal nerves run a more or less horizontal course and are relatively short. The further down the nerve, the more obliquely downward and the longer is its course in the vertebral canal before it emerges from the intervertebral foramen. During development, the spinal cord and spinal canal are equal in length, so that every spinal nerve leaves through the intervertebral foramen of its level. However, as development proceeds, the vertebral canal increases in length much more than the spinal cord, so that the lower end of the cord lies at an

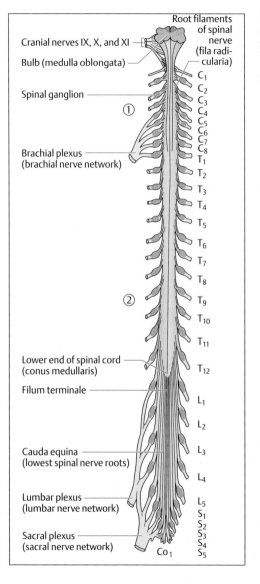

Root filaments
of spinal
nerve
(fila radi-
cularia)

Cranial nerves IX, X, and XI

Bulb (medulla oblongata)

Spinal ganglion

①

Brachial plexus
(brachial nerve network)

②

Lower end of spinal cord
(conus medullaris)

Filum terminale

Cauda equina
(lowest spinal nerve roots)

Lumbar plexus
(lumbar nerve network)

Sacral plexus
(sacral nerve network)

C_1 C_2 C_3 C_4 C_5 C_6 C_7 C_8
T_1 T_2 T_3 T_4 T_5 T_6 T_7 T_8 T_9 T_{10} T_{11} T_{12}
L_1 L_2 L_3 L_4 L_5
S_1 S_2 S_3 S_4 S_5
Co_1

Fig. 13.**16 The spinal cord
and emerging spinal
nerves seen from behind**
1 Cervical enlargement (intumescentia cervicalis)
2 Lumbosacral enlargement (intumescentia
lumbosacralis)

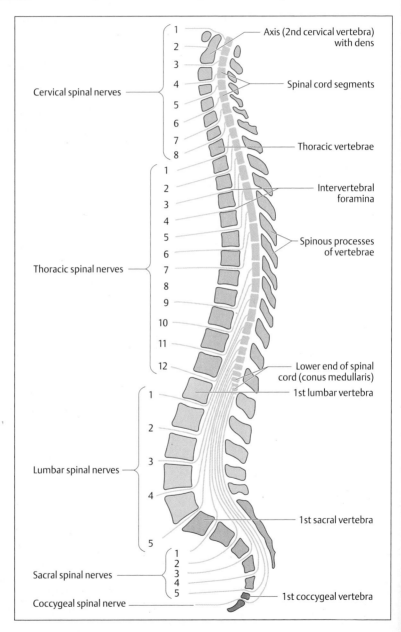

Cervical spinal nerves

1
2
3
4
5
6
7
8

Axis (2nd cervical vertebra) with dens

Spinal cord segments

Thoracic vertebrae

Thoracic spinal nerves

1
2
3
4
5
6
7
8
9
10
11
12

Intervertebral foramina

Spinous processes of vertebrae

Lower end of spinal cord (conus medullaris)

1st lumbar vertebra

Lumbar spinal nerves

1
2
3
4
5

1st sacral vertebra

Sacral spinal nerves

1
2
3
4
5

Coccygeal spinal nerve

1st coccygeal vertebra

ever higher level in relation to the surrounding vertebrae. The lower the point of origin of the roots from the spinal cord, the longer is their course in the vertebral canal (Fig. 13.**17**). Below the end of the spinal cord (*conus medullaris*) at the level of the 1st or 2nd lumbar vertebra, the vertebral canal contains only nerve roots, which are called *cauda equina* (horse's tail) because they resemble the tail of a horse (Fig. 13.**16**). These anatomical relationships make it possible, for instance, to obtain cerebrospinal fluid (CSF, see p. 578) without danger of damaging the spinal cord, either for diagnostic purposes (lumbar puncture) or to inject substances such as local anesthetics in order to attain anesthesia of the lower part of the body (spinal anesthesia).

Gray and White Matter of the Spinal Cord

The spinal cord is divided into two symmetrical halves by the connective tissue *dorsal median septum of the spinal cord* (*septum medianum posterium medullae spinalis*) and a deep *anterior groove* (*fissura mediana anterior medullae spinalis*) (Fig. 13.**19**). In cross-section, two different areas that vary in different regions of the spinal cord can be distinguished: the *gray substance* (*substantia grisea*), shaped like a butterfly in cross-section and varying in size, and the *white substance* (*substantia alba*) surrounding it (Fig. 13.**18**). Exactly as in the cerebral hemispheres, the gray substance is composed primarily of cell bodies and the white substance of myelinated nerve fibers. The dorsal projections of the gray substance are called *dorsal horns* (*cornua posteriora*) and the anterior projections *anterior horns* (*cornua anteriora*). The thoracic region also contains a *lateral horn* (*cornu laterale*) lying between the dorsal horn and the anterior horn. In the middle of the gray substance runs the fluid-filled central canal.

- ■ **Anterior horns:** The anterior horns contain motor nerve cells, the axons of which leave the spinal cord through the anterior root and mainly supply striated muscle.
- ■ **Posterior horns:** The posterior horns contain sensory nerve cells, on which the afferent nerve fibers coming from the periphery end in synapses and are relayed.

◁ Fig. 13.**17**   **Lateral view of the vertebral canal with spinal cord and emerging spinal nerves.** (After Kahle)

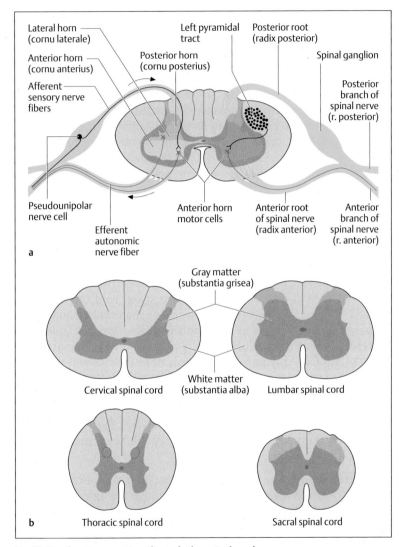

Fig. 13.**18 a, b Cross-section through the spinal cord**
a With anterior and posterior roots; **b** at four different levels

■ **Lateral horns:** The lateral horns contain motor cells of the autonomic system, the axons of which also leave the spinal cord in the anterior roots and run, for example, to smooth muscle or glands.

Ascending and Descending Tracts of the Spinal Cord

The white substance of the spinal cord is composed mainly of ascending (afferent) and descending (efferent) myelinated nerve fibers. These are grouped according to their function in fiber bundles that may be well-defined (fascicles, fasciculi) or more diffuse (tracts, tractus), and that are as a rule named according to their origin and destination. Together the tracts and fascicles form cords (funiculi). The intersegmental fibers of the spinal cord itself run immediately adjacent to the gray substance (fasciculi proprii). They do not leave the spinal cord and subserve especially the spinal reflexes (see below). From the fasciculi proprii outward there follow *dorsal, ventral,* and *lateral funiculi,* the latter two sometimes being known as the anterolateral funiculus (Fig. 13.**19**).

■ **Ascending Tracts**
1. **Tracts of the anterolateral funiculus:** Afferent tracts to the thalamus for coarse touch and tactile sensation as well as pressure, pain, and temperature sensations of the extremities and the trunk (anterior and lateral spinothalamic tracts).
2. **Tracts of the posterior funiculus** (*posterior columns):* Afferent tracts to the thalamus for deep sensation (sensation of joint position and muscle tension = proprioception), vibration, light touch, and tactile discrimination on the limbs and trunk (fasciculus gracilis, fasciculus cuneatus). The fasciculus gracilis and fasciculus cuneatus project to the correspondingly named nuclei in the medulla, which, in turn, project to the thalamus by way of the medial lemniscus, an important fiber bundle in the brainstem (cf. Fig. 13.12).
3. **Spinocerebellar tracts:** Afferent tracts to the cerebellum for unconscious deep sensation (proprioception from muscles, tendons and joints (tractus spinocerebellaris ventralis and tractus spinocerebellaris dorsalis).

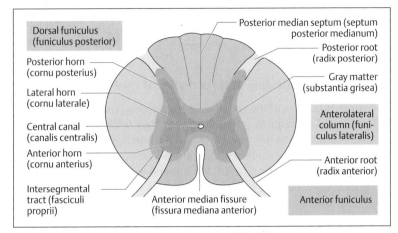

Dorsal funiculus (funiculus posterior)

Posterior horn (cornu posterius)

Lateral horn (cornu laterale)

Central canal (canalis centralis)

Anterior horn (cornu anterius)

Intersegmental tract (fasciculi proprii)

Posterior median septum (septum posterior medianum)

Posterior root (radix posterior)

Gray matter (substantia grisea)

Anterolateral column (funiculus lateralis)

Anterior root (radix anterior)

Anterior funiculus

Anterior median fissure (fissura mediana anterior)

Fig. 13.**19** **Gray and white matter of the spinal cord.** The posterior, lateral, and anterior funiculi together form the white matter. (After Faller)

■ **Descending tracts:**
1. **Pyramidal tract:** Efferent tracts from the motor cortex to the motor cells of the anterior horn for voluntary fine movements of the extremities and the trunk (corticospinal tracts).
2. **Extrapyramidal tracts:** Efferent tract from the brainstem to the motor cells of the anterior horn for involuntary movements, e.g., position and posture, automatic movements, associated movements (synkinesis) (reticulospinal tract, etc.).

Voluntary Motor Tracts (Pyramidal Tracts)

The corticospinal tract is the principal path for the nerves activating all voluntary muscular activity. Its large cell bodies lie in the *precentral gyrus* of the frontal lobe of the cerebrum (Figs. 13.**10** and 13.**20**), where it originates. Because many of the cells have a pyramidal shape, the corticospinal tract is also called the *pyramidal tract*. From these cell bodies the axons leave the cerebral cortex and pass through the *internal capsule*, which is not really a capsule but the principal path for the ascending and descending tracts (see p. 563).

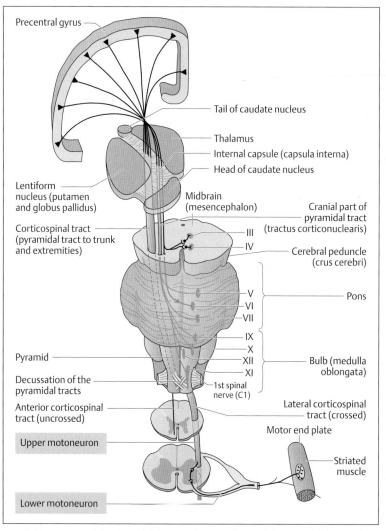

Precentral gyrus

Tail of caudate nucleus

Thalamus

Internal capsule (capsula interna)

Head of caudate nucleus

Lentiform nucleus (putamen and globus pallidus)

Midbrain (mesencephalon)

Cranial part of pyramidal tract (tractus corticonuclearis)

Corticospinal tract (pyramidal tract to trunk and extremities)

III

IV

Cerebral peduncle (crus cerebri)

V

VI

VII

Pons

IX

X

XII

XI

Pyramid

Bulb (medulla oblongata)

Decussation of the pyramidal tracts

1st spinal nerve (C1)

Anterior corticospinal tract (uncrossed)

Lateral corticospinal tract (crossed)

Motor end plate

Upper motoneuron

Striated muscle

Lower motoneuron

Fig. 13.**20** **Course of the pyramidal tract.** The cranial part of the pyramidal tract (corticobulbar tract) ends at the motor areas of the nuclei of the cranial nerves: III, oculomotor nucleus; IV, trochlear nucleus; V, trigeminal nucleus; VI, abducens nucleus; VII, facial nucleus; IX, glossopharyngeal nucleus; X, vagus nucleus; XI, spinal accessory nucleus; XII, hypoglossal nucleus. The tracts to the nuclei of cranial nerves III, IV, and VI have not been determined with certainty. (After Duus)

Voluntary Motor Tracts of the Head

After leaving the internal capsule, the pyramidal axons run through the cerebral peduncles and enter the medulla oblongata (bulb). While passing through the brainstem, the nerve fibers for the cranial voluntary muscles leave the pyramidal tract (*corticobulbar tract, corticonuclear tract*), cross the midline, and end in the motor nuclei of the cranial nerves (Fig. 13.**20**). There they form synapses with the neurons that leave the brainstem with the cranial nerves and supply the cranial striated muscles (e. g., muscles of mastication).

Voluntary Motor Tracts of the Trunk and Extremities

Some 80–90% of the axons of the pyramidal tract cross to the opposite (contralateral) side of the medulla (pyramidal crossing or decussation), and then descend in the spinal cord. Since the descending fibers run in the lateral funiculus of the spinal cord, the tract is called the lateral corticospinal tract. Those axons that do not cross in the medulla descend in the anterior funiculus of the spinal cord of the same (ipsilateral) side and are therefore called the anterior (or ventral) corticospinal tract (Fig. 13.**20**).

The axons of the lateral corticospinal tract lose their myelin sheaths at various levels of the spinal cord and enter the gray substance of the anterior horn, where they end in synapses on the motor cells of the anterior horn. At the corresponding sites in the spinal cord, the axons of the anterior corticospinal tract cross to the opposite side, where they also end in synapses with the motor cells of the anterior horn.

It is important to emphasize that both the anterior and lateral corticospinal tracts in their entire course from the precentral gyrus to the anterior horn consist of individual uninterrupted neurons. These neuron are also known as upper motoneurons. They synapse with lower motoneurons, the axons of which run in the anterior roots and supply the peripheral voluntary muscles. These secondary neurons are called lower motoneurons (Fig. 13.**20**). As we will see, the distinction between upper motoneurons and lower motoneurons is clinically very important (see the sections on lesions of the motoneurons below). In a person 6 feet (184 cm) tall, the axons supplying the toes are almost 36 inches (90 cm) in length. In this case, the upper motoneurons begin in the prefrontal cortex and end in the lower spinal cord, where the axons of the lower motoneurons begin and run to the muscles in the sole of the foot.

Somatotope Organization of the Motor Area

The cell bodies of the upper motoneurons in the gray substance of the precentral gyrus are arranged with the neurons supplying the feet and the muscles of the lower extremity in the upper midline part of the gyrus (Fig. 13.**21**). Arranged from there laterally and downward lie the centers supplying the muscles of the trunk, chest, arms, hands and face. To describe this arrangement more concretely, the distribution resembles a person standing on his head, with the feet in the longitudinal fissure, and

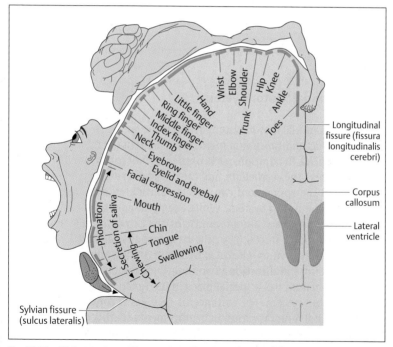

Fig. 13.**21**   **Motor cortex with somatotopic arrangement of the regions of the body.** (After Frick et al)

the head at the border of the lateral sulcus of the cerebral cortex. This is called the somatotopic arrangement of the regions of the body, each of which has an area of different size allocated in the precentral gyrus.

Sections of the body where the muscles must execute very finely adjusted movements are represented over especially large areas of the precentral gyrus. For instance, the area of the neurons supplying the hand is exceptionally large in relation to other areas and reflects the large number of neurons necessary to accomplish the complex fine movements of, say, playing the violin, performing surgery, or writing. Another somatotopic arrangement can be found in the internal capsule, the principal path of the ascending and descending fibers. The internal capsule, with its anterior and posterior limbs and their connecting area, the knee, can be seen in a horizontal section through the cerebral hemispheres (Fig. 13.**6a**, **b**). The motor fibers supplying the face are located in the genu, and those responsible for the rest of the body in the anterior two-thirds of the posterior limb. If the genu is injured, the facial muscles are affected, while if the middle region of the posterior genu is damaged, the muscles of the lower extremity receive no impulses.

Extrapyramidal Motor System

The extrapyramidal motor system includes the *basal ganglia* (see p. 542), the *red nucleus* and *substantia nigra* (see p. 550) in the midbrain, and the *vestibular nuclei*. In addition, parts of the *cerebral cortex* (*premotor* or *associative areas*), the *cerebellum*, and the *descending extrapyramidal motor pathways* to the spinal cord can also be considered components of the extrapyramidal motor system. While the pyramidal tract mainly transmits commands to the voluntary muscles, the extrapyramidal motor system with its motor nuclei (e. g., the basal ganglia) and pathways is responsible for *involuntary muscle movements*. Among other things, it controls the extent and direction of voluntary movements.

The cerebellum has a special place in the functioning of the extrapyramidal motor system. For instance, it receives a copy of information about planned voluntary muscular movements (corticocerbellar tracts, Fig. 13.**14**). Since the cerebellum simultaneously receives information from the muscles through the cerebellar tracts of the lateral funiculus, it can coordinate the planning and execution of a movement. It transmits corrective commands from the cerebellar nuclei (see p. 553) to the motor centers in the brainstem, the basal ganglia, and the cerebral cortex. For instance, fibers that originate in the premotor area of the cerebral cortex (Fig. 3.**10**) do not send stimuli to the voluntary muscles, rather they inhibit the lower motoneuron and so prevent overshooting of the muscles during reflex reactions to sensory stimuli.

However, as a result of current understanding, the division into pyramidal and extrapyramidal systems is often put aside, since the functions of the two systems are closely intertwined.

Lesions of the Lower Motoneuron (Flaccid Paralysis)

Flaccid paralysis ensues when, for instance, a peripheral nerve is severed on its path to the muscle or when the cell bodies in the anterior horn are destroyed selectively by the virus of poliomyelitis (infantile paralysis). In both cases, the muscles are deprived of their direct innervation. They cannot contract and show characteristic signs of flaccid paralysis, i.e., they become soft and flaccid and atrophy. Since the efferent limb of the reflex arc (p. 571) is interrupted, the muscles naturally cannot respond to sensory stimuli.

Lesions of the Upper Motoneuron (Spastic Paralysis)

Lesions anywhere in certain parts of the corticospinal tract (e. g., the cell bodies in the precentral gyrus or the descending fibers in the internal capsule, the brainstem, or the spinal cord) cause *spastic paralysis*. The commonest site of a lesion is within the cerebral hemispheres, before the decussation of the pyramids. Such lesions often occur as a result of arterial occlusions or cerebral hemorrhage, when oxygen deficiency causes destruction of the nerves (cerebral infarct, apoplexy, or stroke). When the lesion is above the decussation of the pyramids, typical paralytic symptoms occur in the muscles of the contralateral side, while after a lesion below the decussation, such as a lesion on the left side of the spinal cord, the resulting paralysis will occur on the same side.

This type of lesion differs from flaccid paralysis in several ways. For one thing, in contrast to a flaccid paralysis, the lower motoneuron is not damaged, so that the reflex arc (see below) remains intact and reflexes can be elicited. Instead, because the inhibiting extrapyramidal motor fibers run in close association with the upper motoneurons, they are affected by the same lesion, and so can no longer exert their influence over the lower motoneuron. The result is an overshoot of muscular reflex response to sensory stimuli, because the impulses sent out by the lower motoneurons are uncontrolled. This condition is known as *hyperreflexia*: if, for instance, the wrist joint of the paralyzed arm is grasped and held, a series of muscle contractions following rapidly one on another ensues (clonus). *Spastic paralysis* is this condition of increased reflex activity resulting from a lesion of the upper motoneuron, combined with increased spastic muscle tone.

Spinal Reflexes

Reflexes are involuntary and unchanging responses of an organism to external or internal stimuli received by the CNS. For instance, a light tap with a reflex hammer on the tendon below the kneecap (patella) leads to a brief contraction of the quadriceps femoris muscle. This is the reflex known as the patellar reflex (knee jerk).

Reflex Arc

The basis of such a spinal reflex is what is called a reflex arc, which is a functional entity with the following components (Fig. 13.**22b**):

- A receptor that registers and transmits the information
- An afferent neuron by which an impulses reach the spinal cord
- A synapse, in which the impulse is relayed to the motor cell in the anterior horn
- An efferent neuron by which the impulses leave the spinal cord
- An effector organ

Proprioceptive or Stretch Reflex

In the patellar reflex, only one synapse is interposed between the afferent and efferent neuron and the receptor and effector are common to the

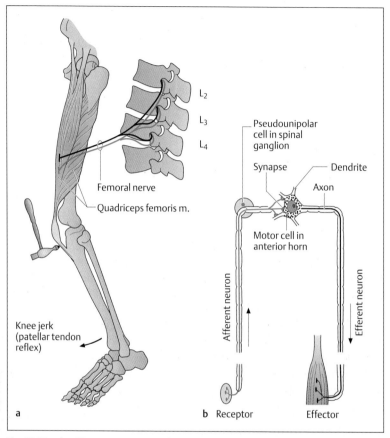

Fig. 13.22 a, b   Monosynaptic proprioceptive or stretch reflex
a Patellar tendon reflex; **b** components of the reflex arc

same organ. Such a reflex is called a *monosynaptic* proprioceptive or stretch reflex (Fig. 13.**22a**, **b**). These reflexes are characterized by a rapid reflex time, i.e., the time from the beginning of the stimulus to the initiation of the contraction (about 20–50 milliseconds), by lack of fatigue, and by the fact that proprioceptive reflexes run their course independently of the strength of the triggering stimulus.

The physiological significance of such a stretch reflex lies in the fact, among others, that it controls the length and tension of a muscle (so-called postural tone) and so balances the effect of gravity. For instance, without postural tone in the quadriceps femoris when standing, our knee joints would constantly give way. The reflex arc therefore ensures that even with slight relaxation of the knee, the corresponding muscle stretch triggers a reflex contraction, thereby restoring the extension of the knee joint.

Sensorimotor or Skin Reflexes

In sensorimotor or skin reflexes, the skin is stimulated and a muscle responds by contracting. When, for instance, the abdominal skin is stroked with a pointed object, the abdominal muscles contract (abdominal reflexes). In contrast to proprioceptor reflexes, in this reflex the receptor and effector are separated and are located in different organs. Moreover, in these reflexes several synapses and intercalated neurons are inserted into the reflex arc. These reflexes are therefore often called *polysynaptic* reflexes. Intercalated neurons allow the involvement of neighboring spinal segments and contralateral organs.

These reflexes are characterized by prolonged reflex times (e. g., 70–150 milliseconds for the eyelid closure reflex), rapid fatigability and accommodation, as well as the phenomenon of summation of subthreshold stimuli. The latter term describes the triggering of a reflex by constant repetition of small stimuli each of which by itself would not elicit a reflex response. As an example, prolonged irritation of the nasal mucosa summates to exceed the threshold for a sneeze. Other examples of such protective reflexes include coughing, tearing, and digestive reflexes such as swallowing and sucking.

Pathological Reflexes

A typical example of a pathological reflex is the *Babinski* reflex, which is the result of a lesion of the pyramidal tract. When the outside edge of the sole of the foot is stroked with a pointed object, all the toes plantarflex reflexly. After a lesion of the pyramidal tract, however, the big toe dorsiflexes, while the other toes open out like a fan and are dorsiflexed.

Membranes of the Brain and Spinal Cord

The tissues of the brain and spinal cord are the most delicate of all the tissues of the body. These organs are essential to life and so are protected by being encased in closed bony chambers—the skull and the vertebral canal.

Membranes of the Brain

Three membranes, the *meninges* (Fig. 13.**23**), surround the brain to protect it from hard bones and blows to the head. The outermost is the densely fibrous and thick *dura mater* (*dura mater cranialis*), which is closely applied to the inside of the bones and tightly adherent to the periosteum. Under the dura mater lies the middle layer, the thin and delicate *arachnoid* (*arachnoidea mater cranialis*). The third and innermost

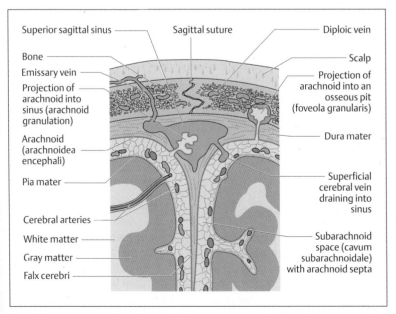

Fig. 13.**23 Coronal section through skull, meninges, and brain.** The area shown is a section at the level of the falx cerebri

layer is the very thin and sensitive *pia mater* (*pia mater cranialis*), rich in capillaries, which is directly applied to the brain and dips into the fissures.

Although the dura is very closely applied to the inside of the skull, it can become detached under certain circumstances (hemorrhage), creating an *epidural space* (*extradural space*; e. g., epidural or extradural hemorrhage after skull fractures). The virtual space between the dura and the arachnoid (subdural space) is traversed by veins and can also be the site of clinically significant hemorrhage. The arachnoid and the pia mater are separated by a relatively wide space, the *subarachnoid space,* which is filled with *cerebrospinal fluid (CSF)*. This clear fluid fills the whole subarachnoid space and so surrounds the brain like a protective cushion. A further layer of protection is added by connective tissue strands, the arachnoid septa, that run between the arachnoid and the pia mater. They attach the brain to the arachnoid and so prevent its excessive movement when the head is exposed to sudden shocks. The cerebral arteries and veins run in the fluid-filled subarachnoid space (Figs. 13.**23**, 13.**27a**, **b** and 13.**28**). The pia mater is so closely adherent to the underlying brain that there is no space between them, the pia mater tightly holding the brain.

The dura dips into the longitudinal cerebral fissure. This fold between the two hemispheres is known as the *falx cerebri* (Fig. 13.**23**). The space between the cerebellum and the occipital lobe of the cerebrum over it is also lined with dura, which thus forms a tentlike cover over the cerebellum, the *tentorium cerebelli*. Finally, the dura dips between the cerebellar hemispheres to form the *falx cerebelli*. The membranes of the brain, the subarachnoid space, and the CSF pass through the foramen magnum in the base of the skull.

Membranes of the Spinal Cord

After passing through the foramen magnum, the membranes of the brain continue into the vertebral canal to become the membranes of the spinal cord, surrounding the spinal cord and the roots of the spinal nerves (Fig. 13.**24**). The *dura mater of the spinal cord* (*dura mater spinalis*) forms a strong sac (dural sac) that is anchored around the foramen magnum and the intervertebral foramina and extends to the second sacral vertebra. In contrast to the dura of the brain, which is closely adherent to the

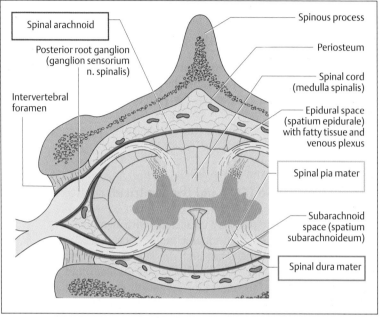

Fig. 13.**24** **Cross-section through the vertebral canal with the spinal cord and spinal meninges**

periosteum of the skull, the dura of the spinal cord is not adherent to the bones of the vertebral canal, but separated from it by a space (*epidural space, extradural space = spatium epidurale*). This space is filled with fatty tissue and contains an extensive venous plexus.

Inside the dura, the arachnoid (*arachnoidea mater spinalis*) is closely adherent to it, and is connected to the *pia mater* (*pia mater spinalis*) by delicate strands of connective tissue. The subarachnoid space, filled with CSF, lies between the arachnoid and the pia mater, which is closely applied to the surface of the spinal cord (Fig. 13.**24**).

The spinal cord in the vertebral canal ends at the level of the 1st or 2nd lumbar vertebra (Fig. 13.**17**), but the pia mater of the spinal cord continues as the *filum terminale*, to be attached to the back of the coccyx

(Fig. 13.**16**). Additionally, the pia mater over the length of the spinal cord has toothlike projections, the *ligamenta denticulata*. These are attached to the dura and the arachnoid and stabilize the spinal cord in the coronal plane.

All spinal roots, including those in the cauda equina, are covered by the pia mater, which simply entrains the other two spinal membranes at the exit of the spinal nerves from the vertebral canal. Thus, the spinal nerves on leaving the vertebral canal are also covered by the dura and the arachnoid, which continue as the perineurium and epineurium (see Chapter 3: The Nerves).

Cerebrospinal Fluid (CSF) and the Ventricular System

The *cerebrospinal fluid (CSF)* is a clear fluid, with a volume of about 130–150 ml, which fills the whole subarachnoid space. It acts as a protective fluid cushion around the brain and the spinal cord, damping shocks caused by blows or falls. The central canal of the spinal cord is also filled with CSF. The CSF is an important diagnostic tool: using a relatively simple procedure (lumbar puncture), the physician can take a sample of CSF and so obtain a picture of events inside the skull and the spinal cord (CSF diagnosis for disorders of the CNS, see p. 578).

Deep inside the brain lies the ventricular system (Fig. 13.**25a, b**). This consists of interconnected chambers in which the CSF is secreted and circulates. Each cerebral hemisphere contains a large cavity, the lateral ventricle, which consists of a frontal (anterior) horn in the frontal lobe of the cerebrum, a central part (pars centralis) in the frontal and parietal lobes, an occipital (posterior) horn in the occipital lobe, and a temporal (inferior) horn in the temporal lobe (Fig. 13.**25a, b**). Each lateral ventricle, as well as the third (diencephalon) and fourth (under the cerebellum) ventricles, contains an arterial network, the choroid plexus. The CSF is produced in the plexus, reaching the ventricle by diffusion and active transport.

From the lateral ventricles, the CSF flows through an opening in each side (interventricular foramen, foramen of Monro) into the single median *third ventricle* between the walls of the left and right diencephalon. Eventually, the CSF produced in the ventricles flows through a narrow canal (*aqueductus mesencephali, cerebral aqueduct, aqueduct of Sylvius*)

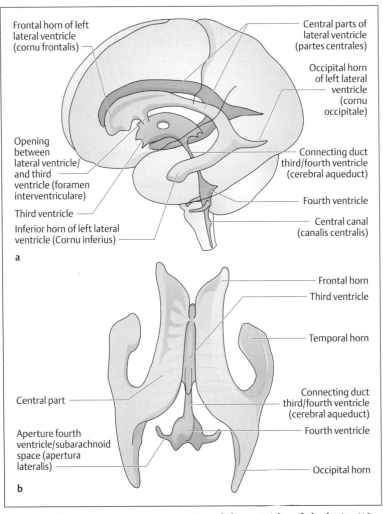

Frontal horn of left
lateral ventricle
(cornu frontalis)

Central parts of
lateral ventricle
(partes centrales)

Occipital horn
of left lateral
ventricle
(cornu
occipitale)

Opening
between
lateral ventricle
and third
ventricle (foramen
interventriculare)

Connecting duct
third/fourth ventricle
(cerebral aqueduct)

Fourth ventricle

Third ventricle

Central canal
(canalis centralis)

Inferior horn of left lateral
ventricle (Cornu inferius)

a

Frontal horn

Third ventricle

Temporal horn

Central part

Connecting duct
third/fourth ventricle
(cerebral aqueduct)

Fourth ventricle

Aperture fourth
ventricle/subarachnoid
space (apertura
lateralis)

Occipital horn

b

Fig. 13.**25 a, b   Diagrammatic representation of the ventricles of the brain.** (After
Duus and Kahle)
a Lateral view with outline of the brain; **b** view from above

in the midbrain into the single *fourth ventricle*, from which it flows through three openings (apertures) in the roof of the fourth ventricle into the *subarachnoid space* (Fig. 13.**26**). In certain areas the subarachnoid space is distinctly enlarged and forms the so-called cisterns, such as the posterior cerebellomedullary cistern (cisterna magna) (Fig. 13.**26**).

CSF Drainage

Since CSF is secreted at 30 ml per hour, the question is: where does it drain? At the superior sagittal sinus, the arachnoid projects through small openings in the dura into the venous sinus. The fluid accumulation exerts pressure, which drives the fluid though *arachnoid villi* into the venous blood. Macroscopically, these arachnoid villi look like grains of salt or sugar, and so are called *arachnoid granulations* (Fig. 13.**23**). In the spinal cord, the CSF drains into a dense venous plexus and lymph vessels where the spinal nerves emerge (Fig. 13.**26**).

Lumbar Puncture

A *lumbar puncture* (puncture of the subarachnoid space with a needle inserted between two lumbar laminae) can be performed to remove CSF for diagnostic or therapeutic purposes, or to introduce substances into the subarachnoid space (medications, radiological contrast media, anesthetics). When properly performed, lumbar puncture does not endanger the spinal cord, because the cord ends at the L1 or L2 level, while the subarachnoid space continues downward to S2. Lumbar puncture can be dangerous under certain circumstances; a complete discussion of its indications, contraindications, and technique would be beyond the scope of this book.

Blood Supply of the Brain

Nerve cells have high oxygen requirements, so that even 3–4 minutes without oxygen can lead to necrosis of the neurons. The nerve cells of the cerebral cortex are the most sensitive, those of the brainstem the most resistant. The significance of an adequate blood supply to the brain can

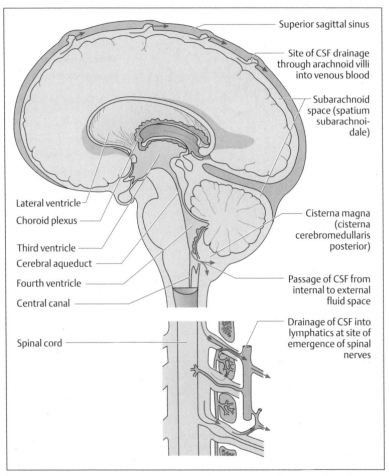

Superior sagittal sinus

Site of CSF drainage through arachnoid villi into venous blood

Subarachnoid space (spatium subarachnoidale)

Cisterna magna (cisterna cerebromedullaris posterior)

Passage of CSF from internal to external fluid space

Drainage of CSF into lymphatics at site of emergence of spinal nerves

Lateral ventricle

Choroid plexus

Third ventricle

Cerebral aqueduct

Fourth ventricle

Central canal

Spinal cord

Fig. 13.**26** **Diagram of the internal (ventricle) and external (subarachnoid space) fluid-filled spaces.** (After Kahle)

be seen by the fact that the brain's weight is only 2% of that of the body but it uses 15–20% of the cardiac output.

The blood supply to the brain is provided by two sets of bilateral arteries, the *internal carotid arteries* and the *vertebral arteries* (Fig. 13.**27a,**

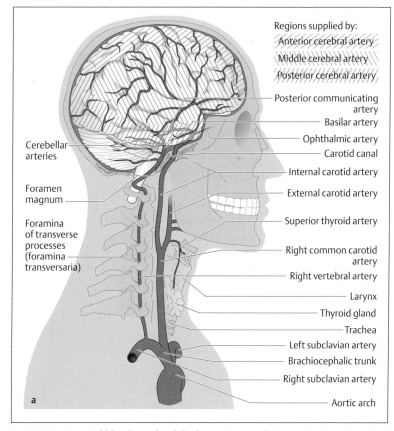

Regions supplied by:
Anterior cerebral artery
Middle cerebral artery
Posterior cerebral artery

Posterior communicating artery
Basilar artery
Ophthalmic artery
Carotid canal
Internal carotid artery
External carotid artery
Superior thyroid artery
Right common carotid artery
Right vertebral artery
Larynx
Thyroid gland
Trachea
Left subclavian artery
Brachiocephalic trunk
Right subclavian artery
Aortic arch

Cerebellar arteries
Foramen magnum
Foramina of transverse processes (foramina transversaria)

a

Fig. 13.**27 a   Arterial blood supply of the brain.** Course of the great arteries (vertebral and internal carotid arteries) supplying the brain and areas of the right cerebral hemisphere supplied by the cerebral arteries (seen from the right side)

b). The left and right internal carotid arteries run from the division of the common carotid artery to the base of the skull, and reach the inside of the cranial cavity through a canal (carotid canal). They have no branches. The left and right vertebral arteries arise from the corresponding subclavian artery and run cephalad to the atlas through the foramina in the transverse processes of the upper six cervical vertebrae. By passing

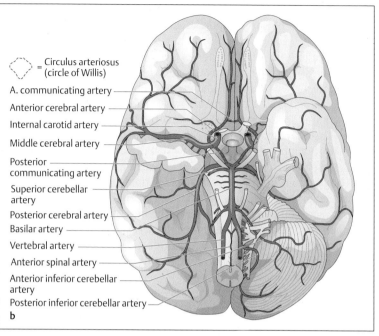

= Circulus arteriosus
(circle of Willis)

A. communicating artery

Anterior cerebral artery

Internal carotid artery

Middle cerebral artery

Posterior
communicating artery

Superior cerebellar
artery

Posterior cerebral artery

Basilar artery

Vertebral artery

Anterior spinal artery

Anterior inferior cerebellar
artery

Posterior inferior cerebellar artery

b

Fig. 13.**27 b**   **Arteries of the base of the brain and circle of Willis** (the right cerebellar hemisphere and the right temporal lobe have been removed; the circle of Willis (circulus arteriosus) is marked by the interrupted line)

through the foramen magnum they also reach the inside of the cranial cavity. The four arteries anastomose with each other in an arterial ring (circulus arteriosus, circle of Willis) (Fig. 13.**27b**). The circle of Willis and all arteries arising from it run in the subarachnoid space.

After passing through the foramen magnum, the two vertebral arteries run on the anterior side of the medulla oblongata, each giving rise to an *inferior posterior cerebellar artery* to the cerebellum and the *spinal arteries* (e. g., *anterior spinal artery*) to supply the spinal cord (Fig. 13.**27b**). At the lower edge of the pons, the two vertebral arteries join to form the *basilar artery*, which gives rise to the *inferior anterior* and the *superior cerebellar arteries*. At the upper edge of the pons, the basilar artery divides into the left and right posterior cerebral arteries; these run backward to supply the posterior part of the hemispheres, especially the inferior surface of the temporal lobe and both occipital lobes (Fig. 13.**27a**).

The two internal carotid arteries give rise to the two *ophthalmic arteries* (each supplying one eye and part of the nose) immediately after entering the base of the skull, and in their subsequent course divide into the *anterior* and *middle cerebral arteries* (*aa. cerebri anterior* and *media*). The two anterior cerebral arteries at first run forward in the longitudinal fissure (fissura longitudinalis cerebri), then run backward on the corpus callosum to supply the medial side of the two hemispheres. The two middle cerebral arteries run laterally between the temporal and frontal lobes and fan out in the lateral sulcus to supply the greater part of the lateral side of the cerebral hemispheres (Fig. 13.**27a**). In their course between the frontal and temporal lobes, the middle cerebral arteries give off important branches to supply the internal capsule (*striate arteries, aa. centrales anteromediales*). The middle cerebral artery is the largest of the three cerebral arteries and represents the direct continuation of the internal carotid artery.

The two anterior cerebrtal arteries are connected by the *anterior communicating artery*. The two *posterior communicating arteries* connect the middle and posterior cerebral arteries (Fig. 13.**27b**). They form an arterial circle (circle of Willis, circulus arteriosus cerebri) between the vertebral and carotid arteries at the base of the brain. This is of clinical significance, since after occlusion of one of the four contributing vessels the remaining three can supply the affected region. The circle of Willis is often the site of aneurysms, i.e., saccular dilatations of the vessel wall. These weak places in the vascular wall may rupture as a result of a brief rise in blood pressure, with consequent hemorrhage into the subarachnoid space (subarachnoid hemorrhage).

If a blood clot (*thrombus*) forms along the course of an artery supplying the brain (usually because of atherosclerosis of the arterial wall), or if a thrombus arises elsewhere (e. g., in the heart) and is transported into a cerebral artery by way of the bloodstream (anything transported in this manner is called an *embolus*), blockage of the artery can result, depriving the tissue normally supplied by the artery of its blood flow. This hypoperfusion (*ischemia*) results in an inadequate supply of oxygen and nutrients, causing cell death (*necrosis*). Ischemic necrosis is called *infarction*, and the area of dead tissue is called an *infarct*. Cerebral infarction is

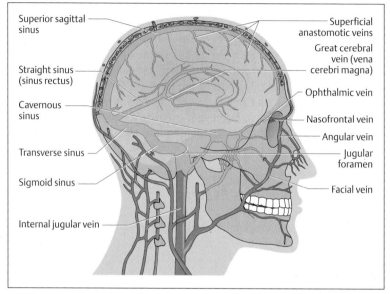

Superior sagittal sinus

Straight sinus (sinus rectus)

Cavernous sinus

Transverse sinus

Sigmoid sinus

Internal jugular vein

Superficial anastomotic veins

Great cerebral vein (vena cerebri magna)

Ophthalmic vein

Nasofrontal vein

Angular vein

Jugular foramen

Facial vein

Fig. 13.**28**   **Veins of the brain and venous sinuses in lateral view**

one of the two most common types of *stroke* (also called *cerebrovascular accident*; i.e., any event affecting the blood vessels of the brain that produces a sudden, usually irreversible, or only partially reversible, neurological deficit). *Cerebral hemorrhage* (bleeding) due to rupture of an artery causes the death of cells adjacent to the hemorrhage; this is the other common type of stroke. (Note: subarachnoid hemorrhage, discussed above, is also a type of stroke according to strict definition, but is nevertheless usually not considered as such.)

Venous drainage occurs essentially through superficial and deep cerebral veins and venous sinuses. The veins from the cerebral capillaries run to the surface and drain into larger veins. These run in the subarachnoid space like the arteries and give off anastomotic veins (Fig. 13.**28**) that drain into large venous sinuses (e. g., *superior sagittal sinus*) formed by the dura mater. The blood from the interior of the brain flows through the deep cerebral veins and eventually through the *great cerebral vein* (*vena cerebri magna*) into the *straight sinus* (*sinus rectus*).

The superior sagittal sinus and the straight sinus join on the internal surface of the occipital bone (*confluence of the sinuses*), after which they drain into the *right and left transverse sinuses*; each of these in turn is continued as a *sigmoid sinus* (Fig. 13.**28**). Eventually these drain into the internal jugular vein through the jugular foramen, an opening in the base of the skull at the side of the foramen magnum. The *cavernous sinus*, located around the sella turcica, receives, among others, the drainage of the superficial facial veins (facial vein–angular vein–nasofrontal vein); it also drains through the jugular foramen into the internal jugular vein (Fig. 13.**28**).

■ Peripheral Nervous System

The peripheral nervous system includes the *pathways* (*peripheral nerves*) running through the spinal nerves and the cranial nerves to the periphery of the body, and in the reverse direction, as well as some *collections of nerve cell bodies* (*ganglia*).

Peripheral Nerves

A peripheral nerve is a mixed nerve, since it carries afferent as well as efferent somatic and autonomic nerve fibers (p. 608). Somatic fibers are those that run from a receptor (e. g., skin or pain receptor) to the spinal cord (somatic afferent) or from the motor cells in the anterior horn of the spinal cord to skeletal muscles (somatic efferent). Autonomic fibers are afferent and efferent fibers connected to internal organs, blood vessels, and glands.

Ganglia

Ganglia are knotlike enlargements in nerves and nerve roots, a few millimeters thick, containing collections of nerve cell bodies. *Ganglia* may be *sensory* or *autonomic*. Sensory ganglia (e. g., spinal ganglia or cranial nerve ganglia) contain the cell bodies of the primary afferent nerves of both the somatic and autonomic nervous systems. The cell bodies have a peripheral process that may come, for instance, from a pain receptor in the skin or an internal organ, and a central process that connects the ganglion with the spinal cord.

Autonomic ganglia (see Chapter 14: The Autonomic Nervous System), contain cell bodies of the second-order efferent neurons (e. g., cranial parasympathetic ganglia or ganglia of the sympathetic chain). The ganglia relay information transmitted synaptically by autonomic nerve fibers from the spinal cord or the brainstem (*preganglionic fibers = first-order efferent neurons*) to the cell bodies of *second-order efferent neurons*. The latter send nerve fibers (*postganglionic fibers*) to the effector organ in the periphery (e. g., glands or smooth muscle).

Spinal Nerves

The spinal nerves divide into four branches (rami) after leaving the vertebral canal (Fig. 13.**29**):

- A *posterior branch* (*r. posterior*), supplying sensory innervation to the skin of the back and motor branches to a large part of the musculature of the vertebral column (segmental back muscles)
- An *anterior branch* (*r. anterior nervi spinalis*), supplying sensory and motor innervation to the rest of the trunk and the limbs
- A sensory branch to supply the spinal membranes and the ligaments of the vertebral column (*r. meningeus*)
- A branch that connects the sympathetic part of the autonomic nervous system (see Fig. 14.**2**) with the somatic nervous system (*white communicating branch of the spinal nerve, r. communicans albus*)

Networks of Nerves (Plexus or Plexuses)

The anterior branches of the spinal nerves form nervous networks in the cervical, lumbar, and sacral regions: the *cervical plexus* (C1–C4), the *brachial plexus* (C5–T1), the *lumbar plexus* (T12–L4), and the *sacral plexus* (L5–S4).

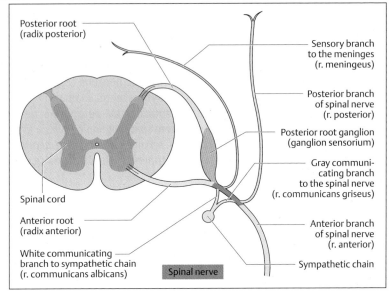

Posterior root
(radix posterior)

Sensory branch
to the meninges
(r. meningeus)

Posterior branch
of spinal nerve
(r. posterior)

Posterior root ganglion
(ganglion sensorium)

Gray communi-
cating branch
to the spinal nerve
(r. communicans griseus)

Spinal cord

Anterior root
(radix anterior)

Anterior branch
of spinal nerve
(r. anterior)

White communicating
branch to sympathetic chain
(r. communicans albicans)

Spinal nerve

Sympathetic chain

Fig. 13.**29** **Spinal nerve roots, a spinal nerve, and its branches.** (After Faller)

Cervical Plexus

The nerves of the cervical plexus supply sensory innervation to the regions of the neck and shoulder and provide motor innervation to the hyoid muscles and the diaphragm (phrenic nerve).

Brachial Plexus

From the brachial plexus arise motor nerves to the muscles of the shoulder girdle and the upper limb, and sensory nerves to the skin in the region of the shoulder and upper limb. The most important nerves supplying the upper limb are (Figs. 13.**30a**, **b** and 13.**31**):

- The ulnar nerve (n. ulnaris)
- The musculocutaneous nerve (n. musculocutaneus)
- The median nerve (n. medianus)
- The radial nerve (n. radialis)

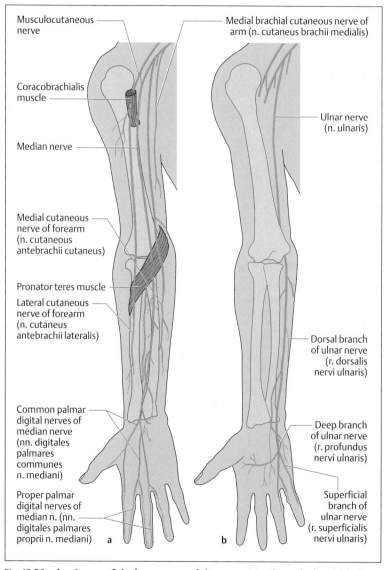

Musculocutaneous nerve

Medial brachial cutaneous nerve of arm (n. cutaneus brachii medialis)

Coracobrachialis muscle

Median nerve

Ulnar nerve (n. ulnaris)

Medial cutaneous nerve of forearm (n. cutaneous antebrachii cutaneus)

Pronator teres muscle

Lateral cutaneous nerve of forearm (n. cutaneus antebrachii lateralis)

Dorsal branch of ulnar nerve (r. dorsalis nervi ulnaris)

Common palmar digital nerves of median nerve (nn. digitales palmares communes n. mediani)

Deep branch of ulnar nerve (r. profundus nervi ulnaris)

Proper palmar digital nerves of median n. (nn. digitales palmares proprii n. mediani) **a**

Superficial branch of ulnar nerve (r. superficialis nervi ulnaris)

b

Fig. 13.**30 a, b   Course of the long nerves of the arm arising from the brachial plexus and running along the anterior aspect of the upper extremity.** (After Feneis)
a   The ulnar nerve is not marked
b   Course of the ulnar nerve

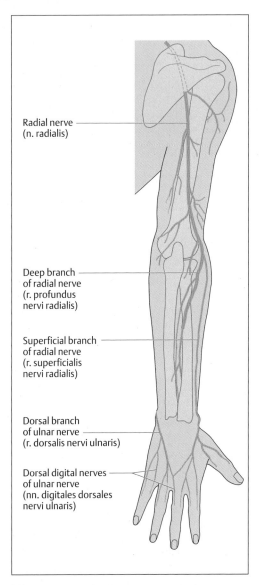

Fig. 13.**31 Course of the radial nerve from the brachial plexus on the back of the upper extremity.** (After Feneis)

Radial nerve
(n. radialis)

Deep branch
of radial nerve
(r. profundus
nervi radialis)

Superficial branch
of radial nerve
(r. superficialis
nervi radialis)

Dorsal branch
of ulnar nerve
(r. dorsalis nervi ulnaris)

Dorsal digital nerves
of ulnar nerve
(nn. digitales dorsales
nervi ulnaris)

Lumbar Plexus

The sensory branches of the lumbar plexus supply the skin of the abdomen, the genital region, and the anterior thigh (Fig. 13.**32a**, **b**). The motor branches supply chiefly the muscles of the hip, and through the femoral nerve the quadriceps femoris muscle.

Sacral Plexus

Finally, the sacral plexus supplies sensory and motor innervation for the muscles of the pelvic floor, the muscles of the lower extremity, as well as the skin of the posterior genital region (perineum) and the lower limbs. It also gives rise to the largest nerve of the whole body (Fig. 13.**32a**, **b**), the sciatic nerve (n. ischiadicus).

Cranial Nerves

The 12 *pairs of cranial nerves* (Fig. 13.**33**) can be grouped in various ways, e. g., by their central location: cranial nerves I and II, the *olfactory nerve* and the *optic nerve* are not true nerves, but extensions of the cerebrum and diencephalon respectively. The *oculomotor* and *trochlear nerves*, cranial nerves III and IV, are related to the midbrain. The *trigeminal nerve* (V), the *abducens* (VI), and the *facial nerve* (VII) are located at the level of the pons. The remaining cranial nerves, the *auditory nerve* (VIII, *vestibulocochlear nerve*), the *glossopharyngeal nerve* (IX), the *vagus nerve* (X), the *spinal accessory nerve* (XI), and the *hypoglossal nerve* (XII) arise from the medulla.

Another way of classifying the cranial nerves is by the function of their components. A few nerves are composed exclusively of *sensory neurons*. These include:

- **Olfactory nerve (I),** for the sense of smell
- **Optic nerve (II),** for vision
- **Vestibulocochlear nerve (VIII),** which conducts the sensations of hearing and equilibrium
  Other cranial nerves contain exclusively motoneurons supplying voluntary muscles. They include:
- **Trochlear nerve (IV),** which supplies one of the external muscles of the eye, the superior oblique muscle

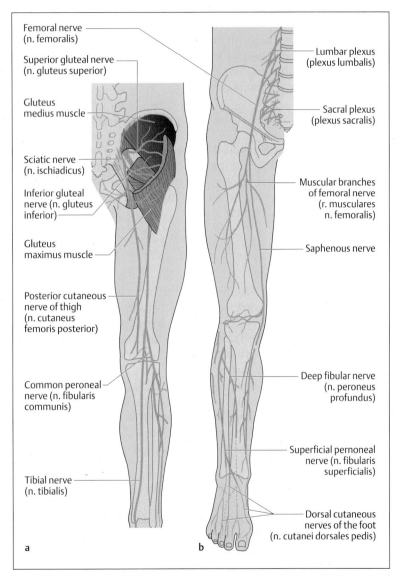

Femoral nerve
(n. femoralis)

Superior gluteal nerve
(n. gluteus superior)

Gluteus
medius muscle

Sciatic nerve
(n. ischiadicus)

Inferior gluteal
nerve (n. gluteus
inferior)

Gluteus
maximus muscle

Posterior cutaneous
nerve of thigh
(n. cutaneus
femoris posterior)

Common peroneal
nerve (n. fibularis
communis)

Tibial nerve
(n. tibialis)

a

Lumbar plexus
(plexus lumbalis)

Sacral plexus
(plexus sacralis)

Muscular branches
of femoral nerve
(r. musculares
n. femoralis)

Saphenous nerve

Deep fibular nerve
(n. peroneus
profundus)

Superficial pernoneal
nerve (n. fibularis
superficialis)

Dorsal cutaneous
nerves of the foot
(n. cutanei dorsales pedis)

b

Fig. 13.**32 a, b** Course of the most important nerves of the leg from the lumbar and sacral plexus, on the back (a) and the front (b) of the lower extremity. (After Feneis)

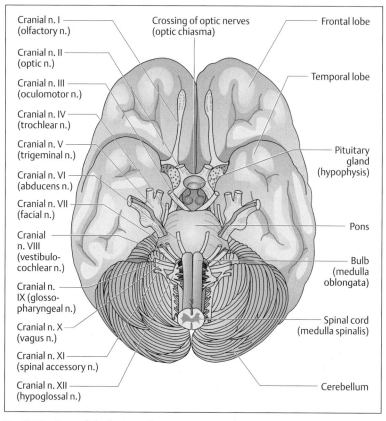

Fig. 13.**33** **Base of the brain with emerging cranial nerves**

- **Abducens (VI),** which also supplies one external eye muscle, namely, the lateral rectus muscle
- **Spinal accessory nerve (XI),** which supplies two important muscles outside the head, namely, the trapezius and the sternocleidomastoid
- **Hypoglossus (XII),** which supplies all the muscles of the tongue
  The remaining cranial nerves have mixed functions. They are:
- **Oculomotor nerve (III),** which includes motor and parasympathetic components (see Chapter 14: The Autonomic Nervous System, p. 605):

1. Voluntary motor fibers to four of the external ocular muscles (superior, inferior, and medial rectus muscles and the inferior oblique) and the levator palpebrae superioris muscle
2. Parasympathetic nerve fibers to the pupillary sphincter (m. sphincter pupillaris, constricts the pupil) and the ciliary muscle (accommodation)

■ **Trigeminal nerve (V),** with its three terminal branches, the ophthalmic, maxillary, and mandibular nerves, which have sensory as well as motor components.

1. Sensory fibers transmit pain, temperature, touch, pressure, and proprioceptive sensation from the face, the cornea, the mouth, the nasal sinuses, the tongue, the teeth, the meninges, the external surface of the ear drum, and the jaw joint.
2. Motor components to the muscles of mastication (masseter, temporalis, lateral and medial pterygoid muscles) and the muscles of the floor of the mouth (anterior belly of the digastric muscle, mylohyoid muscle), the soft palate (m. tensor veli palati), and the eustachian tube (m. tensor tympani).

■ **Facial nerve (VII),** a complex nerve with three main components:

1. Special fibers for taste sensation in the anterior two-thirds of the tongue (chorda tympani)
2. Parasympathetic fibers to the salivary glands (lingual and submandibular glands), the lacrimal gland (tear gland), and the glands of the mouth and nose (palatine and nasal glands)
3. Motor fibers to the voluntary muscles of expression, as well as the muscles of the hyoid bone (stylohoid muscle), the floor of the mouth (posterior belly of the digastric muscle), and the middle ear (m. stapedius)

■ **Glossopharyngeal nerve (IX),** which also has three main components:

1. Special fibers for taste sensation in the posterior third of the tongue
2. Parasympathetic fibers to the parotid gland through the autonomic otic ganglion
3. Sensory neurons (pain, temperature, pressure, and touch sensation) to the eustachian tube, the palatine end of the tongue, the internal surface of the ear drum, the throat, and the carotid sinus (changes in blood pressure)

■ **Vagus nerve (X),** a nerve essential to life, with three main components:

1. Parasympathetic neurons to all the autonomic structures of the thoracic and abdominal cavities as far as the left flexure of the transverse colon (e. g., heart, coronary arteries, bronchi, stomach, arteries and arterioles of the small bowel, and glands)
2. Motor fibers to those muscles of the larynx and the throat that are involved in swallowing and speech
3. Sensory nerves from the larynx, the internal organs, the carotid body (a chemoreceptor), the carotid sinus, the meninges of the posterior cranial fossa, and the lower part of the throat

Summary **The Central and Peripheral Nervous Systems**

■ **Classification and Role**

According to its spatial arrangement the nervous system is divided into a central and a peripheral nervous system:

- *Central nervous system (CNS):* brain and spinal cord
- *Peripheral nervous system:* peripheral nerves (spinal and cranial nerves, collections of nerve cells = ganglia)

Functionally the CNS and peripheral nervous systems can be divided into a somatic and an autonomic (= vegetative) nervous system:

- *Somatic nervous system* (organism–environment): responsible for (1) conscious perception, (2) voluntary movements, and (3) rapid processing of information
- *Autonomic* (*vegetative*) *nervous system* (organism–internal organs): responsible for (1) maintaining a constant internal milieu (homeostasis) and (2) regulation of organic functioning in response to environmental demands

The somatic and autonomic nervous systems both include afferent and efferent impulses:

- *Afferents:* all impulses transmitted from the periphery (e. g., skin, internal organs) centrally (to brain, spinal cord)
- *Efferents:* all impulses reaching the periphery (e. g., striated skeletal muscle, smooth muscle of the internal organs and blood vessels, glandular cells) from the center (brain, spinal cord)

■ Development
The central and peripheral nervous systems develop from the outer germ layer (ectoderm) of the three-layered embryonic disk. The rudiment appears at the end of the third week as an ectodermal thickening (neural plate = neural ectoderm) above the notochord (chorda dorsalis). Lateral folds in the neural plate (neural folds) lead to the formation of the neural groove, which eventually closes to form the *neural tube*. Parts of the neural folds become the *neural crests*. The neural tube develops into the CNS, the neural crests into the peripheral nervous system.

■ Central Nervous System (CNS)
The central nervous system consists of the brain (encephalon) and the spinal cord (medulla spinalis); both parts develop from the neural tube. The wall of the neural tube develops into the gray and white substance of the brain and spinal cord, while the anterior part of the lumen develops into the ventricles of the brain and the posterior part into the central canal of the spinal cord. The cranial part of the neural tube (primary brain vesicles) becomes the brain, the caudal part forms the spinal cord.

● *Derivatives of the three primary brain vesicles (prosencephalon, mesencephalon, and rhombencephalon):*
  – Prosencephalon (anterior brain vesicles): telencephalon (cerebrum) and diencephalon
  – Mesencephalon (middle brain vesicle): mesencephalon (midbrain)
  – Rhombencephalon (posterior brain vesicle): pons, cerebellum, and medulla oblongata

The Brain
Average weight: in women 1245 g, in men 1375 g, in the newborn 400 g; definitive weight is reached at age 5–7 years Weight in relation to body weight (b.w.): women 22 g/kg b.w., and men 20 g/kg b.w.

Cerebrum (Telencephalon)
This most highly developed part of the brain consists of the two cerebral hemispheres, the basal ganglia, the two lateral ventricles, and the limbic system. The surface of the cerebrum is extended by convolu-

tions (gyri) and fissures (sulci). The central fissure (sulcus centralis) and the lateral fissure (sylvian fissure, sulcus lateralis) divide each hemisphere into four lobes: the frontal, parietal, temporal, and occipital lobes. The **cerebral cortex** (*cortex cerebri*) contains primarily cell bodies (gray matter, gray substance); the inner white matter (white substance) contains nerve fibers or axons. Nerve fibers may connect the two hemispheres (commissural fibers), begin and end within a hemisphere (association fibers), or run from the cerebral cortex to other parts of the CNS (projection fibers). The largest commissure, with about 200 million axons, is the corpus callosum; the most important projection tract is the pyramidal tract (corticospinal tract). Almost all projection fibers are closely bundled with the tracts ascending to the cortex as they pass through the internal capsule, which is bounded by the basal ganglia and parts of the diencephalon (thalamus).

Within the cerebral cortex are located highly developed **functional cortical areas** with specific functions: primary areas (where the projection tracts begin and end) and secondary areas (association areas, which process information and make up about 80% of the cortical surface).

- The most important *primary areas* are:
  - The precentral gyrus (primary motor cortex): origin of large parts of the pyramidal tract (execution of voluntary movements)
  - The postcentral gyrus (primary sensory cortex): terminal area of somatic sensory tracts for conscious perception
  - The calcarine fissure (primary visual cortex): terminal area of the optic pathways
  - The transverse temporal gyrus (primary auditory cortex): terminal area of the acoustic pathways.

- The most important *association areas* are:
- The inferior frontal gyrus (motor speech center = Broca's area): coordination of speech (80–90% located in the left, dominant hemisphere; lesions cause motor aphasia.
- The superior temporal gyrus (secondary auditory center/sensory language center = Wernicke's area: auditory association area; lesions cause sensory aphasia.

Essentially the left hemisphere is responsible for the right half of the body and the right hemisphere for the left half of the body (crossover of the afferent and efferent pathways). Certain functions are located preferentially in one hemisphere (hemispheric dominance); left hemisphere: reading, speech, writing; right hemisphere: memory, language comprehension, visual/spatial imagination and musical comprehension.

The **basal ganglia** are collections of nerve cell bodies in the white matter. They have an important role in the extrapyramidal motor system (control of extent and direction of voluntary movements). They include the globus pallidus, the putamen, and the caudate nucleus: The globus pallidus and the putamen together are known as the lentiform nucleus, while the caudate nucleus and the lentiform nucleus together form the corpus striatum (striate body).

The **limbic system** runs along the corpus callosum like a hem. It takes part in creating memories and in triggering and processing emotional reactions. It is formed from phylogenetically older parts of the telencephalon: paleocortex and archicortex; those parts of the brain that are phylogenetically younger (essentially the cerebral hemispheres) are called the neocortex (isocortex, neopallium). The limbic system includes: (1) derivatives of the paleocortex—olfactory brain; (2) derivatives of the archicortex—amygdala, hippocampus, dentate gyrus (gyrus dentatus), cingulate gyrus (gyrus cinguli), indusium griseum (supercallosal gyrus), and the most important fiber tract to the hypothalamus, the fornix.

Diencephalon

The diencephalon lies between the cerebral hemispheres under the corpus callosum and surrounds the third ventricle. It includes:

- *The thalamus:* central relay station of the sensory tracts (pain, temperature, pressure, touch)
- *The metathalamus (medial and lateral geniculate bodies):* central relay station of the visual and auditory pathways
- *The hypothalamus:* center controlling the autonomic nervous system (e. g., body temperature, water balance, nutrition)
- *The hypophysis* (pituitary gland): principal organ controlling the endocrine system

- The *epithalamus* (pineal body): biological clock controlling the circadian rhythm

Brainstem

The brainstem includes the midbrain, the pons, and the medulla oblongata and contains the reticular formation and the nuclei of the cranial nerves.

Midbrain (Mesencephalon)

The midbrain is the smallest part of the brain and lies between the diencephalon and the pons. It contains the tectum, the tegmentum, the cerebral aqueduct (conduit between the third and fourth ventricles), and the two crura cerebri. The tectum is formed by the corpora quadrigemina (superior and inferior colliculi = relay stations of the visual and auditory reflex pathways). The tegmentum contains two basal ganglia (red nucleus and the substantia nigra) and the nuclei of cranial nerves III and IV (oculomotor and trochlear nerves). The ascending tracts to the cortex pass through the tegmentum, the descending tracts through the crura cerebri.

Pons

The pons lies between the midbrain and the medulla and is separated from the cerebellum by the superior part of the fourth ventricle. Besides the ascending and descending tracts the pons contains the nuclei of cranial nerves V, VI and VII (trigeminal, abducens and facial nerves).

Medulla Oblongata

The medula oblongata forms the transition from the brain to the spinal cord and extends to the foramen magnum. The medulla contains the respiratory and circulatory centers and the nuclei of cranial nerves VIII–XII (vestibulocochlear, glossopharyngeal, vagus, spinal accessory, and hypoglossal nerves). Anteriorly, the pyramids lie on either side of the median fissure, and a little below them is the decussation of the pyramidal tract. The posterior side of the medulla is partly covered by the cerebellum, and together with the rhomboid fossa forms the floor of the fourth ventricle (the upper part of the rhomboid fossa is considered part of the pons). Below the rhomboid fossa lie two raised areas which are relays for the tracts of the posterior funiculus (fasciculus cuneatus and fasciculus gracilis).

Cerebellum

The cerebellum lies in the posterior cranial fossa under the tentorium (tentorium cerebelli). It consists of the vermis and two cerebellar hemispheres, the surface of which is greatly extended by parallel folia (gyri). The cerebellum weighs 130–140 g and is connected to the brainstem by the peduncles. The parts of the cerebellum can be classified by their phylogenetic age: an oldest part (archicerebellum) a second oldest part (paleocerebellum), and a new part (neocerebellum).

- *The archicerebellum:* includes the nodulus and the bilateral flocculus (flocculonodular lobe). It is responsible for maintaining the equilibrium.
- *The paleocerebellum:* formed by the anterior lobes of the cerebellar hemispheres and part of the vermis. It regulates muscle tone.
- *The neocerebellum:* includes the posterior lobe of the cerebellar hemispheres and the rest of the vermis. It is responsible for the coordination of voluntary muscles.

Spinal Cord (Medulla Spinalis)

The spinal cord represents an extracranial part of the central nervous system and lies in the vertebral canal, extending from the foramen magnum to the 1st–2nd lumbar vertebra. The spinal cord contains ascending and descending bundles of nerve fibers through which the brain communicates with the peripheral nervous system.

Spinal Nerves

The 31 pairs of spinal nerves each are formed from an anterior and a posterior root (radix anterior and radix posterior). They leave the vertebral canal through the intervertebral foramina. The spinal nerves arise in pairs, of which there are eight cervical (from the cervical cord C1–C8), 12 thoracic (from the thoracic cord T1–T12), five lumbar (from the lumbar cord L1–L5), five sacral (from the sacral cord S1–S5) and 1–2 coccygeal (from the coccygeal cord Co1–Co2).

Gray Matter of the Spinal Cord

The gray matter (substantia grisea) of the spinal cord, in cross-section shaped like a butterfly, lies in the middle of the spinal cord. It contains the bodies of the nerve cells and contains:

- *The anterior horn (anterior column):* contains motoneuron cells, the axons of which leave the spinal cord by the anterior root and supply the striated skeletal muscles.
- *The posterior horn (dorsal column):* contains the sensory nerve cells, where some of the peripheral afferent nerve cells entering through the posterior root end in synapses.
- *The lateral horn (intermediate column):* contains motor nerve cells of the autonomic system, the efferent axons of which leave the spinal cord by the anterior roots to innervate among others the smooth muscle of the internal organs.

White Matter of the Spinal cord

The gray matter is surrounded by the white matter (substantia alba), which contains the ascending and descending myelinated fibers. It is divided into dorsal, lateral (or anterolateral), and ventral funiculi. The intersegmental (intercalated) fibers of the spinal cord itself (fasciculi proprii) run next to the gray substance.

- *Ascending tracts.* tracts of the ventral funiculus (afferent tracts to the thalamus for pressure, coarse touch and tactile discrimination, as well as pain and temperature sensation from the extremities and the trunk). tracts of the dorsal funiculus (afferent pathways to the thalamus for deep sensation, vibration, light touch, and tactile discrimination on the limbs and trunk); spinocerebellar tracts of the lateral funiculus (afferent tracts to the cerebellum for unconscious deep sensations from muscles, tendons, and joints).
- *Descending tracts:* pyramidal tract (efferent tract from the motor cortex to the anterior horn cells carrying voluntary motor fibers to the extremities and the trunk); extrapyramidal tracts (efferent tracts for involuntary movements, such as position, posture and automatic movements, from the brainstem, the basal ganglia, and the premotor areas to the anterior horn cells).

Spinal Reflexes

The basis for all spinal reflexes (e. g., the patellar reflex) is the reflex arc, consisting of the following components: (1) receptor, (2) afferent neuron, (3) synapse, (4) efferent neuron, and (5) effector organ. Reflexes include proprioceptive or stretch reflexes, sensorimotor or skin reflexes, and pathological reflexes.

Tracts for the Voluntary Innervation of Muscles (Pyramidal Tracts)

Pyramidal Tracts

Principal pathway for all voluntary muscular activity. It begins in the precentral gyrus of the frontal lobe and runs through the internal capsule in the brainstem, ending either in the nuclei of the cranial nerves (corticobulbar tract) or in motor cells of the anterior horn of the spinal cord (corticospinal tract). Hence these tracts include:

- *The corticobulbar tract (corticonuclear tract) for the innervation of the cranial voluntary muscles:* the efferent axons of the corticobulbar tract leave the pyramidal tract in the brainstem, cross to the opposite side and end in synapses in the motor nuclei of the cranial nerves.
- *The corticospinal tract for the innervation of the muscles of the trunk and extremities:* 80–90% of the axons cross in the medulla in the decussation of the pyramidal tracts to the opposite side. They run as the lateral corticospinal tract to the corresponding cells in the spinal cord; the uncrossed axons descend through the anterior corticospinal tract of the same side and do not cross until they reach the level of the anterior horn cells.

The axons of the pyramidal tract are called upper motoneurons regardless of their target area; axons to the striated skeletal muscles arising after relay in the nuclei of the cranial nerves or the anterior horn cells are called lower motoneurons. Lesions of the upper motoneuron cause spastic paralysis; lesions of the lower motoneuron flaccid paralysis.

Extrapyramidal Motor System

The extrapyramidal motor system includes among others the basal ganglia of the cerebrum (globus pallidus, putamen, caudate nucleus) and the midbrain (red nucleus, substantia nigra), the vestibular nuclei, the premotor areas of the cerebral cortex, the cerebellum, and the extrapyramidal descending motor tracts of the spinal cord. It is responsible for involuntary muscular activity and controls the extent and direction of voluntary movements.

Membranes of the Brain and Spinal Cord

To protect them from external influences, the brain and spinal cord are surrounded by connective tissue membranes (meninges) as well as bony structures (skull and vertebral canal). The membranes include a dense fibrous outer dura mater of the brain and spinal cord (*dura mater cranialis and spinalis*) a thin and delicate middle arachnoid (*arachnoidea cranialis and spinalis*) and a soft inner membrane (*pia mater cranialis and spinalis*) directly applied to the surface of the brain and spinal cord. Between the arachnoid and the pia mater lies the subarachnoid space, which is filled with CSF and contains the cerebral and spinal vessels as well as the cranial nerves and the roots of the spinal nerves. While the dura mater is directly adherent to the bony skull, an epidural space filled with fatty tissue and veins lies between the vertebrae and the spinal dura.

Cerebrospinal Fluid (CSF) and the Ventricular System

- *Cerebrospinal fluid:* the CSF is contained in the internal (ventricles of the brain) and external (subarachnoid space) fluid-filled spaces (total amount: 130–150 ml). About 500–600 ml of CSF is secreted daily from the choroid plexus of the ventricles; it reaches the subarachnoid space through three openings in the fourth ventricle and is reabsorbed through the arachnoid villi (projections from the arachnoid into the superior sagittal sinus) and where the spinal nerves emerge (fluid is replaced 3–4 times a day).
- *The ventricular system:* includes one lateral ventricle for each cerebral hemisphere (first and second ventricles), each connected to the third ventricle through an interventricular foramen (foramen of Monro) (in the diencephalon). A fourth ventricle between the brainstem and the cerebellum is connected to the third ventricle by the cerebral aqueduct (of Silvius), which runs through the midbrain. The apertures to the subarachnoid space lie at the level of the fourth ventricle, which also contains an aperture to the central canal of the spinal cord.

Blood Supply of the Brain

- *Arterial supply* is provided by the vertebral arteries (through the foramen magnum) and the internal carotid arteries (through the carotid canal), the branches of which form the circulus arteriosus (of Willis) at the base of the brain, which supplies blood to the brain. The larger vessels run at first in the subarachnoid space, and from there they pass into the brain. The most important are the anterior, posterior, and middle cerebral arteries.

- *Venous drainage* is by the deep (great cerebral vein) and superficial (e. g., superior cerebral) veins that give off anastomotic branches to the venous sinuses: superior sagittal, straight, transverse, sigmoid, and cavernous sinus. Each sinus collects venous blood and channels it through the sigmoid sinus to the jugular foramen, where it drains into the two internal jugular veins.

■ Peripheral Nervous System

The peripheral nervous system includes the nerves that originate in the spinal cord (spinal nerves) and those that originate in the brainstem (cranial nerves III through XII) to run to the peripheral body, those running in the reverse direction (peripheral nerves), and collections of nerve cells bodies (ganglia).

- *Peripheral nerves* are mixed nerves, that is, they contain efferent and afferent somatic as well as autonomic axons.
- *Ganglia* are knotlike enlargements, a few millimeters thick, in peripheral nerves or nerve roots. They include:
  - Sensory ganglia: e. g., spinal root ganglia, containing the cell bodies of primary afferent neurons (somatic and autonomic)
  - Autonomic ganglia: e. g., parasympathetic ganglia, containing the cell bodies of secondary efferent neurons (autonomic)
- *Spinal nerves* are formed by the junction of the posterior and anterior roots to continue as mixed nerves (afferent and efferent nerve fibers):
  - The *posterior root* contains exclusively afferent nerve fibers, the cell bodies of which lie in a knot (spinal ganglion, dorsal root ganglion) in the root.
  - The *anterior root* contains exclusively efferent nerve fibers, the cell bodies of which are located in the anterior and lateral horns.

Spinal nerves divide into four branches:

  - A posterior branch (r. posterior): sensory and motor supply to the skin of the back and the segmental muscles of the back

- An anterior branch (r. anterior): sensory and motor supply for the rest of the trunk and the extremities
- A recurrent branch (r. meningeus): sensory supply to the spinal meninges and the ligaments of the vertebral column
- A communicating branch (r. comunicans albus): a communication from the sympathetic part of the autonomic nervous system to the somatic nervous system
- *Nervous networks (plexuses)* are formed by the anterior branches of the spinal nerves (except T2–T11); cervical plexus (C1–C4), brachial plexus (C5–T1), lumbar plexus (T12–L4), and sacral plexus (L5–S4).
- *Cranial nerves:* there are 12 pairs of cranial nerves:

(I)	olfactory n.	(VII)	facial n.
(II)	optic n.	(VIII)	vestibulocochlear n.
(III)	oculomotor n.	(IX)	glossopharyngeal n.
(IV)	trochlear n.	(X)	vagus n.
(V)	trigeminal n.	(XI)	spinal accessory n.
(VI)	abducens n.	(XII)	hypoglossal n.

14

The Autonomic Nervous System

Contents

■ Function and Components

The autonomic nervous system, also known as the vegetative or visceral nervous system, stimulates and regulates involuntary and unconscious functioning of organs. For instance, the functioning of the heart, circulation and respiration, digestion, metabolism, and excretion as well as heat and energy exchange are constantly being regulated by the autonomic nervous system. It stimulates the striated cardiac muscle, most glands, and all of the smooth muscle found in many organs. The autonomic nervous system is divided into three parts:

- **The sympathetic nervous system (thoracolumbar outflow)**
- **The parasympathetic nervous system (craniosacral outflow)**
- **The enteric plexus**

As a rule, both sympathetic and parasympathetic fibers innervate an organ (Fig. 14.**1a**), and the two systems function as *antagonists*. For example, sympathetic stimulation raises the heart rate, while parasympathetic stimulation reduces it; sympathetic impulses dilate the pupils, while parasympathetic impulses constrict them. Hence *equilibrium* between the *sympathetic* and *parasympathetic systems* is a prerequisite for the *optimal functioning of organs*.

The enteric nervous system of the gastrointestinal tract is often regarded as an independent third part of the autonomic nervous system. Arguments in favor of such a special position are the relatively independent functioning of the enteric nervous system, the extremely large number of cells involved (10–100 million), and a different functional organization. The independent activity of the enteric nervous system can be shown by the fact that dilation of the gastric or intestinal wall is itself an adequate stimulus to trigger peristalsis.

Fig. 14.**1 a, b**   **Simplified representation of the autonomic nervous system**
a   Origins of the sympathetic and parasympathetic nervous systems and organs they innervate. The origins are bilateral. Only one side is shown for each system
b   Relay systems of the efferent sympathetic and parasympathetic nerve fibers

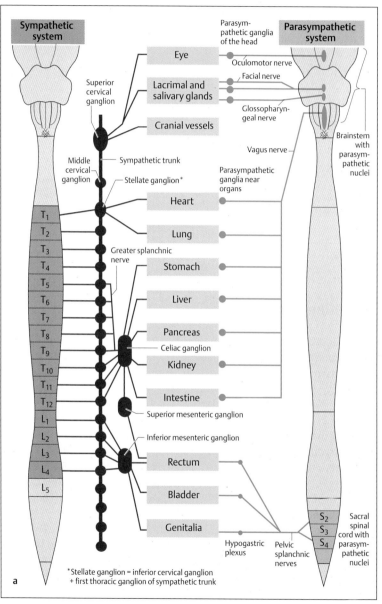

Fig. 14.**1 a**

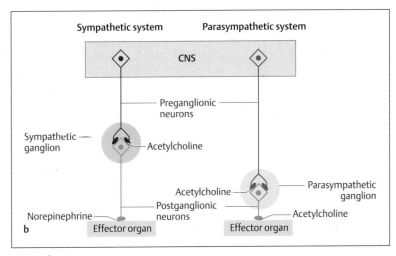

Fig. 14.**1 b**

■ Outline of the System

The sympathetic and parasympathetic systems include an *efferent* and an *afferent pathway*. The efferent path is distinguished by the serial arrangement of two neurons. The first neuron conducts impulses from the central nervous system (spinal cord and brainstem) to a synaptic relay, an *autonomic ganglion* containing the cell bodies of the second neuron (Figs. 14.**1a**, **b** and 14.**2**). The latter continue to the effector organ. From its relation to the relay in the ganglion, the first neuron is called *preganglionic*, the second *postganglionic*. Preganglionic fibers are usually myelinated, while postganglionic fibers are unmyelinated. Despite the essentially similar structures of the sympathetic and parasympathetic systems, they differ in the origin of the preganglionic fibers in the CNS, the location of the autonomic ganglia, and their chemical transmitter substances.

The afferent nerve fibers transmit information, e. g., the degree of filling of organs (pressure or tension), from the viscera back to the CNS. The cell bodies of these fibers lie in the dorsal root ganglia, similarly to those of the somatic sensory fibers. Thus, in contrast to the efferent fibers, there is only one neuron.

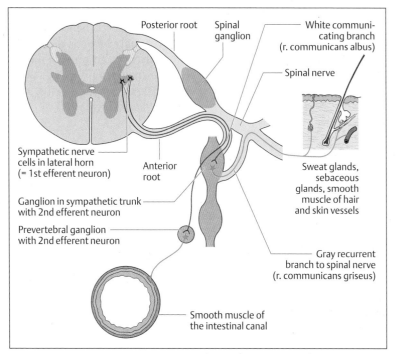

Fig. 14.**2** **Preganglionic and postganglionic fibers of the sympathetic nervous system.** Preganglionic fibers are shown in pink, postganglionic fibers in red

■ Sympathetic Nervous System

Function

The sympathetic system is dominant during *physical* and *psychic* stress. In both cases there is a feeling of threat and the body reacts automatically with preparation for flight or fight. Under such circumstances the muscles begin to work harder, thus requiring more oxygen and energy. The respiratory rate rises while the bronchi open to allow a more rapid respiration and increased respiratory volume, the heart rate and force increase in order to increase the ejection of blood from the heart and raise the blood pressure. The arteries of the heart and the voluntary muscles

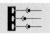

dilate, in order to increase blood flow, while at the same time the arteries to the skin and peripheral regions of the body constrict (hence in stressful situations the skin feels cold). In this way, more blood is directed to the active muscles. The liver metabolizes glycogen to provide energy rapidly, and intestinal peristalsis ebbs, since the body provides neither time nor energy for digestion. The pupils dilate to provide a better view of the situation, hair becomes erect, and the person sweats.

Structure

The cell bodies of the preganglionic neuron are located in the lateral horn of the spinal cord (Fig. 14.**2**), but only between the 1st thoracic and 4th lumbar segments (T1–L4) (Fig. 14.**1a**). Hence this system is often called the "*thoracolumbar outflow*." The nerve fibers leave the spinal cord through the anterior root and by way of a communicating branch (*r. communicans albus*) reach the *sympathetic trunk*. This consists of a number of ganglia and nerve fibers and extends from the neck to the sacrum along each side of the vertebral column. The sympathetic trunks of the two sides join in front of the sacrum in the ganglion impar ("unpaired ganglion").

The myelinated preganglionic axons innervating the *sweat glands*, the *hair*, and the *smooth muscle of the vessels* of the skin leave the spinal cord through the anterior root and enter the sympathetic trunk through the white rami communicantes (white communicating branches, which are white because they contain myelinated axons). After being relayed in the sympathetic ganglion of the chain, the unmyelinated postganglionic fibers return to the spinal nerve by way of the gray rami communicantes grisei (gray communicating branches, which are gray because they contain unmyelinated axons) and reach their effector organs with the peripheral nerves.

The cell bodies responsible for the innervation of *heart* and *lung* are located in the lateral (intermediate) horn of the spinal cord in segments T1–T4. The axons leave the spinal cord and after passing through the white communicating branches enter the sympathetic ganglia, where they synapse with the postganglionic neuron. The latter leave the ganglion as specific nerves to the heart and lung. The *preganglionic neuron* is myelinated, while the *postganglionic* neuron has no myelin sheath.

The sympathetic nerve fibers supplying the *glands* (e.g., salivary glands) and *smooth muscle* of the *head* (e.g., in vessel walls, piloerector muscles, pupilloconstrictor muscle) leave the spinal cord as preganglionic fibers in the first thoracic nerve (T1) and travel by way of the white ramus communicans to the cervical portion of the sympathetic trunk, which contains three sympathetic ganglia—the inferior, middle, and superior cervical ganglia. The inferior cervical ganglion is fused with the first thoracic ganglion of the sympathetic trunk to form the stellate ganglion (Fig. 14.**1a**). The preganglionic neurons synapse onto the postganglionic neurons mainly in the superior cervical ganglion; postganglionic fibers leave the spinal cord as preganglionic fibers in the first thoracic segment (T1) and enter the sympathetic trunk by white communicating branches. They then ascend to the highest sympathetic ganglion in the neck (*superior cervical ganglion*) (Fig. 14.**1a**). Here they synapse with postganglionic neurons, the fibers of which leave the ganglion and innervate the glands and other structures. The postganglionic axons reach their effector organs by winding around the arteries on their way to supplying the innervated structures. In this way the neurons reach and supply the glands and smooth muscles together with the arteries.

The sympathetic cells responsible for the innervation of the *abdominal organs* are located in the lateral horns of the 5th to 12th thoracic segments. Their axons pass through the sympathetic trunk, form the *greater* and *lesser splanchnic nerves* (*nn. splanchnici major* and *minor*) and do not synapse with the postganglionic neuron until they reach the prevertebral ganglia (*celiac ganglion* and *superior mesenteric ganglion*) (Fig. 14.**1a**, **b**). The postganglionic axons form networks or plexuses (e.g., the *solar plexus* originating in the celiac ganglion) (Fig. 14.**3**) and run with the vessels to the effector organs.

Some of the preganglionic fibers run directly to the *adrenal gland*. The cells of the adrenal medulla are *altered nerve cells* (cell bodies of postganglionic neurons), specialized to secrete epinephrine (80%) and norepinephrine (20%). Both hormones are secreted into the circulation and supplement the sympathetic effect of the neurons on organs. They ensure, for instance, that substances such as glucose and fatty acids are readily available for combustion in situations involving physical stress. However, epinephrine and norepinephrine are also secreted into the blood during emotional stress, and it is easy to imagine that during constantly repeated physical and emotional stress (e.g., in traffic or in the

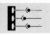

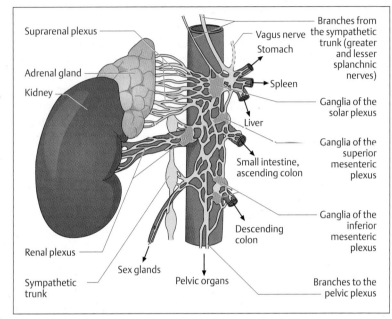

Fig. 14.**3** **The abdominal autonomic plexuses**

workplace) the long-term elevation of the blood epinephrine level could favor the development of various diseases.

Most of the preganglionic neurons for the *pelvic organs* are located in the lateral horns of spinal segments L1–L4. Their axons reach the sympathetic trunk through white communicating branches, but descend without synaptic contact to the inferior mesenteric ganglion. From here the postganglionic fibers spread fanwise (inferior mesenteric plexus) to supply the urogenital organs, as well as the descending colon, the sigmoid colon, and the rectum (Fig. 14.**3**).

Chemical Neurotransmitters

The *neurotransmitter* of the preganglionic neuron is *acetylcholine*, while the transmitter of the postganglionic fibers is *norepinephrine* (*noradrenaline*) and small amounts of *epinephrine* (*adrenaline*) (exception!: acetylcholine for the sweat glands of the skin).

Postsynaptic Receptors on Effector Organs

To understand the action of the two neurotransmitters norepinephrine and epinephrine, it is important to know that sympathetically innervated organs have two types of receptors: α-*adrenergic* and β-*adrenergic receptors*. Differences in the effect of norepinephrine, which is chiefly present at the postganglionic sympathetic nerve endings, and of epinephrine, which is chiefly liberated from the adrenal medulla, can be attributed to the differences in their reaction to different sympathetic receptors. While α-adrenergic receptors respond especially well to norepinephrine, β-adrenergic receptors respond best to epinephrine. In general α-adrenergic receptors transmit the stimulatory action, while β-adrenergic receptors transmit the inhibitory action of the sympathetic system.

Stimulation of α-adrenergic receptors in the vessel walls, for instance, provokes vasoconstriction, and with it a rise in blood pressure. An exception to this action is provided by the gastrointestinal tract, where stimulation of α receptors is inhibitory. This results in relaxation of the muscle. On the other hand, stimulation of β receptors in the vascular walls leads to dilatation of the blood vessels, and in the bronchi it leads to dilatation of the bronchi. The heart provides an exception to this action, as stimulation of β receptors is activating, resulting in an increase in heart rate.

Pharmacological substances that block one or the other of these receptors are of therapeutic importance. These are the α- and β-blockers. For instance, the blood pressure of a hypertensive patient can be lowered by slowing the heart rate with a β-blocker. However, the patient should not have comorbid bronchial asthma, since blocking the β receptors would prevent relaxation of the bronchial musculature and hence dilatation of the bronchi (see above). Such an effect would increase the respiratory distress of the patient.

■ Parasympathetic Nervous System

Function

While the sympathetic nervous system is dominant in situations of stress and its actions are catabolic in nature, the parasympathetic system is dominant when we are quiet and relaxed. In such situations the heart

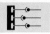

beats more slowly, peristalsis and other digestive functions are active, the pupils are constricted, and respiratory frequency is slowed. These metabolic processes have anabolic characteristics (building the substance of the body).

Structure

Turning to the anatomy of the system, the preganglionic cell bodies are located in the *brainstem* and in the *lateral horns of the sacral region.* Hence this system is also known as the "*craniosacral outflow.*"

Chemical Neurotransmitters

The chemical transmitter of the parasympathetic system is *acetylcholine* in both preganglionic and postganglionic neurons.

Cranial Parasympathetic System

The cell bodies in the brainstem lie in various specific nuclei, the parasympathetic axons of which join cranial nerves III, VII, IX, and X.

Cranial Nerve III (Oculomotor Nerve)

Preganglionic cell bodies lie in the midbrain in the Edinger–Westphal nucleus, a parasympathetic nucleus. The axons join the motor fibers of the lower motor neurons of the oculomotor nerve and leave the brainstem with them to run to the orbit (Fig. 14.**4**). Just before the nerve terminates in the eye muscles, the preganglionic parasympathetic fibers leave it and enter the ciliary ganglion, where they form a synapse with the postganglionic neurons. These send short axons (short ciliary nerves, nn. ciliares breves) to the sphincter of the pupil (m. sphincter pupillae; constricts the pupil = miosis) and the ciliary muscle (m. ciliaris; accommodation = distance adaptation).

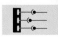

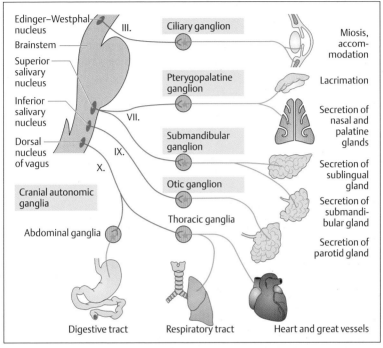

Fig. 14.**4** **Cranial parasympathetic.** The parasympathetic fibers leave the brainstem with cranial nerves III (oculomotor nerve), VII (facial nerve), and IX (glossopharyngeal nerve) and are relayed from preganglionic to postganglionic in the cranial autonomic ganglia. The fibers of cranial nerve X (vagus nerve) are relayed in ganglia near the thoracic and abdominal organs

Cranial Nerve VII (Facial Nerve)

The preganglionic cell bodies associated with the facial nerve are located in the superior salivatory nucleus (n. salivatorius superior) and their axons run first to the pterygopalatine and submandibular ganglia (Fig. 14.**4**). From there, postganglionic axons run to the tear gland (lacrimal gland), the nasal and palatine glands, the submandibular gland, and the sublingual gland.

Cranial Nerve IX (Glossopharyngeal Nerve)

The preganglionic nerve cells of the parasympathetic part of the glossopharyngeal nerve lie in the inferior salivatory nucleus. The axons run to the otic ganglion, from which postganglionic fibers run to the parotid gland (Fig. 14.**4**).

Cranial Nerve X (Vagus Nerve)

The vagus nerve is the most important cranial nerve, for most of its fibers are parasympathetic neurons supplying the heart, lungs, and all abdominal organs to the left colic flexure (flexura coli sinistra). The preganglionic cell bodies lie in the dorsal nucleus of the vagus nerve (nucleus posterior nervi vagi). The axons run with the vagus nerve to the periphery, ending in ganglia that lie in the walls of the above-mentioned organs (intramural ganglia) or near them (parasympathetic ganglia of the chest and abdomen) (Fig. 14.**5**). Postganglionic fibers leave these ganglia to innervate the target structures.

Sacral Parasympathetic Outflow

The large intestine below the *left colic flexure*, and the urogenital system are innervated by the sacral outflow of the parasympathetic system. The preganglionic cell bodies lie in the lateral horn of spinal cord segments S2–S4. The axons pass through the anterior root to the spinal nerve. After a short course they leave this in the *pelvic splanchnic nerves* (*radices parasympathetica gangliorum pelvicorum*) and end in the parasympathetic ganglia of the *hypogastric plexus*. After relaying there, the axons of the postganglionic fibers run to the descending and sigmoid colon, the rectum, the ureter, the bladder, and the genital organs (Fig. 14.**1a**).

■ Nervous System of the Intestinal Wall

The enteric nervous system (enteric plexus) regulates essential *digestive*, *endocrine*, and *immune* functions of the gastrointestinal tract. This system includes all the neuronal elements of the gastrointestinal tract from

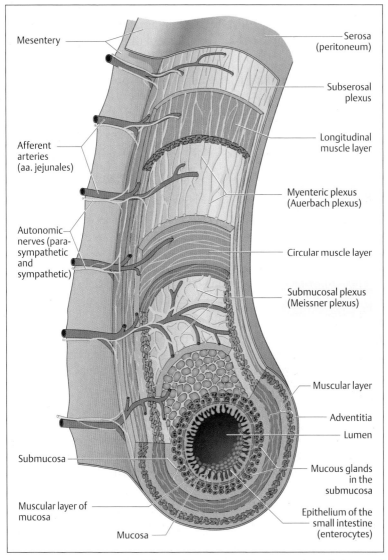

Fig. 14.5 Nervous networks of the small intestine. In this diagram the wall of the small intestine is shown as somewhat larger in proportion to the lumen than is actually the case. (After Netter)

the esophagus to the internal anal sphincter. It consists of several nervous networks (plexuses) that extend into different layers of the intestinal wall. The nerve cells are principally located in the ganglia of two great plexuses:

- The myenteric plexus (p. myentericus) (Auerbach plexus)
- The submucosal plexus (p. submucosus) (Meissner plexus)

The myenteric plexus lies between the outer longitudinal and inner circular muscle layers, while the submucosal plexus lies in the submucosa (Fig. 14.**5**). There is also a subserosal plexus just under the peritoneum.

Summary   **The Autonomic Nervous System**

The autonomic (= vegetative or visceral) nervous system regulates organ functions the execution of which is not consciously initiated or completed (e. g., functioning of the heart, circulation, or repiration). There are three parts:

- The sympathetic nervous system (thoracolumbar outflow)
- The parasympathetic nervous system (craniosacral outflow)
- The enteric plexus (nervous system of the intestinal wall)

The *sympathetic* and *parasympathetic* nervous systems with few exceptions innervate all organs and are antagonists, i.e., they have opposite effects (e. g., on the heart: sympathetic system raises, parasympathetic lowers heart rate). The enteric plexus functions as an independent system in the whole gastrointestinal tract, but is influenced by the sympathetic and parasympathetic systems.

■ **Outline of the System**
The sympathetic and parasympathetic systems both include efferent and afferent neurons.

- *Efferent:* consist of two neurons in series, the cell bodies of the first efferent neuron are located within the CNS, those of the second efferent neuron in an autonomic ganglion (synaptic relay station).

These neurons are also called preganglionic (first efferent neuron) and postganglionic (second efferent neuron).

● *Afferent:* consist of a neuron the cell body of which lies in the sensory ganglion of the spinal nerve; i.e., there is no relay on the way from the receptor (e. g., in the internal organs) to the central nervous system.

■ Sympathetic Nervous System

Function

The sympathetic nervous system promotes increased performance and predominates during physical and psychological stress by, for example, raising blood pressure, accelerating heart and respiratory rate, dilating the bronchi, increasing perfusion of skeletal muscle, dilating the pupils, erecting hair, increasing sweat secretion, inhibiting intestinal peristalsis, reducing secretion in the intestinal glands, and increasing energy metabolism.

Structure

The cell bodies of the preganglionic efferent neurons lie in the lateral horns of spinal cord segments T1–L4. The axons leave the spinal cord with the anterior root and run through a white communicating branch (ramus commuincans albus) to the ganglia of the bilateral sympathetic chains. Here they synapse with postganglionic efferent fibers. The latter send axons through a gray communicating branch back to the spinal nerve, which they accompany to their effector organ (heart, lung, sweat glands, smooth muscle of skin vessels and hair). The synapses for the salivary glands and the smooth muscle of the head are located in the uppermost ganglion of the sympathetic chain in the neck (superior cervical ganglion). The synapses for the abdominal and pelvic organs are located in the unpaired prevertebral ganglia (abdominal organs—celiac ganglion and superior mesenteric ganglion; pelvic organs—inferior mesenteric ganglion). The adrenal medulla receives direct sympathetic innervation by preganglionic neurons that synapse with the cells of the adrenal medulla (altered postganglionic neurons) and elicit the secretion of the two medullary hormones epinephrine and norepinephrine (elicit sympathetic responses in effector organs by stimulating α- and β-adrenergic receptors) directly into the bloodstream.

Chemical Neurotransmitters

Acetylcholine (sympathetic and prevertebral ganglia) and norepine-phrine (effector organ). Exception: sweat glands (acetylcholine).

■ The Parasympathetic Nervous System

Function

The parasympathetic system regenerates and builds the reserves of the body, e. g., it lowers the blood pressure, slows the heart and respiratory rate, increases intestinal peristalsis and other digestive functions, increases the secretion of saliva, promotes the emptying of the rectum and bladder, and constricts the pupils.

Structure

The cell bodies of the preganglionic efferent neurons lie in the brainstem (cranial parasympathetic system) and in the lateral horns of spinal cord segments S2–S5 (sacral parasympathetic system).

- *Cranial parasympathetic system:* the preganglionic axons leave the brainstem with cranial nerves III, VII, IX, and X and relay in the intracranial autonomic ganglia. Exception: vagal relays (ganglia near the organs in the chest and abdomen). With the exception of the vagus, their postganglionic neurons innervate the intrinsic eye muscles and the glands of the head.
  - *Oculomotor n. (III):* ciliary ganglion (intrinsic eye muscles)
  - *Facial n. (VII):* pterygopalatine ganglion (lacrimal gland, nasal and palatine glands) and submandibular ganglion (sublingual and submandibular glands)
  - *Glossopharyngeal n. (IX):* otic ganglion (parotid gland)
  - *Vagus n. (X):* thoracic ganglia (respiratory tract, heart) and abdominal ganglia (digestive tract).
- *Sacral parasympathetic system:* Preganglionic neurons originate in the lower end of the spinal cord (pelvic splanchnic nerves), and synapse with postganglionic nerves in the ganglia of the hypogastric plexus in the vicinity of the organs. They supply the following organs: descending and sigmoid colon, rectum, bladder, ureter, and genitalia.

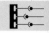

Chemical Neurotransmitter

Acetylcholine (preganglionic and postganglionic).

■ Enteric Plexus (Nervous System of the Intestinal Wall)

Consists of about 10–100 million nerve cells located in the ganglia of the intestinal wall. Their axons are connected in nervous networks (plexuses):

- *Myenteric plexus (Auerbach plexus):* between circular and longitudinal fibers
- *Subserosal plexus:* under the serosal surface
- *Submucosal plexus (Meissner plexus):* submucosa

15
Sense Organs

Contents

■ Receptors and Sensory Cells

Sensation results from the excitation of sensors (receptors) by internal or external stimuli and the ensuing processing of nerve impulses in the peripheral and central nervous systems. *Superficial, deep, and visceral sensation* are respectively subserved by receptors in the skin and mucous membranes (e. g., of the oral and nasal cavities), in the muscles, tendons, and joints, and in the internal organs. These types of sensation are known collectively as *somatovisceral sensation,* in distinction to the special senses: sight, hearing, smell, and taste.

The function of a sensory receptor is to convert (transduce) a physical or chemical stimulus into an electrical excitation (receptor potential). Receptors can be classified according to the type of stimulus that excites them as *mechanoreceptors, thermoreceptors,* and *chemoreceptors,* and according to their sensitivity as low-threshold or high-threshold receptors (i.e., relatively sensitive or relatively insensitive receptors). *Nociceptors* (receptors that subserve pain), for example, are high-threshold receptors responding only to stimuli that cause actual, or threatened, tissue damage.

The neural output of a receptor cell is a measure of the intensity of the corresponding type of stimulus in the area of tissue for which the cell is responsible (its receptive field). The graded receptor potential is translated into nerve impulses (action potentials) of higher or lower frequency, which travel, either *directly* or after *synaptic transmission,* through an afferent nerve fiber toward the central nervous system.

Receptors can be classified according to their structure as follows:

- Primary sensory receptors
- Secondary sensory receptors
- The axon terminals of afferent fibers (as a "free nerve terminal" or as a specialized receptor organ with an encapsulated nerve terminal)

Primary sensory receptors are specialized nerve cells possessing both a receptor process and a neural process (neurite, axon) that transmits impulses toward the central nervous system. Olfactory receptor cells and the rod and cone photoreceptors of the retina are of this type.

Secondary sensory receptors make synaptic contact with the terminal of an afferent nerve fiber. When stimulated, the receptor releases a neurotransmitter that excites an action potential in the afferent fiber. The receptors found in taste buds and in the organs of hearing and equilibrium are of this type.

Sometimes the *axon terminal of the afferent fiber* is itself the site at which the receptor potential originates. This may be a free nerve terminal (by far the commonest type of receptor for somatovisceral sensation) or a specialized receptor organ (e. g., muscle spindles, Golgi tendon organs, Vater–Pacini corpuscles).

■ The Eye

The actual organ of seeing includes the eyeball with the optic nerve and accessories including eyelids, the lacrimal apparatus, and the extraocular (outside the eye) muscles.

The Eyeball (Globe, Bulbus Oculi)

Location of the Globe and Structure of its Wall

The approximately spherical eyeball lies in the bony eye socket (orbit), embedded in fatty tissue. The wall of the eyeball consists of three layers, which have different tasks in the anterior and posterior halves of the globe. They are, starting from the from outside (Fig. 15.**1**):

- The fibrous tunic (tunica fibrosa bulbi), which forms the sclera posteriorly and the cornea and conjunctiva anteriorly.
- The vascular tunic (tunica vasculosa bulbi) or uvea, which forms the choroid in the posterior half of the eyeball and the iris as well as the ciliary body in the anterior half.
- The internal tunic of the eye (tunica interna bulbi), whose posterior half is the retina, composed of a photoreceptor layer (stratum nervosum) and a layer of pigment epithelium (stratum pigmentosum), and whose anterior half is the pigment epithelium of the ciliary body and iris.

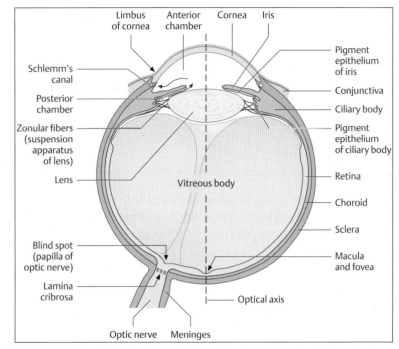

Fig. 15.1 Horizontal section through the eyeball. Different colors indicate the three tunics of the eyeball: internal (yellow), middle (red), and external (green). The egress of fluid from the anterior chamber is marked with red arrows

Anterior Part of the Globe

The anterior part of the globe contains the optical (refractory) apparatus, which projects an image onto the retina and is composed of the following structures:

- The *anterior* and *posterior chambers* of the eye
- The *lens* and *ciliary body*
- The iris with a *central opening (pupil)*
- The *cornea*
- The *vitreous body*

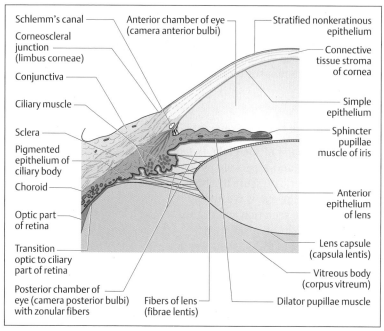

Schlemm's canal — Anterior chamber of eye — Stratified nonkeratinous
(camera anterior bulbi)   epithelium

Corneoscleral   — Connective
junction   tissue stroma
(limbus corneae)   of cornea

Conjunctiva —

Ciliary muscle —   — Simple
                                                                 epithelium

Sclera —   — Sphincter
                                                                 pupillae
Pigmented   muscle of iris
epithelium of —
ciliary body

Choroid —   — Anterior
                                                                 epithelium
                                                                 of lens
Optic part —
of retina

Transition —   — Lens capsule
optic to ciliary   (capsula lentis)
part of retina
                                                              — Vitreous body
Posterior chamber of —   (corpus vitreum)
eye (camera posterior bulbi)   Fibers of lens —   — Dilator pupillae muscle
with zonular fibers   (fibrae lentis)

Fig. 15.**2**   **Horizontal section through the anterior part of the eyeball.** (After Faller)

Anterior and Posterior Chamber of the Eye

The eye can be divided into three spaces (Figs. 15.**1** and 15.**2**): the anterior chamber, the posterior chamber, and the cavity of the eye containing the vitreous body (corpus vitreum). The anterior chamber lies behind the cornea. It is filled with aqueous humor, and extends posteriorly to the pupil and the iris. At the iridocorneal angle lies a meshwork of connective tissue trabeculae. The aqueous humor flows through its spaces to reach a circular vein, the *Schlemm canal (sinus venosus sclerae)*. At the pupil the anterior chamber is connected to the posterior chamber, where the aqueous humor is secreted. The posterior chamber is bounded by the posterior surface of the iris and the ciliary body (ciliary muscle and zonular fibers) together with the anterior part of the vitreous body (vit-reous humor). The vitreous body contains neither vessels nor nerves and is composed of a clear glassy gelatinous substance (98% water) that is essentially composed of collagen and hyaluronic acid (binds water). It stabilizes the bulb and takes up about two-thirds of the total volume of the eyeball.

Intraocular (inside the eye) Pressure

The external shape of the globe is maintained by its connective tissue coat, the sclera, and especially by an internal pressure that is elevated above atmospheric pressure by about 15–20 mmHg (2–3 kPa). The internal pressure of the eye is created by the aqueous humor, and the equilibrium between secretion and drainage of the aqueous humor plays an important role in its maintenance. If, for instance, drainage from Schlemm's canal (see above) is impeded, the internal pressure of the eyeball can rise dangerously (*glaucoma*). The rise in pressure must be treated with medication, since an elevated pressure can reduce perfusion, thereby damaging the retina and leading to blindness.

Lens and the Process of Accommodation

Light falling on the lens is focused because the posterior surface of the lens is more curved than the anterior surface. The lens consists of a nucleus, epithelium, and fibers, and it is completely transparent. It is suspended from the circular *ciliary muscle* (*m. ciliaris*) by a similarly circular arrangement of fibers (zonular fibers) (Figs. 15.**1** and 15.**2**). By changing its shape, the lens can vary its refraction (see below). By this mechanism the eye can bring objects at varying distances into sharp focus (accommodation).

When the ciliary muscle contracts, the zonular fibers relax, because the distance between the muscle and the lens becomes smaller (muscle contraction shortens the muscle and thickens its belly). Hence the zonular fibers no longer pull on the lens, which now becomes increasingly spherical as a result of its own elasticity, i.e., its radius of curvature decreases. Consequently, the incident light rays are more strongly refracted and the eye accommodates to near vision. When the parasympathetically innervated ciliary muscle relaxes, the distance between lens

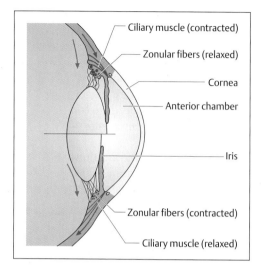

Fig. 15.**3** **Simplified diagram of the process of accommodation**
Upper half: near setting (ciliary muscle is contracted, zonular fibers are relaxed) Lower half: distance setting (ciliary muscle is relaxed, zonular fibers are stretched)

and muscle increases, and the lens is flattened by the pull of the zonular fibers. By this means the eye accommodates to distant vision (Fig. 15.3). These complex relations cn be seen at a glance below:

Ciliary muscle	Zonular fibers	Lens	Refraction	Accommodation
Contracts	Relaxed	Spherical	Increases	Near
Relaxes	Tensed	Flattened	Decreases	Distant

With increasing age, the lens loses its elasticity and hardens (scleroses). This reduces its ability to accommodate and it cannot focus on close objects (presbyopia, see p. 637).

Iris and Pupillary Reflexes

The iris forms a sort of variable aperture (pupil), the opening of which can be constricted or dilated by two smooth muscles (*m. sphincter pupillae* and *m. dilator pupillae*) in the connective tissue of the iris (Fig. 15.2). The contraction of the parasympathetically innervated m. sphincter pupillae leads to *miosis* (*constriction*), while the sympathetically innervated m. dilator pupillae dilates the pupil (*mydriasis*). The width of the pupil is reflexly controlled and depends on the intensity of the light falling on it, among other factors. It varies between 1.5 mm (miosis) and 8 mm (mydriasis). The pupillary light reflex can also be triggered when light does not fall on the eye. If, for instance, the light from a flashlight enters one eye, the pupils of both eyes constrict, the so-called *consensual light reflex.* Failure to trigger this reflex suggests a serious condition in the CNS. Fixing a nearby object also leads to constriction of the pupil (increasing depth of focus) as well as *convergence* of the axes of the two eyes.

The color of the iris depends on the quantity and location of pigments in the connective tissue and the pigment epithelium behind the iris. If the iris is completely devoid of pigment, it appears red, because blood vessels can be seen through it (as in albinos).

Cornea

The cornea, the most anterior portion of the outer coat of the eye, is more strongly curved than the sclera, like a flattened dome inserted into the anterior aspect of the globe (Fig. 15.**2**). It is devoid of blood vessels and receives nutrients by diffusion through the aqueous humor. The outer surface of its connective tissue stroma is covered by a stratified *noncornified* (i.e., the name cornea is misleading) squamous epithelium, while its inner surface is covered by a single epithelial layer. Its transparency rests on a certain fluid content and the degree of swelling of the lamellar collagen fibers of the stroma. If this specific degree of swelling changes, the cornea becomes cloudy.

Posterior Part of the Globe

The posterior part of the globe consists of the sclera, the uvea, and the perceptive parts in the form of the sensory cells of the retina, the processes of which leave the posterior wall as the optic nerve.

Sclera

The opaque sclera is made up of tough bundles of collagen fibers, and its inelastic connective tissue capsule maintains the shape of the eyeball, supported by the internal pressure of the globe and the pull of the extraocular muscles. At the *corneoscleral junction* or *corneal limbus* (Fig. 15.**2**) anteriorly, the sclera blends into the cornea, which represents about one-sixth of the surface of the eyeball. Where the optic nerve leaves the eyeball, the sclera is pierced like a sieve (*lamina cribrosa*) and continues as the dura mater and arachnoid covering the optic nerve (Fig. 15.**1**).

Vascular Tunic (Uvea)

The vascular tunic is 0.2 mm thick and consists of the iris, the ciliary body, and the choroid. It is applied to the inside of the sclera. In front of the corneal limbus it forms the ciliary body which, in contrast to the smooth choroid, is covered with ridges, folds, and processes. Its connective tissue stroma is continued into the iris. The choroid consists of delicate pigmented connective tissue and contains numerous blood vessels (Fig. 15.**5**), which supply nutrition to the adjacent layers, especially the avascular outer layers of the retina.

Retina

The retina is composed of a posterior *light-sensitive segment* (*pars optica retinae*) and an anterior *light-insensitive part* (*pars ciliaris* and *pars iridica*). The boundary between the two parts of the retina is a serrated line (*ora serrata*) at the posterior border of the ciliary body. The pars ciliaris and the pars iridica are simple epithelia covering the ciliary body and the posterior surface of the iris respectively. Where it covers the iris, the epithelium is densely pigmented.

The optical part of the retina coats the entire posterior area of the globe and consists of two layers, an outer pigmented epithelium (*pars pigmentosa*) and an inner light-sensitive layer (*pars nervosa*). The simple pigmented epithelium directly adjoins the choroid and contains elongated brown pigment granules. With cellular processes of varying shapes, the pigmented layer extends to the photoreceptors of the nervous layer. Its main function is the nutrition of the photoreceptors.

The light-sensitive part of the retina contains three layers of neurons of the visual pathway. These layers, from outside inward, contain (Figs. 15.**4** and 15.**5**):

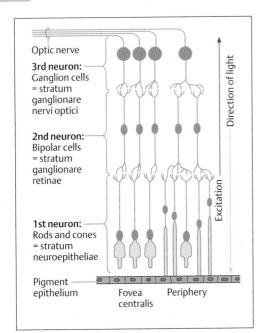

Optic nerve

3rd neuron: Ganglion cells = stratum ganglionare nervi optici

2nd neuron: Bipolar cells = stratum ganglionare retinae

1st neuron: Rods and cones = stratum neuroepitheliae

Pigment epithelium

Fovea centralis

Periphery

Direction of light

Excitation

Fig. 15.**4** **Neuronal connections in the retina.** In the region of the fovea centralis of the macula lutea, the only sensory cells are cones; outside the fovea centralis (periphery), they include rods. Note the direction of the light. (After Duus)

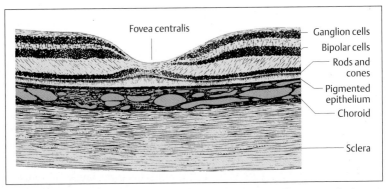

Fovea centralis

Ganglion cells

Bipolar cells

Rods and cones

Pigmented epithelium

Choroid

Sclera

Fig. 15.**5** **Longitudinal section through the macula lutea (yellow spot) of a human eye.** In the fovea centralis the light impinges directly on the cones

- The first neurons, i.e., photoreceptors (rods and cones; stratum neuroepitheliale retinae)
- The second neurons, i.e., bipolar retinal ganglion cells (ganglionic layer of retina, stratum ganglionicum retinae)
- The third neurons, i.e., the ganglion cells of the optic nerve (stratum ganglionare nervi optici)

The retina is divided by anatomists into 10 layers, though the borders between adjacent layers are admittedly somewhat indistinct. The pattern of layers is produced by the various components of the types of neurons listed above lying at characteristic depths within the retina.

Rods and Cones

The light-sensitive photoreceptors, the rods and cones, lie in the outermost layer overlying the pigmented layer, and are covered by the nerve cells of the two inner layers. Hence, the light-sensitive cells are turned away from the incident light, i.e., the light must first penetrate the inner layers of the retina before reaching the rods and cones. Hence the eye is sometimes called "inverted."

The light-sensitive sensory cells consist of about 120 million rods (light and dark sensitive, as well as vision in dim light) and about 6 million cones (color vision). They synapse with relay cells (bipolar retinal ganglion cells, 2nd neuron), the axons of which end in synapses on the ganglion cells of the optic nerve (3rd neuron) (Fig. 15.**5**). There are considerably fewer retinal and optic nerve ganglion cells than sensory cells. The result is that the impulses from several sensory cells are conducted to only one retinal or optic ganglion cell (*convergence of impulse conduction*).

Optic Disk (Discus Nervi Optici)

Finally, the central axons of the optic ganglion cells reach a point in the posterior pole of the eyeball where they collect (optic disk, papilla nervi optici, discus nervi optici) and leave the eye through a sievelike interruption in the sclera (lamina cribrosa). They then continue as the optic nerve (n. opticus) to the diencephalon. The disk is devoid of sensory cells (blind spot). The vessels of the optic nerve (central artery of the retina) enter here (Fig. 15.**6**).

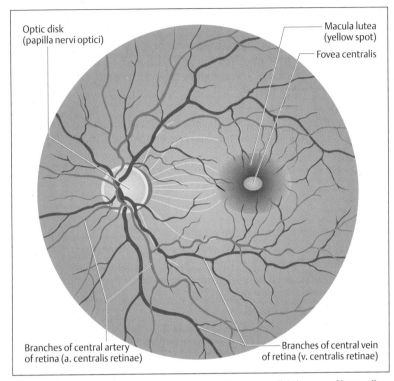

Optic disk
(papilla nervi optici)

Macula lutea
(yellow spot)

Fovea centralis

Branches of central artery
of retina (a. centralis retinae)

Branches of central vein
of retina (v. centralis retinae)

Fig. 15.**6** **Normal fundus of a left eye.** At the optic disk (papilla) the nerve fibers collect to become the optic nerve and the central artery of the retina enters

Macula Lutea (Yellow Spot)

The retina is almost devoid of blood vessels in the macula lutea, a depression lying about 4 mm lateral to the optic disk (Figs. 15.**5** and 15.**6**). It contains a depression (*fovea centralis*) in which only cones are found. The remaining retinal layers are pushed aside at this point, so that light falling on it reaches the sensory cells directly. The macula and fovea are therefore the points where vision is most acute.

Eye Ground (Fundus)

The red- to orange-colored fundus can be viewed directly with an oph-thalmoscope (Fig. 15.**6**). The optic disk, where all the nerve fibers con-verge to leave the eye, lies in the nasal half. The *central retinal artery* ent-ers in the middle of the disk and divides into several branches, of which some run toward the macula. The somewhat darker and wider veins join in a central retinal vein and also leave the retina through the papilla. Ophthalmoscopic examination allows an examiner to view the vessels and to determine retinal changes.

The Optic System

The optical (dioptric) apparatus projects an inverted, markedly reduced image of the world on the retina. *Visible light* entering the eye is com-posed of wavelengths between 400 and 700 nm (1 nm = one billionth of a meter = 10^{-9} m). These waves induce a photochemical excitation in the sensory cells, which the visual pathways conduct to the visual cortex of the cerebrum (see The Visual Pathway below).

Power of Refraction

The image on the retina is formed by the refraction of light rays by the curved surfaces (e. g., cornea, lens). For sharp vision, all the rays coming from a specific point on an object must reunite in a point on the retina. Thus the optic system of the eye functions as a focusing lens. The more curved the lens (i.e., the more convex) the more strongly the rays are re-fracted (refraction increases) and the shorter their focal length. When looking at close objects (positive accommodation), refraction must be increased; when viewing distant objects (negative accommodation), it must be reduced, and the lens flattens.

The measure of the refractive power of the optic system of the eye is the *diopter* (D). Refractive power is calculated as follows:

■ Refractive power (D) = 1/focal length (m)

For a human eye with maximal negative accommodation (lens flat-tened), the whole optical system has an anterior focal length of 0.017 m

(17 mm); the total power of refraction is therefore 1/0.017 = 59 D. For an eye with maximal positive accommodation (lens curved), the power of refraction increases by about 10 D. This increase in power of refraction is also known as the power of accommodation. Because the lens becomes less and less elastic with increasing age (the ability to relax is lost), the power of accommodation decreases, leading to presbyopia (old sightedness). Here the ability to see distant objects is unimpeded, but for close viewing (e.g., reading) glasses with convex lenses are necessary.

Cloudiness of the lens (cataract), a condition most often encountered in the elderly but which may occur at any age, can be treated by surgical removal of the lens if necessary. The loss in refractory power of the lens must be replaced either by the use of strong convex glasses (cataract lens) or by replacing the lens that has been removed with a plastic lens.

Errors of Refraction

Apart from the refractive error of old age (presbyopia), congenital malformations of the globe can cause visual defects. The anterior surface of the cornea is normally exactly 24.4 mm distant from the retina. A distance that is too short or too long results in an error of refraction. If the eyeball is too long the result is *nearsightedness* (*myopia*); when the distance is too short the result is *farsightedness* (*hyperopia*) (Fig. 15.**7a**, **b**).

Nearsightedness

In cases of nearsightedness, light rays originating at infinity come together before reaching the retina and then diverge again. Thus the refractive power of the eye is too great relative to the length of the eye, and the image projected on the retina will be blurred. Hence myopic people, having eyeballs that are too long, can only focus on nearby objects. In order to be able to focus on distant objects, they must wear glasses with concave lenses (diverging lenses) (Fig. 15.**7b**).

Farsightedness

Because the eyeball is too short in cases of farsightedness, light rays originating at infinity would converge behind the retina. In order to see

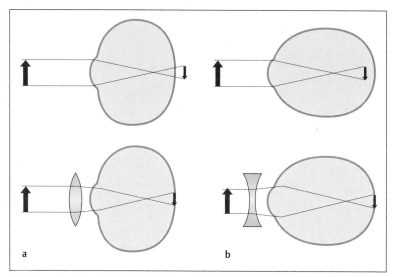

Fig. 15.**7 a, b   Farsightedness (hyperopia) and nearsightedness (myopia).**
a When the globe is too short (farsightedness): correction by convex lens (+ diopters)
b When the globe is too long (nearsightedness) correction by concave lens (− diopters)

distant objects clearly in spite of this, hyperopic persons must constantly accommodate, i.e., increase the power of refraction. In this way, farsighted people can bring distant objects into focus even though their eyeball is too short. However, their power of refraction is not sufficient to see close objects, and they need correction with a convex lens (converging lens) (Fig. 15.**7a**). This is also required for distant vision, in order not to tire the eye by constant contraction of the ciliary muscle (producing headaches).

Astigmatism

In astigmatism an irregular curvature of the cornea results in a point being projected not as a point but as a line. This error is corrected by cylindrical glasses that are curved in the appropriate direction.

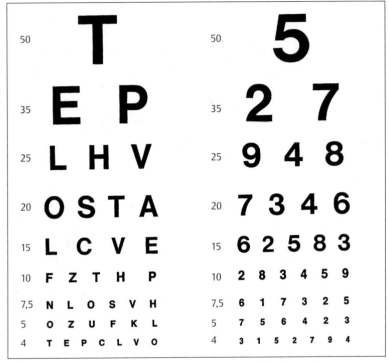

Fig. 15.8 Eye charts. If the chart is placed at a distance of 20 feet, the person tested should be able to read the lowest line prescribed for that distance. Vision is then said to be 20/20. If the line read is that which would normally be legible at 40 feet, vision would be 20/40

Visual Acuity

The ability of the eye to distinguish between two points at a certain distance is called resolution or visual acuity. Visual acuity is tested with special test charts that are usually read at a distance of 20 feet (Fig. 15.**8**). In good lighting conditions, the normal eye should be able to see two points separated by 1.5 mm as distinct points.

The Visual Pathway

Each eye has a *lateral* (*temporal*) and *medial* (*nasal*) *visual field*. The incident light from the temporal field falls on the nasal part of the retina, and the nasal visual field is projected on the temporal part of the retina (Fig. 15.**9**).

The visual pathway begins at the retina and ends in the *visual cortex* in the *calcarine fissure* of the occipital lobe. It comprises *four successive neurons*, the cell bodies of the first three of these being located in the retina (Fig. 15.**4**).

- The photoreceptors (1st neuron)
- The retinal ganglion cells (2nd neuron)
- The ganglion cells of the optic nerve (3rd neuron), the axons of which run posteriorly in the optic nerve

At the *crossing of the optic nerves* (*optic chiasma*) below the diencephalon, the axons of the nasal halves of the retina cross to join the uncrossed axons of the temporal halves of the retina. Together they continue backward as the *optic tract* and end in the *lateral geniculate body* of the diencephalon. There they synapse with the 4th neurons, the axons of which form the optic radiations, ending in the visual cortex (Fig. 15.**9**).

Thus the left visual field of each eye is represented in the cortex of the right hemisphere, while the right visual fields are projected to the visual cortex of the left hemisphere. The area with greatest visual acuity, the macula lutea with the fovea centralis, is projected to by far the largest area in the visual cortex.

Visual Field Defects

During the examination of the eye, the visual fields of both eyes are tested and recorded. If, for instance, the left optic nerve is injured (example **a** in Fig. 15.**9**), both visual fields in that eye are affected, resulting in *blindness* (*amaurosis*) in the left eye. If, on the other hand, a pituitary tumor presses on the nasal axons of the two optic nerves where they cross in the chiasma (example **b** in Fig. 15.**9**), this leads to blindness in the temporal visual fields of both eyes (*bitemporal hemianopsia*). An injury to the left optic tract (example **c** in Fig. 15.**9**) leads to a defect of the right visual field, known as *right homonymous hemianopia* (blindness in

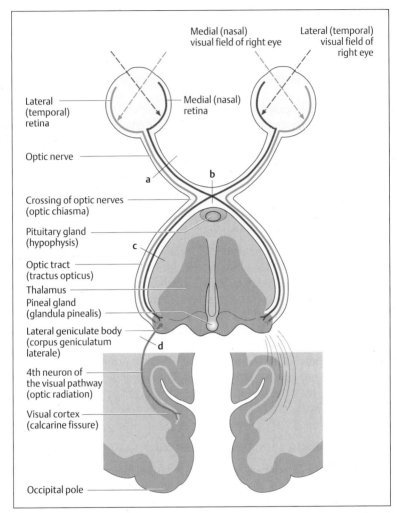

Fig. 15.**9 The visual pathway.** The medial (nasal) visual field is projected to the lateral (temporal) half of the retina. The lateral (temporal) visual field is projected to the medial (nasal) half of the retina. Fibers of the optic nerve from the temporal retina (green) do not cross. Fibers from the medial half of the retina (pink) cross to the opposite side. For description of defects following lesions of the optic nerve (**a**), inside the crossing of the optic fibers (**b**), the optic tract (**c**), and the 4th neuron in the optic radiation (**d**), see Visual Field Defects in the text

the temporal visual field of the right eye and the nasal visual field of the left eye). A similar visual disturbance can be due to injury to e. g., the left optic radiation (example **d** in Fig. 15.**9**).

Accessory Structures

Eyelids (Palpebrae)

In front, the cover of the eyelids protects the eyeball (Fig. 15.**10**). The *upper* and *lower lids* bound the *palpebral fissure*, and each is made more rigid by a *connective tissue plate* (*tarsal plate, tarsus*). Sebaceous glands embedded in the margin of the lid grease this margin, from which grow several rows of *eyelashes*. The outer part of the lid is covered by keratinous stratified squamous epithelium, while the inner side is lined by the *conjunctiva*. This consists of a stratified squamous epithelium, which is reflected from the sclera at the upper and lower conjunctival fornix (fold).

The most important muscles of the eyelids are the *m. levator palpebrae superioris*, supplied by the oculomotor nerve (cranial III), and the *m. orbicularis oculi*, supplied by the facial nerve (cranial VII), which closes the palpebral fissure. Both muscles are voluntary muscles.

Lacrimal Apparatus

The lacrimal apparatus includes the *lacrimal gland* (*glandula lacrimalis*), and the pathways by which the tears drain. The lacrimal glands lies laterally and above the eyeball (Fig. 15.**10**), and drain through several ducts into the outer part of the fornix. The lacrimal fluid constantly moistens the anterior surface of the globe and cleans and nourishes the cornea. It is distributed evenly by blinking and accumulates in the inner canthus (angle) of the eye.

The pathways by which the tears drain begin with the lacrimal punctum (punctum lacrimale), from which the lacrimal fluid drains through the lacrimal canal (canaliculus lacrimalis) into the lacrimal sac (Fig. 5.**10**). From there the tears drain through the lacrimonasal duct (ductus nasolacrimalis) into the inferior nasal meatus of the nasal cavity.

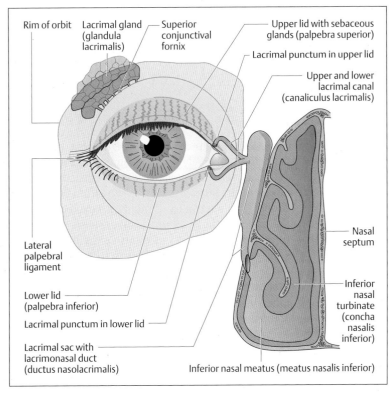

Rim of orbit — Lacrimal gland (glandula lacrimalis) — Superior conjunctival fornix — Upper lid with sebaceous glands (palpebra superior)

Lacrimal punctum in upper lid

Upper and lower lacrimal canal (canaliculus lacrimalis)

Nasal septum

Inferior nasal turbinate (concha nasalis inferior)

Lateral palpebral ligament

Lower lid (palpebra inferior)

Lacrimal punctum in lower lid

Lacrimal sac with lacrimonasal duct (ductus nasolacrimalis)

Inferior nasal meatus (meatus nasalis inferior)

Fig. 15.**10**   **The lacrimal apparatus**

Extraocular Muscles

The eyeball lies in the fatty tissue of the orbit, in the space of which it can be moved in all directions by six striated extraocular muscles (Figs. 15.**11** and 15.**12a**, **b**). The eye movements are functionally coordinated (*conjugate eye movements*). The muscles include four rectus muscles (*superior, inferior, medial* and *lateral rectus muscles*) and two oblique muscles (*superior* and *inferior oblique muscles*), supplied by cranial nerves III, IV, and VI (see p. 589).

The recti originate from a tendinous ring (anulus tendineus) in the region of the optic canal (canalis opticus) and run to the inner and outer

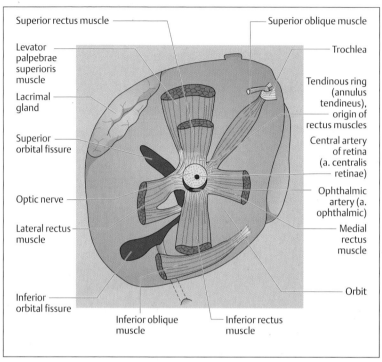

Fig. 15.**11   Origin of the extraocular muscles.** Posterior wall of the orbit viewed from in front. (After Faller)

side, as well as the upper and lower side, of the eyeball, where their tendons are inserted into the sclera near the cornea. Because of their course they can raise or lower the eyeball around a horizontal axis, and turn it inward or outward around a vertical axis.

The superior oblique muscle also arises from the tendinous ring and runs along the inner wall of the orbit obliquely forward. Near the rim of the orbit it passes through a *connective tissue sling* (*trochlea*) (Figs. 15.**11** and 15.**12a**, **b**), is reflected backward at an acute angle, and is inserted below the tendon of the superior rectus muscle. The inferior oblique muscle arises from the lower orbital rim and runs to the outer side of the eyeball. Both muscles move the globe around a sagittal axis.

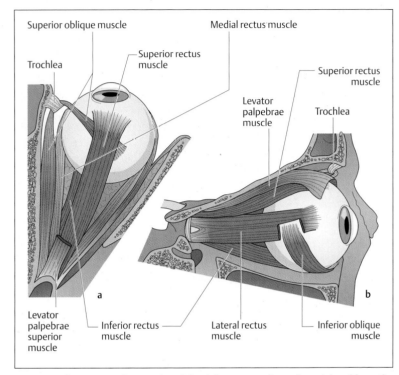

Fig. 15.**12 a**, **b** **Extraocular muscles of the right eye seen from above (a) and from the side (b).** In **a** the anterior portion of the levator palpebrae superioris muscle has been removed. (After Kahle)

■ The Ear

The ear contains two sensory organs with different functions (organs of *hearing* and of *equilibrium*) that nevertheless form an anatomical unit, the *inner ear*. It lies in the petrous pyramid of the temporal bone and consists of the *cochlea* and the vestibular apparatus (labyrinth), the latter including two fluid-filled *pouches* (*utricle* and *saccule*) and three *semicircular canals*, also fluid-filled. The organ of hearing, in contrast to the vestibular apparatus, has accessory structures to conduct sound waves: the *external ear* and the *middle ear*.

The Organ of Hearing

External Ear

The external ear includes the *auricle* or *pinna* (*auricula*), the *external auditory meatus* (*meatus acusticus externus*), about 3 cm long, and the eardrum (*membrana tympani*). The pinna consists mainly of elastic cartilage, which continues into the outer end of the external auditory meatus. This then continues as the bony part of the external auditory canal, which is somewhat S-shaped. The cartilaginous part contains numerous *ceruminous glands* that secrete the "*earwax*" (*cerumen*). The eardrum stretches across the inner end of the bony canal and forms the boundary of the middle ear.

Middle Ear

The middle ear (Fig. 15.**13a**, **b**) includes the *tympanic cavity*, lined with mucous membrane and containing the *auditory ossicles* (*ossicula auditus*) (*malleus*, *incus* and *stapes*); its continuation anteriorly into the pharynx, the *eustachian tube* (*tuba auditiva*); as well as numerous mucosa-lined cavities in the mastoid process. The eardrum is nearly circular with a diameter of about 1 cm and forms the outer wall of the tympanic cavity. It is made up of three layers. The mainly tense connective tissue framework of the eardrum (*membrana tensa, pars tensa*) is weaker in only a small section at its upper end (*membrana flaccida, pars flaccida*) (Fig. 15.**14**). Its inner surface is lined with a mucous membrane, its outer surface with skin. The long handle of the malleus is fastened to the tympanum, bulging it inward like a funnel (Fig. 15.**15**).

The auditory ossicles, together with the tympanum, form the sound-conducting apparatus. *Malleus* (*hammer*), *incus* (*anvil*), and *stapes* (*stirrup*) form a jointed chain between the eardrum and the *oval window* (*fenestra vestibuli*), into which the footplate of the stapes is inserted. The auditory ossicles conduct vibrations elicited by sound waves in the eardrum through the oval window to the inner ear. The latter, together with the first turn of the cochlea, forms the inner bony boundary of the tympanic cavity (promontory). The plate of the stapes in the oval window transmits the vibrations to the fluid of the inner ear. The malleus and stapes are also stabilized by two muscles, the m. tensor tympani, and the m. stapedius. Both can influence sensitivity to the transmission.

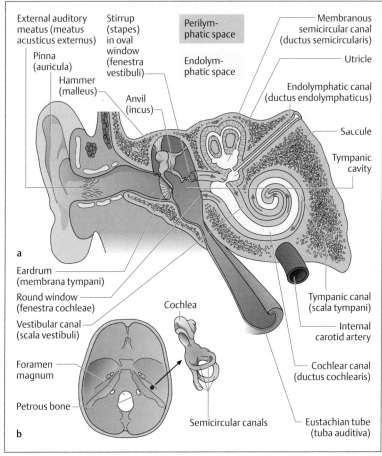

External auditory meatus (meatus acusticus externus)

Pinna (auricula)

Hammer (malleus)

Anvil (incus)

Stirrup (stapes) in oval window (fenestra vestibuli)

Perilym-phatic space

Endolym-phatic space

Membranous semicircular canal (ductus semicircularis)

Utricle

Endolymphatic canal (ductus endolymphaticus)

Saccule

Tympanic cavity

a

Eardrum (membrana tympani)

Round window (fenestra cochleae)

Vestibular canal (scala vestibuli)

Foramen magnum

Petrous bone

Cochlea

Semicircular canals

Tympanic canal (scala tympani)

Internal carotid artery

Cochlear canal (ductus cochlearis)

Eustachian tube (tuba auditiva)

b

Fig. 15.**13 a, b Diagrammatic view of the external ear, the middle ear, and the inner ear** (coronal section). (After Kahle)
a External ear (to the eardrum), middle ear (auditory ossicles and eustachian tube), and inner ear (labyrinth and cochlea)
b Position of the inner ear in the skull (base of skull seen from above), with a cast of the organs of hearing and equilibrium

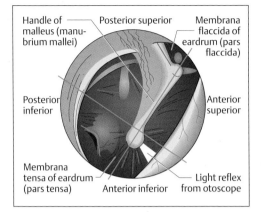

Fig. 15.**14 The right eardrum seen from outside**.
The posterior superior,
posterior inferior, anterior
superior, and anterior inferior quadrants have been
drawn over the mirror
image of the ear; ca. 4×
magnification

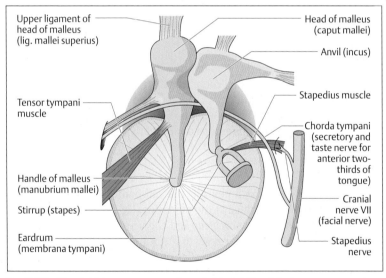

Fig. 15.**15 The right tympanum seen from behind.** (After Faller)

Inner Ear

The inner ear (Fig. 15.**13**) is surrounded by a hard bony capsule, and consists of a fluid-filled (*perilymph*) labyrinthine system of passages and cavities (*bony labyrinth*). The membranous labyrinth, also fluid-filled (*endolymph*), lies inside the bony labyrinth. Perilymph and endolymph differ chiefly in their sodium and potassium contents. The membranous labyrinth contains the organs of hearing and equilibrium.

The *bony spiral* (*cochlea*) of the inner ear, about 3 cm long, makes up a passage that in humans winds about $2^1/2$ times around a bony axis, the *central pillar* or *columella* (*modiolus*). A cross-section of the cochlea (Fig. 15.**16** and 15.**17**) shows three separate cavities: *the cochlear canal* (*ductus cochlearis*) in the middle, the *vestibular canal* (*scala vestibuli*) above it, and the *tympanic canal* (*scala tympani*) below. The scala tympani and the scala vestibuli join at the apex of the cochlea (helicotrema). They are filled with perilymph and end at the round window (fenestra cochleae) and the oval window (fenestra vestibuli), respectively (Fig. 15.**13a**).

The cochlear duct is filled with endolymph and abuts the scala tympani by the *basilar lamina* (*lamina basilaris*), and the scala vestibuli by *Reissner's membrane* (*paries vestibularis*). The *organ of Corti* (*spiral organ*) (Fig. 15.**17**) rests on the basilar membrane. It contains some 15 000 auditory sensory cells arranged in rows (inner and outer hair cells) as well as numerous support cells. The sensory hairs of the hair cells are connected to a *gelatinous layer* (*membrana tectoria*) overlying it.

Auditory Pathway

The hair cells synapse with neurons the cell bodies of which lie in the spiral ganglion of the cochlea at the modiolus (Fig. 15.**17**). From here the central axons run with the *cochlear* and the *vestibular nerves* in cranial nerve VIII (vestibulocochlear nerve) to the brainstem. There the axons of the cochlear nerve end in the nuclei of the cochlear nerve (nucleus cochlearis), while those of the vestibular nerve terminate in the vestibular nuclei. On the way to the auditory area in the anterior transverse gyrus of the temporal lobe, the auditory pathway synapses several times, including synapses in the medial geniculate body of the diencephalon.

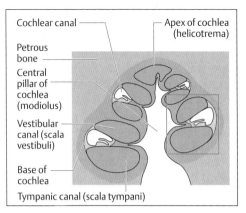

Cochlear canal

Apex of cochlea (helicotrema)

Petrous bone

Central pillar of cochlea (modiolus)

Vestibular canal (scala vestibuli)

Base of cochlea

Tympanic canal (scala tympani)

Fig. 15.**16 Cross-section through a human cochlea.** Apex of the cochlea (helicotrema) with transit from the vestibular canal (scala vestibuli) to the tympanic canal (scala tympani). (Blue box indicates section for Fig. 15.**17**)

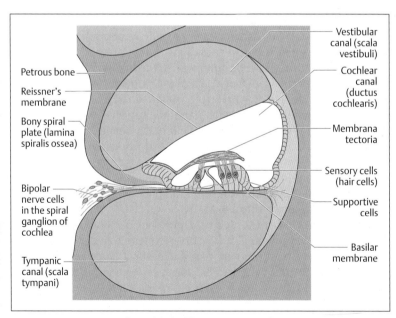

Petrous bone

Reissner's membrane

Bony spiral plate (lamina spiralis ossea)

Bipolar nerve cells in the spiral ganglion of cochlea

Tympanic canal (scala tympani)

Vestibular canal (scala vestibuli)

Cochlear canal (ductus cochlearis)

Membrana tectoria

Sensory cells (hair cells)

Supportive cells

Basilar membrane

Fig. 15.**17 Cross-section through a cochlear turn.** Section from Fig. 15.**16.** Purple: perilymph. White: endolymph

Mechanism of Hearing

Vibrations (sound waves) impinging on the oval window, after transmission by the eardrum and the auditory ossicles, create pressure waves in the perilymph of the vestibular canal. These pressure waves continue to the apex of the cochlea and then return through the tympanic canal (Fig. 15.**13a**). The opposing flows of the perilymph in the vestibular and tympanic canals create vibrations in the endolymph of the cochlear duct, and this excites the sensory cells by moving the sensory hairs in the membrana tectoria (Fig. 15.**17**). Since the basilar membrane is narrow at the base of the cochlea, and broader at its apex, the frequency of the pressure waves decreases toward the apex. By this mechanism, high-pitched tones are heard at the base of the cochlea, low-pitched tones at the apex.

Pure tones or musical notes are produced by regularly recurring (periodic) vibratory processes of a defined frequency and intensity, while noises are characterized by nonperiodic (irregular) auditory events. In general it can be said that sound waves with frequencies between 20 and 16 000 hertz (1 Hz = one vibration per second) excite the hair cells in the inner ear and so elicit sound sensations (tones, notes, or noises). The higher the frequency of the sound waves, the higher pitched the tone that is experienced (see above). Frequencies below 20 Hz (infrasonic frequencies) and above 16 000 Hz (ultrasound) do not elicit excitations in the human inner ear. On the other hand, auditory events must exceed a certain intensity (minimal pressure) before they can be heard. The auditory threshold, that is the sound pressure that just elicits sound perception, for a tone with a frequency of 1000 Hz would be about (2×10^{-5} Newton/m^2 (N/m^2 = Pascal). The ear is most sensitive in a range between 2000 and 5000 Hz, where even very low sound pressures are sufficient to exceed the auditory threshold.

The *reference power level* has been introduced to obtain an objective measure of sound pressure. It is usually expressed in *decibels (dB)*. By convention, the sound pressure that just elicits a perceived sound has been pegged at 0 dB. Every tenfold increase in sound pressure corresponds to an increase in the reference power level of 20 decibels.

Hearing Problems

Hearing problems are a widely distributed phenomenon affecting millions of people. In general they may be divided into two kinds. The first is *middle ear* or *conduction deafness*, in which there is a mechanical impediment to the tone reaching the cochlea. This impediment may, for example, be a torn drum or blockage of the auditory meatus by earwax. The commonest cause of conduction deafness, however, is otosclerosis, in which the stapes in the middle ear is ankylosed (fixed) and so cannot transmit vibrations. The second type of hearing problem is *inner ear deafness,* caused, for example, by lesions of the cochlea or the auditory nerve. An infection with German measles during the first four months of pregnancy can often lead to the birth of a completely deaf infant.

The Organ of Equilibrium

The organ of equilibrium (*vestibular organ*) includes three semicircular ducts with their dilatations (*ampullae*), in which lie the acoustic crests (*cristae ampullares*) with their sensory cells, and the *utricle* and *saccule*, each with a *sensory area* (*macula utriculi* and *macula sacculi*). They are filled with endolymph and form the membranous labyrinth (Figs. 15.**13** and 15.**18**). They register *acceleration* and *changes in position*, and so determine spatial orientation. Specialized sensory cells project into the endolymph, and these react to fluid movements, which they sense. The endolymph moves with shifts in posture or changes in position of the head. The sensory cells so stimulated send information to the cerebellum, which responds reflexly to the changes.

Macula of Utricle and Saccule

The two sensory areas of the larger and smaller vestibular pouches register primarily straight-line accelerations, especially when they are horizontal (e. g., the braking of an automobile) or vertical (e. g., traveling in an elevator).

The epithelium lining the saccule and utricle is thickened in certain areas, where it is differentiated into special sensory and support cells. These sensory areas (maculae) are covered with a gelatinous substance

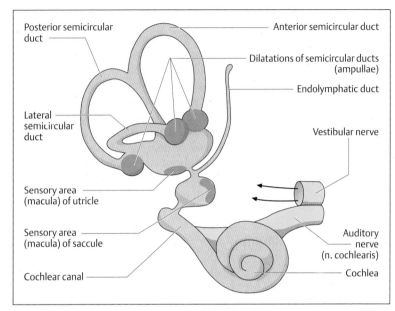

Posterior semicircular duct

Anterior semicircular duct

Dilatations of semicircular ducts (ampullae)

Endolymphatic duct

Lateral semicircular duct

Vestibular nerve

Sensory area (macula) of utricle

Sensory area (macula) of saccule

Auditory nerve (n. cochlearis)

Cochlear canal

Cochlea

Fig. 15.**18** **Right membranous labyrinth**

(*membrana statoconiorum macularum*), which is weighted down by tiny calciferous granules (otoliths, statoconia, otoconia). From below, processes of the sensory cells, the sensory hairs or cilia, project into the gelatinous membrane (Fig. 15.**19**). When the sensory epithelium and the statoconic membrane move against each other, the shear force displaces the cilia. Since the macula in the floor of the utricle is oriented almost horizontally, its sensory cells are stimulated mainly by *horizontal acceleration*. On the other hand, the macula of the saccule is oriented nearly vertically on the anterior wall of the saccule and so responds mainly to vertical acceleration.

Acoustic Crest (Crista Ampularis)

The *acoustic crests* (*cristae ampullares*) in the dilatations (*ampullae*) of the semicircular ducts register especially rotary acceleration moving the endolymph. They lie in the three principal spatial planes and are essentially connected to reflex eye movements.

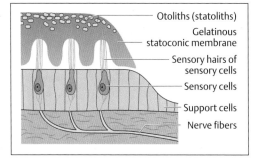

Fig. 15.**19** **Simplified representation of a sensory area (macula)**

- Otoliths (statoliths)
- Gelatinous statoconic membrane
- Sensory hairs of sensory cells
- Sensory cells
- Support cells
- Nerve fibers

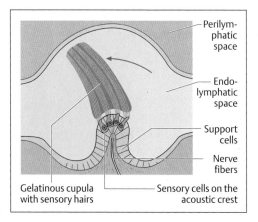

Fig. 15.**20** **Simplified representation of a semicircular canal.** The gelatinous cupula is distorted by movements of the endolymph in the endolymphatic space (arrow)

- Perilymphatic space
- Endolymphatic space
- Support cells
- Nerve fibers

Gelatinous cupula with sensory hairs — Sensory cells on the acoustic crest

Each semicircular duct contains an acoustic crest (crista ampullaris), which contains sensory and support cells. The sensory cells send sensory hairs into a gelatinous *cap* (*cupula*) that caps each acoustic crest (Fig. 15.**20**). If the cupula with its sensory hairs is displaced, the sensory cells are excited.

The peripheral axons of the vestibular nerve synapse with the sensory cells of the maculae and crests. Their cell bodies lie in the *vestibular ganglion* in the internal auditory meatus. The central axons run toward the brainstem, join with the neurons of the cochlear nerve, and form cranial nerve VIII (vestibulocochlear nerve). They terminate in four vestibular nuclei from which connections run principally to the cerebellum, the nuclei of the extraocular muscles, and the spinal cord.

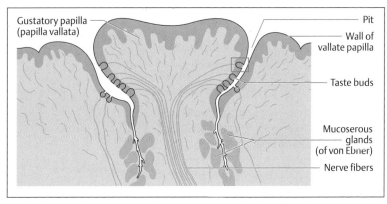

Fig. 15.**21** **Longitudinal section through a taste papilla (papilla vallata).** For the indicated section see Fig. 15.**22**

■ The Sense of Taste

The sensory cells for the perception of various tastes lie together with support cells in the taste buds, which are arranged in the taste papillae of the tongue (see Chapter 9: The Oral Cavity, The Tongue). The taste buds are shaped like tulip buds and lie in the stratified squamous epithelium of the tongue (Figs. 15.**21** and 15.**22**). On the epithelial surface they are provided with a depressed pit with an opening, the *taste pore*, into which the sensory cells project with *taste hairs*. Each taste bud is supplied with several nerve fibers, which connect to fibers supplying other taste buds. The anterior two-thirds of the tongue are supplied by neurons of the facial nerve (cranial nerve VII) whose fibers travel in the chorda tympani), the posterior part by sensory neurons from the glossopharyngeal nerve (cranial nerve IX). The four taste sensations (*sweet, sour, salty*, and *bitter*) are perceived in different areas of the tongue and probably registered by different receptors in individual taste buds. Sour is perceived especially at the lateral border of the tongue, salty at the borders and the tip of the tongue, bitter at the base of the tongue, and sweet especially at the tip of the tongue (see Fig. 9.**5**). The grooves adjacent to the taste papillae contain mucoserous glands (of von Ebner) (Fig. 15.**21**) that secrete a watery fluid thought to have a "rinsing" function.

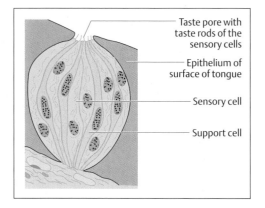

Taste pore with taste rods of the sensory cells

Epithelium of surface of tongue

Sensory cell

Support cell

Fig. 15.**22 Longitudinal section through a taste bud.** Section from Fig. 15.**21**

■ The Sense of Smell

The human olfactory mucous membrane encompasses an area of about 500 mm² in the superior nasal turbinate and on each side of the upper nasal septum (*regio olfactoria*, see Fig. 8.**1**). It can be distinguished from the remaining nasal mucosa (regio respiratoria) by an epithelium that is distinctly higher, containing mostly basal cells (proliferative cells), supportive (sustentacular) cells, and sensory cells (Fig. 15.**23**). In humans there are about 10 million sensory cells (olfactory cells). These bipolar nerve cells (fila olfactoria) are the 1st neurons of the olfactory pathway. At their upper end (dendrite) they project a small knob, the olfactory rod, with numerous olfactory hairs. Their axons pass into the anterior cranial fossa through a bony plate, which is perforated like a sieve (cribroid plate of the ethmoid bone, lamina cribrosa) (Fig. 4.**55,** p. 192). They synapse with the nerve cells (2nd neurons) of the olfactory bulb, an enlargement of the olfactory nerve. The olfactory nerve runs to the olfactory cortex, where the corresponding perceptions are generated.

Under the olfactory mucosa lie numerous mucous glands (Bowman's glands), the ducts of which end on the surface of the epithelium and the secretions of which dissolve and remove olfactory substances.

Sense Organs

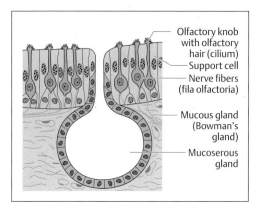

Fig. 15.**23 Longitudinal section through the olfactory mucosa**

Olfactory knob with olfactory hair (cilium)
Support cell
Nerve fibers (fila olfactoria)
Mucous gland (Bowman's gland)
Mucoserous gland

Summary **Sense Organs**

The classic sense organs are the eye, the ear, the nose, and the organs of touch and taste. In addition, there are numerous specialized receptors, e. g., in the skin (pain and temperature receptors) and in the internal organs (chemoreceptors and osmoreceptors). With the aid of sensory cells and receptors, they receive objective sense impressions from the environment or from within the body and conduct them to the central nervous system, where the incoming impulses are processed. Eventually this leads to a subjective perception of the sensory stimulus. Sensory cells may be primary (altered nerve cells) or secondary (epithelial cells altered to include a receptor function).

■ **The Eye**

The organ of sight includes the eyeball (bulbus oculi) and the optic nerve, as well as the accessory structures (eyelids, lacrimal apparatus, extraocular muscles).

Location and Structure of the Wall of the Globe

The globe is embedded in fatty tissue in the bony orbit. Its wall consists of three layers, each with different tasks in the anterior and posterior halves of the globe:

- *Outer coat:* sclera (posteriorly) and cornea (anteriorly)
- *Middle coat:* choroid (posteriorly) and iris and ciliary body (anteriorly)
- *Inner coat:* retina (posteriorly) and pigmented epithelium of the ciliary body (anteriorly).

Anterior Part of the Globe

The anterior part of the globe contains the optical apparatus and is made up of the following structures:

- *Anterior and posterior chambers of the eye:* contain the aqueous humor, which is secreted in the posterior chamber and reaches the anterior chamber by the opening in the iris (pupil). It drains through Schlemm's canal in the iridocorneal angle. The aqueous humor generates the intraocular pressure (15–20 mmHg = 2–3 kPa). A rising intraocular pressure leads to glaucoma, with danger of retinal damage.
- *Cornea:* bounds the anterior chamber of the eye. Consists of an avascular, transparent, stratified nonkeratinous (!) epithelium.
- *Vitreous body:* Consists of a clear, glassy, gelatinous substance (collagen and hyaluronic acid).
- *Lens:* consists of nucleus, epithelium, and fibers and is completely transparent (clouding of the lens = cataract). The perfectly round lens is attached along its entire circumference to the ciliary muscle by the zonular (zonula = belt) fibers (zonular fibers + ciliary muscle = ciliary body). The curvature of the lens, and hence its refractive power, is changed by contraction and relaxation of the ciliary muscle (accommodation).
- *Iris:* forms a variable aperture (pupil) in front of the lens, controlling the amount of light entering the eye (color of the iris depends on the density of its pigments). The sphincter of the pupil (m. sphincter pupillae) is innervated by the parasympathetic, and constricts the pupil (miosis), while the dilator of the pupil (m. dilator pupillae) dilates it (mydriasis). Pupillary reflexes: consensual light reflex (when the incident light hits only one eye, both eyes are reflexly constricted); convergence (internal rotation of the axes of both eyes and constriction of the pupils when fixating close objects).

The optical apparatus acts like a convex lens and projects an inverted and markedly reduced image of the world on the retina. The more curved the lens, the greater its power of refraction (measured in diopters) and the shorter the focal length: refractive power (D) = 1/focal length (m). When the eye is maximally accommodated for distance (flattened lens with a focal length of 0.017 m) the power of refraction 1/0.017 m = 59 D. When accommodation is maximal for close vision (curved lens), the power of refraction increases by about 10 D (increase in refractive power = range of accommodation). Because the lens becomes less elastic, the range of accommodation decreases with aging, resulting in presbyopia (convex glasses needed for close vision).

Posterior Part of the Globe

The posterior part of the globe includes the sclera, the choroid and the retina.

- *Sclera:* forms an inelastic connective tissue capsule, into which the extraocular muscles are inserted. It is pierced like a sieve where the optic nerve exits.
- *Choroid:* consists of delicate pigmented connective tissue containing numerous blood vessels.
- *Retina:* separates the choroid and the vitreous and consists of two layers, the outer pigmented layer (stratum pigmentosum) and the inner light-sensitive layer (stratum nervosum), which consists of three layers (starting from the outside):
  1. Layer of photoreceptors (1st neuron) with rods and cones: light-sensitive photoreceptors (about 120 million rods for dark and light vision, and 6 million cones for color vision)
  2. Layer of bipolar retinal ganglion cells (2nd neuron)
  3. Ganglionic layer of optic nerve (3rd neuron), the axons of which form the optic nerve

Optic disk (papilla nervi optici): area where the central axons of the ganglion cells of the optic nerve collect and pierce the sclera, origin of the optic nerve, and point of entry of the central artery of the retina.

Macula lutea (yellow spot): with the fovea centralis, the site of maximal visual acuity, 4 mm lateral to the optic disk. Contains only cones, and the overlying retinal layers are pushed aside (light reaches sensory cells directly).

Eye ground (fundus): examination of the fundus with an ophthalmoscope allows direct examination of vessels (central artery and vein of the retina).

The Visual Pathway

The visual pathway starts at the retina and ends in the primary visual cortex at the calcarine fissure (occipital lobe); it consists of four successive neurons, the first three neurons being located in the retina. The axons of the 3rd neurons (ganglion cells) of the optic nerve form the optic nerve, which crosses at the optic chiasma to continue as the optic tract to the diencephalon, where it synapses with the 4th neuron in the lateral geniculate body. The axon of the 4th neuron form the optic radiation, which ends in the visual cortex of the cerebrum.

- *Visual fields:* the visual field for each eye can be divided into an inner (nasal) and outer (temporal) field. The image from the inner field projects on the temporal, that from the outer field on the nasal half of the retina. The optic nerve fibers from the nasal halves of the retina then cross to the opposite side at the optic chiasma, while the fibers from the temporal side remain uncrossed. By this mechanism, the left visual field of each eye is represented in the right hemisphere and the right visual field in the left hemisphere.
- *Visual field defects:* lesions of the neurons at various points may create partial or total visual field defects.

Accessory Structure of the Eye

These include the eyelids, the lacrimal apparatus, and the extraocular muscles.

- *Eyelids:* the upper and lower lids protect the anterior surface of the eyeball and form the edges of the palpebral fissure. They are reinforced by connective tissue plates, and their outside is covered with stratified keratinous epithelium, their inside with conjunctiva. The levator palpebrae superior muscle is innervated by cranial nerve III, the circular muscle (orbicularis orbis muscle) that closes the palpebral fissure by cranial nerve VII.
- *Lacrimal apparatus:* this includes the lacrimal gland and the pathways by which the tears drain. The tears secreted by the lacrimal gland clean and nourish the cornea. They flow through the lacrimal

puncta and the lacrimal canal into the lacrimal sac, and from there through the nasolacrimal duct into the nasal cavity.

- *Extraocular muscles:* striated muscles that move the two bulbs. There are four rectus muscles on each side (superior rectus, inferior rectus, medial rectus, and lateral rectus) and two oblique muscles (superior oblique and inferior oblique), innervated by cranial nerves III, IV, and VI.

■ The Ear

The ear contains two sensory organs, the organ of hearing and the organ of equilibrium. Both lie in the petrous pyramid of the temporal bone. They form the inner ear, consisting of the cochlea and the vestibular apparatus (labyrinth consisting of two vestibular pouches and three semicircular canals). Their afferent nerves run to the brainstem by way of the vestibulocochlear nerve (cranial nerve VIII) and continue to the auditory cortex in the temporal lobe or to the cerebellum.

The Organ of Hearing

The organ of hearing includes the inner ear and its accessory structures, the external ear and the middle ear:

- *External ear:* this includes the pinna, the external auditory meatus, which is about 3 cm long, and the eardrum, which separates it from the middle ear.
- *Middle ear:* this includes the tympanic cavity, the eustachian tube (connects it to the pharyngeal cavity), and the auditory ossicles (hammer, anvil, and stirrup). Together with the tympanum, the latter form the sound-conducting apparatus. Vibrations elicited by sound waves in the tympanum are conducted by the auditory ossicles to the oval window of the inner ear and so transmitted to the perilymph. Two muscles, the stapedius muscle and the tensor tympani muscle can influence the sensitivity of the transmission.
- *Inner ear:* this is a fluid-filled (perilymph) labyrinthine system of cavities and spaces (bony labyrinth), which contains the membranous labyrinth (contains the actual organs of hearing and equilibrium) filled with endolymph. Endolymph and perilymph differ principally in their sodium and potassium contents. The cochlea, a spiral about 3 cm long, contains a passage winding about $2^{1}/_{2}$ turns around its bony axis (modiolus); in cross-section it contains three

separate cavities: the middle cochlear canal (ductus cochlearis), the vestibular canal (scala vestibuli) above it, and the tympanic canal (scala tympani) below it. The scala tympani begins at the oval window, the scala vestibuli ends at the round window. They are connected at the apex of the cochlea (helicotrema) and are filled with perilymph. The cochlear duct is filled with endolymph and contains the organ of Corti, which is fitted with the sensory auditory cells (hair cells).

The Mechanism of Hearing and the Auditory Pathway

Sound waves traveling along the sound-conducting apparatus impinge on the oval window and create continuous pressure waves in the perilymph of the scala vestibuli; these waves then run in the opposite direction in the scala tympani. They initiate vibrations in the endolymph of the cochlear duct, creating frequency-dependent excitations in the hair cells of the organ of Corti (high-pitched tones are heard at the base of the cochlea, low-pitched at the apex). The action potentials are transmitted to the cochlear nucleus of the brainstem through the cochlear part of the vestibulocochlear nerve (cranial nerve VIII), and eventually through the auditory pathway to the primary acoustic cortex (anterior transverse temporal gyrus).

The Organ of Equilibrium

This includes the three semicircular ducts with their dilatations (ampullae) and the two vestibular pouches, the utricle (larger) and the saccule (smaller), all filled with endolymph. The ampullae and the utricle and saccule contain the sensory areas and their hair cells (acoustic crests, macula utriculi, and macula sacculi) that register acceleration and changes in position:

- *Acoustic crests:* rotational acceleration in the three principal spatial axes
- *Macula utriculi:* horizontal accelerations
- *Macula sacculi:* vertical accelerations

The action potentials reach the vestibular nuclei in the brainstem by the vestibular part of the vestibulocochlear nerve (cranial nerve VIII). From there they run to the cerebellum and to the nuclei of the extraocular muscles.

■ The Sense of Taste

The secondary sensory cells (altered epithelial cells for the sense of taste lie with supportive cells in the intraepithelial taste buds of the tongue. These taste buds lie in depressed pits in the epithelium at the edge of taste papillae, into the bottom of which drain mucoserous glands. The innervation of the sensory cells is by the facial nerve (anterior two-thirds of tongue) and the glossopharyngeal nerve (posterior two-thirds of the tongue). The four taste sensations (sweet, sour, salty, and bitter) are sensed by different receptors in taste buds in different parts of the tongue.

■ The Sense of Smell

The olfactory mucosa (about 500 mm^2) in the superior nasal turbinates and the upper portion of the nasal septum contains about 10 million olfactory cells (bipolar nerve cells), which form the 1st neuron of the olfactory pathway in the form of the olfactory nerve. They pass through the lamina cribrosa of the ethmoid bone to the olfactory bulb, where they synapse with the 2nd neuron, the afferent axons of which run in the olfactory nerve (cranial nerve I) to the olfactory cortex.

16

The Skin and Its Appendages

Contents

■ Skin (Cutis) and Subcutaneous Tissue (Tela Subcutanea)

Layers of the Skin

The skin is the *common integument* (*integumentum commune*) forming the external surface of the body. It is differentiated in various ways in different regions of the body. The term appendages comprises specific derivatives of the skin such as the sensory organs of the skin, the glands of the skin, nails, and hair.

In an adult the integument has a surface area of about 1.7 m²; it is composed of the *skin* (*cutis*) and the *subcutaneous tissue* (*tela subcutanea*). The skin includes the *epidermis*, a stratified squamous keratinous epithelium, and the *dermis*, a dense network of collagen and elastic fibers (Fig. 16.**1**). The subcutaneous tissue is firmly attached to the dermis and laced with dense white connective tissue fibers.

Epidermis

The epidermis with its epithelium forms the surface layer of the body surface. It is a *stratified squamous keratinized* (*horny*) *epithelium*, and is in most areas of the body 0.1–0.2 mm thick. On the palms of the hands and the soles of the feet, the epidermis is distinctly thickened (0.8–1.5 mm) (Fig. 16.**2a**, **b**). It forms a genetically determined pattern of papillary ridges.

The cells divide constantly in the lowest cellular layers (collectively called *germinative stratum*, *stratum germinale*), the *basal* and *prickle* (or *spinous*) *cell layers* (*stratum basale* and *stratum spinosum*) (Fig. 16.**1**). In this process, one daughter cell migrates to the surface, while the other divides again. As the cells migrate toward the surface to become cornified, they form granules (*stratum granulosum*). In the palms of the hands and the soles of the feet, they then lose their nuclei and cell boundaries to form an extra layer, the clear layer (*stratum lucidum*). After reaching the surface, they are shed from the *horny layer* (*stratum corneum*) as keratinous scales.

Three other types of cell can be found within the epithelial complex: *Merkel cells*, *melanocytes*, and *Langerhans cells*. Merkel cells are secondary mechanosensory cells mostly found in sensitive areas of the skin (e. g., fingertips). Melanocytes are large cells with long processes (den-

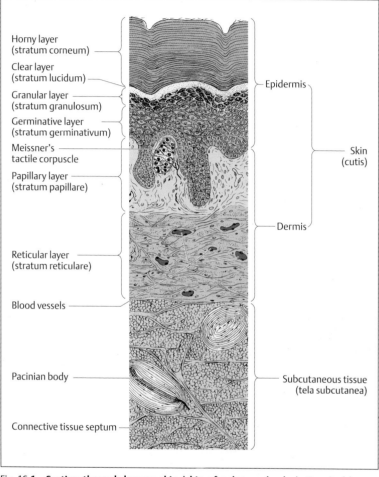

Fig. 16.**1** **Section through human skin (skin of palms and soles).** Germinal layer = basal layer + spinous layer. (After Feneis)

drites) and contain pigment (melanin) formed under the influence of strong sunlight (Fig. 16.**3**). Finally, Langerhans cells are cells of the specific immune system and can ingest antigens (see p. 283) to present to T-helper cells.

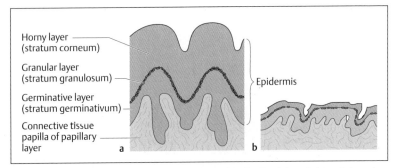

Horny layer
(stratum corneum)

Granular layer
(stratum granulosum)

Germinative layer
(stratum germinativum)

Connective tissue
papilla of papillary
layer

Epidermis

a   b

Fig. 16.**2a, b**   **Epidermis of skin surface of palms and soles (a) and skin of the other body regions (b)**

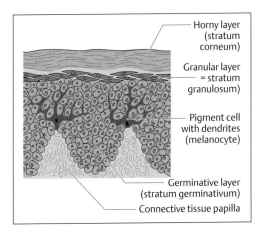

Horny layer
(stratum
corneum)

Granular layer
= stratum
granulosum)

Pigment cell
with dendrites
(melanocyte)

Germinative layer
(stratum germinativum)

Connective tissue papilla

Fig. 16.**3**   **Pigment cells (melanocytes) in the epidermis.** (After Leonhardt)

Dermis

The dermis (or corium) gives skin its resistance to tearing and its plasticity. It consists of a thick network of collagen and elastic fibers and contains blood vessels, lymphatics, nerve fibers, connective tissue cells, and immune cells. It is divided into a *papillary layer* (*stratum papillare*) and a *reticular layer* (*stratum reticulare*), distinguished by the arrangement of their fibers.

The papillary layer is directly adjacent to the epidermis and interdigitates with it by its *dermal papillae*. The height and number of these papillae depends on the mechanical demands of their location. Elastic fiber networks arranged in various ways in the reticular layer give the skin its resilience. They are responsible for the gaping of a wound.

Subcutaneous Tissue

The subcutaneous tissue (tela subcutanea) consists of loose, adipose connective tissue, which is subdivided by bands of connective tissue. It connects the skin with the superficial fascia covering the body and enables the skin to slide over it. The subcutaneous fatty tissue is quite variable between individuals and different regions of the body. It serves as a store for fat. *Structural fat* (e. g., on the soles of the feet) is distinguished from *depot fat* (e. g., abdominal fat pads). Between the subcutaneous tissue and the skin runs a network of arteries and veins, which sends branches as far as the dermal papillae of the dermis (Fig. 16.**1**).

Sensory Organs of the Skin

The sensory organs of the epidermis, the dermis, and the subcutaneous tissue include the *encapsulated nerve endings* (mechanoreceptors) and the *free nerve endings* (mechanical, pressure, pain, and temperature receptors). Their afferent nerve fibers run in skin nerves, together with autonomic efferent axons that supply the blood vessels, glands and hair muscles.

In addition to the Merkel disks (tactile menisci) in the epidermis, touch receptors occur as tactile cells (Meissner's tactile corpuscles) in the connective tissue papillae of the dermis, and as lamellar corpuscles (pacinian bodies, Vater–Pacini corpuscles) in the subcutaneous tissues (Fig. 16.**1**). Free nerve endings can be seen especially in the dermis and in the basket networks of nerves around the hair follicles (Fig. 16.**4**).

Tasks of the Skin

The skin is an organ the individual layers of which have multiple functions:

- Protection: through its keratinized epithelium and the secretions of its glands the skin protects from mechanical, thermal and chemical damage.
- Temperature regulation: body temperature is regulated by constriction and dilation of the skin vessels and by secretion of fluid by the glands of the skin.
- Water balance: protection against fluid loss and regulation of the secretion of fluid and salts by glands.
- Sensory function: sensory organs of the skin in the form of pain, temperature, pressure, and touch receptors.
- Immune function: high number of specific immune cells.
- Communication: e. g., expressing autonomic responses by blushing or turning pale.

■ Skin Appendages

The epithelial appendages of the skin include dermal glands, hair, and nails. The surrounding connective tissue takes part in their formation.

Glands of the Skin

The glands of the skin include *eccrine* and *apocrine sweat glands* and *sebaceous glands*. There are a total of about 2 million eccrine sweat glands, and they are clustered especially in the skin of the forehead, the palms of the hands, and the soles of the feet. Their acid secretion forms an *acid protective coat* on the surface of the skin, inhibiting bacterial growth. Apocrine sweat glands are especially associated with hair (axillary, head, and pubic hair). Their secretion is rather alkaline and is triggered by sex hormones. Sebaceous glands, like apocrine sweat glands, occur mainly in hairy skin (sebaceous glands of hair follicles) (Fig. 16.**4**). Their secretion, sebum, is rich in fatty acids; it combines with sweat to make the skin pliant and contributes to the gloss of hair.

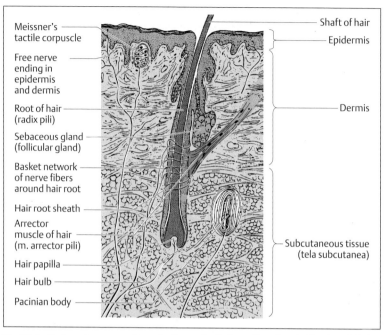

Meissner's tactile corpuscle

Free nerve ending in epidermis and dermis

Root of hair (radix pili)

Sebaceous gland (follicular gland)

Basket network of nerve fibers around hair root

Hair root sheath

Arrector muscle of hair (m. arrector pili)

Hair papilla

Hair bulb

Pacinian body

Shaft of hair

Epidermis

Dermis

Subcutaneous tissue (tela subcutanea)

Fig. 16.**4** **Hair and nerve endings in the scalp** (hair papilla + hair bulb = hair follicle). (After Leonhardt)

Hair

Hair is seen as *lanugo hair* in the newborn and *terminal hair* in the adult. It serves as a cover for warmth and for touch sensation. A terminal hair sits in a root sheath, into which opens a sebaceous gland. The *arrector muscle of hair* (*m. arrector pili*) originates under the sebaceous gland on the side toward which the hair inclines and runs to the epidermis (Fig. 16.**4**). It erects the hair (sympathetic reaction) while pulling the epidermis into a little pit (goose bumps).

The hair includes a keratinous hair shaft with an epithelial root sheath and a root that is attached to a connective tissue hair papilla by an epithelial hair bulb. Hair bulb and hair papilla together form the *hair fol-*

licle, which is supplied by blood vessels and from which hair growth originates. While lanugo originates in the dermis, the roots of terminal hairs lie in the superficial part of the subcutaneous tissue (Fig. 16.**4**). The color of hair depends among other things on its pigment (melanin) content. If melanin production ceases, or after the deposition of small air bubbles, the hair appears gray or white.

Nails

Nails, like hair, are special epidermal formations. They are horny plates (*nail plates*) anchored in the nail bed. The *nail bed* is the epithelial tissue from which the nail grows continuously. The proximal edge of the nail plate lies under the *nail sinus* (*sinus unguis*), the lateral edge in the *lateral nail fold* (Fig. 16.**5a–c**). Distal to the sinus unguis, the nail-forming

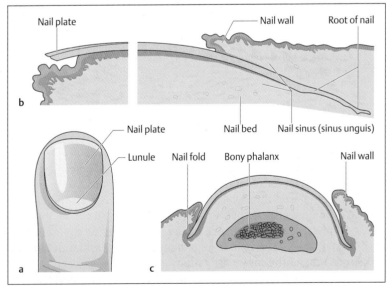

Fig. 16.**5 a–c** **Finger nail.** (After Rauber-Kopsch)
a View from above; **b** longitudinal section through nail bed; **c** cross-section through nail bed

epithelial tissue gleams through the nail as a semilunar whitish area (*lunule*). Capillaries showing through the nail give it its pink color.

The nails protect the terminal phalanges of the fingers and toes and form a backstop for pressure exerted on the pulp. This makes the nails important accessories to the sense of touch.

Summary **The Skin and Its Appendages**

■ **Structure of the Skin**

The skin is the cover of the body and forms its outer surface (ca. 1.7 m²). It includes the actual skin (cutis) and the subcutaneous tissue (tela subcutanea). The cutis is divided into epidermis and dermis:

● **Cutis**
  - *Epidermis:* stratified keratinous squamous epithelium with germinative layer (stratum germinativum = stratum basale and stratum spinosum), granular layer (stratum granulosum), and horny layer (stratum corneum). Its thickness varies: in general skin (e. g., back, abdomen, arms, legs) it is 0.1–0.2 mm thick; in skin of the soles of the feet and palms of the hands it is 0.8–1.5 mm). It contains three other kinds of cell: Merkel receptors (mechanoreceptors), melanocytes (pigment cells), and Langerhans cells (immune cells).
  - *Dermis* (also called corium): consists of a dense network of collagen and elastic fibers as well as nerves and blood vessels. It makes the skin resistant to tears and makes it pliable. The dermis includes a papillary layer (stratum papillare) next to the epidermis and a reticular layer (stratum reticulare) next to the subcutaneous tissue.
● **Subcutis (tela subcutanea, subcutaneous tissue):** Consists of loose connective tissue rich in fatty tissue (subcutaneous fat) with numerous blood vessels. It allows the skin to slide over the underlying tissue and serves as a store for fat: structural fat (e. g., in soles of feet) and depot fat (e. g., abdominal fat pad).
● **Sensory organs of the skin** occur in all its layers. They include encapsulated nerve endings (mechanoreceptors: Merkel cells in the epidermis, Meissner's tactile corpuscles in the stratum papillare,

and pacinian corpuscles in the subcutaneous tissue) and free nerve endings (pain, pressure, and temperature receptors).

Tasks of the Skin
- *Protection:* by cornification and glandular secretions
- *Temperature regulation:* by dilation and constriction of blood vessels and evaporation of fluids
- *Water balance:* by the regulation of fluid and salt secretion
- *Sensory function:* by the presence of various kinds of receptor
- *Immune function:* by the presence of immune cells
- *Communication:* by the expression of autonomic responses.

Skin Appendages
- *Skin glands:* these include eccrine and apocrine sweat glands and sebaceous glands:
  - Eccrine sweat glands (especially on forehead, palms of hands, soles of feet) form an acid secretion (acid protective coat) that inhibits bacterial growth.
  - Apocrine sweat glands (axillary, head and pubic hair) form an alkaline secretion and are triggered by sex hormones.
  - Sebaceous glands (associated with hair) form sebum that is rich in fatty acids and keeps the skin pliant.
- *Hair:* keeps the body warm and serves the sensation of touch (lanugo hair of the newborn and terminal hair of the adult). Terminal hair sits in a root sheath, into which a sebaceous gland opens. A hair muscle erects it. The hair consists of a horny hair shaft with an epithelial hair root sheath and a root (epithelial hair bulb and connective tissue hair papilla = hair follicle).
- *Nails:* 0.5 mm thick horny plates (nail plates) anchored in an epithelial nail bed (growing zone). They protect the terminal phalanx of the fingers and toes and are an important accessory for the sense of touch (backstop for pressure on the pulp of the finger tip).

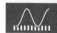

17

Quantities and Units of Measurement

Contents

■ Abbreviations

a.	=	artery or arteria	aa.	=	arteries or arteriae
v.	=	vein or vena	vv.	=	veins or venae
m.	=	muscle or musculus	mm.	=	muscles or musculi
n.	=	nerve or nervus	nn.	=	nerves or nervi
r.	=	ramus	rr.	=	rami
lig.	=	ligament or ligamentum			

■ The SI System of Units

The international system of units (SI = *Système International*) was introduced in many countries as a unified standard of measurement, in view of the many different units used in medicine, especially in physiology (for example, units of pressure include mmHg, cmH_2O, torr, atm, or kg/cm^2).

The SI Base Units

Base quantity	Name	Symbol
Length	meter	m
Mass	kilogram	kg
Time	second	s
Electric current	ampere	A
Thermodynamic temperature	kelvin	K
Amount of substance	mole	mol
Luminous intensity	candela	cd

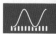

Some Derived SI Units

Other quantities, the *derived quantities*, may be derived from these seven base quantities, mostly by multiplying or dividing one by another. For instance, area = length × length $(m \cdot m)$ = m^2; velocity = distance/time = m/s (or $m\,s^{-1}$).

Derived quantity	Unit	Definition
Frequency	hertz (Hz)	s^{-1}
Force	newton (N)	$m \cdot kg \cdot s^{-2}$
Pressure, stress	pascal (Pa)	$m^{-1} \cdot kg \cdot s^{-2} = N \cdot m^{-2}$
Energy, work, quantity of heat	joule (J)	$m^2 \cdot kg \cdot s^{-2} = N \cdot m$
Power, radiant flux	watt (W)	$m^2 \cdot kg \cdot s^{-3} = J \cdot s^{-1}$
Electric charge	coulomb (C)	$s \cdot A$
Quantity of electricity		
Electric potential difference	volt (V)	$m^2 \cdot kg \cdot s^{-3} \cdot A^{-1} = W \cdot A^{-1}$
Electrical resistance	ohm (Ω)	$m^2 \cdot kg \cdot s^{-3} \cdot A^{-2} = V \cdot A^{-1}$

In addition to the SI base units and their derived units, a number of other units may still be used: gram (g), liter (l), minute (min), hour (h), day (d), and degree centigrade/Celsius (°C).

■ Multiples and Fractions (Powers of Ten)

When numbers are much larger or smaller than 1 they are difficult and cumbersome to write. Hence these numbers are expressed as powers of 10. For example:

$100 = 10 \times 10 = 10^2$
$1000 = 10 \times 10 \times 10 = 10^3$
$10\,000 = 10 \times 10 \times 10 \times 10 = 10^4$

$1 = 10 : 10 = 10^0$
$0.1 = 10 : 10 : 10 = 10^{-1}$
$0.01 = 10 : 10 : 10 : 10 = 10^{-2}$

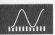

Combining Forms

To improve clarity, it is customary to use certain combining forms to designate multiples and fractions of ten.

Multiples

Power of ten	Prefix	Symbol
10^1	deka (or deca) (tenfold)	da
10^2	hecto (one hundred times)	h
10^3	kilo (one thousand times)	k
10^6	mega (one million times)	M
10^9	giga (one billion times)	G
10^{12}	tera (one trillion times)	T
10^{15}	peta (one quadrillion times)	P
10^{18}	exa (one quintillion times)	E

Submultiples

Power of ten	Prefix	Symbol
10^{-1}	deci (one-tenth)	d
10^{-2}	centi (one-hundredth)	c
10^{-3}	milli (one-thousandth)	m
10^{-6}	micro (one-millionth)	μ
10^{-9}	nano (one-billionth)	n
10^{-12}	pico (one-trillionth)	p
10^{-15}	femto (one-quadrillionth)	f
10^{-18}	atto (one-quintillionth)	a

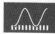

■ Concentrations and Equivalent Values

In the SI system, concentrations can be written as amount of substance (moles) per volume (mol/l) or as mass per volume (g/l). The concentration in terms of amount of substance, formerly known as molar concentration, is proportional to the number of molecules contained in a solution (e. g., blood plasma). Amount-of-substance concentrations are most commonly used when the molecular weight of a chemically pure substance is known.

Equivalents of Older ("Conventional") Concentration Units in SI Units

Substance	Value in conventional unit	Value in SI unit
Sodium	1 mg% (10 mg/l)	0.4350 mmol/l
Potassium	1 mg%	0.2558 mmol/l
Calcium	1 mg%	0.2495 mmol/l
Magnesium	1 mg%	0.4114 mmol/l
Chloride	1 mg%	0.2821 mmol/l
Glucose	1 mg%	0.0555 mmol/l
Urea	1 mg%	0.1660 mmol/l
Cholesterol	1 mg%	0.0259 mmol/l
Uric acid	1 mg%	59.48 µmol/l
Creatinine	1 mg%	88.40 µmol/l
Bilirubin	1 mg%	17.10 µmol/l
Plasma proteins	1 g%	10 g/l

Equivalents of Older Units of Power, Pressure, and Energy in SI Units

Quantity	Derived equation	SI equivalent
Force	1 dyne = 10^{-5} N	1 N = 10^5 dyne
Pressure	1 cmH$_2$O = 98.1 Pa	1 Pa = 0.0102 cmH$_2$O
	1 mmHg (1 torr) = 133.3 Pa	1 Pa = 0.0075 mmHg
	1 atm = 101 kPa	1 kPa = 0.0099 atm
	1 bar = 100 kPa	1 kPa = 0.01 bar
Energy	1 erg = 10^{-7} J	1 J = 10^7 erg
Energy in terms of heat	1 cal = 4.19 J	1 J = 0.239 cal

■ Eponyms (Proper Names) in Medical Anatomy and Physiology

Eponyms are a common part of anatomical terms, especially in clinical usage. The following list includes the dates and sites of activity of some of the scientists named in the text. These names are those most familiar in medical anatomy and physiology. Most of the information derives from the following sources:

Debson J.: *Anatomical Eponyms,* 2nd ed. Livingstone: Edinburgh and London, 1962.

Dorland's Illustrated Medical Dictionary, 29th ed. Saunders: Philadelphia, 2000.

Faller, A.: *Die Fachwörter der Anatomie, Histologie und Embryologie.* Bergmann: Munich, 1978.

Herrlinger, R.: *Eigennamen in Anatomie, Physiologie, Embryologie und physiologischer Chemie.* G. Fischer: Jena, 1947.

Arey, Lesley Brainerd (1891–1988): American anatomist. Originator of Arey's rule to determine the length (in inches) of a fetus from the duration of gestation.

Auerbach, Leopold (1828–1897): German anatomist. Described Auerbach's myenteric plexus.

Bartholin, Caspar Secundus (1655–1738): Physician, anatomist, and administrator in Copenhagen, Denmark. Described the glands of the female vestibule.

Bowman, Sir William (1816–1892): London anatomist, physiologist, and ophthalmologist. Described the capsule of the glomerulus.

Broca, Paul (1824–1860) Paris surgeon and anthropologist. Broca's speech area is named after him.

Corti, Marchese Alphonso (1822–1867): Anatomist active at Vienna, Würzburg, Pavia, Utrecht, and Turin. Described Corti's organ in the cochlea.

Cowper, William (1666–1709): Anatomist and surgeon in London. Described the bulbourethral or Cowper's glands in men.

Döderlein, Gustav (1893–1980): Gynecologist at Jena and Munich. The vaginal Döderlein bacillus is named after him.

Douglas, James (1675–1742): London anatomist and gynecologist. Described Douglas's pouch, the lowest point of the abdominal cavity.

Down, John Langdon Haydon (1828–1896): English physician, who described the Down syndrome.

Edinger, Ludwig (1855–1918): Frankfurt neuroanatomist. He is named in the Edinger–Westphal nucleus, the parasympathetic nucleus of cranial nerve X (vagus nerve).

Eustachio, Bartholomeo (1513–1574): Anatomist and personal physician to the Pope in Rome. The eustachian tube, running between middle ear and oral cavity, is named after him.

Fallopio, Gabriele (1523–1562): Italian anatomist. Described the fallopian tube among other structures.

Golgi, Camillo (1844–1926): Anatomist at Siena and Pavia. Described the Golgi aparatus.

Graaf, Reijnier (Regnier) de (1641–1673): Physician and anatomist in Delft and Paris. The ovulation-ready graafian follicle is named after him.

Haase, Karl Friedrich (1788–1865): Dresden gynecologist. The Haase rule combined with the duration of gestation allows calculation of fetal length in centimeters.

Hassal, Arthur Hill (1817–1894): Physician active in London, the Isle of Wight, and San Remo. The Hassal corpuscles of the thymus are named after him.

Havers, Clopton (1650–1702): London anatomist. The haversian canals in lamellar bone are named after him.

Henle, Friedrich Gustav Jakob (1864–1936): Anatomist and pathologist at Zurich, Heidelberg, and Göttingen. Henle's loop in the medullary portion of the nephron is named after him.

His, William (1863–1934): Internist in Göttingen and Berlin. The cardiac conducting bundle of His is named after him.

Kerckring, Theodor (1640–1693): Physician and anatomist at Amsterdam and Hamburg. Kerckring's folds in the small intestine are named after him.

Kohlrausch, Otto Ludwig Bernhardt (1811–1854): Hannover physician. The Kohlrausch fold of the rectum is named after him.

Korotkoff, Nicolai Sergeeivich (1874–1920): Russian physician. The Korotkoff sounds heard when taking a blood pressure are named after him.

Kupffer, Karl Wilhelm von (1829–1903): Anatomist at Kiel, Königsberg, and Munich. The phagocytosing Kupffer cells in the liver are named after him.

Kussmaul, Adolph (1822–1902): German physician who described Kussmaul breathing seen in diabetic coma.

Langerhans, Paul (1849–1888): Freiburg pathologist. The islets of Langerhans in the pancreas and the Langerhans cells in the skin were described by him.

Leydig, Franz von (1821–1908): Physiologist and anatomist at Würzburg and Bonn. The testicular Leydig cells are named after him.

Lieberkühn, Johann Nathanael (1711–1756): Berlin physician. The crypts in the wall of the small intestine are named after him.

Malpighi, Marcello (1628–1694): Professor of Medicine at Bolgna, Pisa, and Messina. The malpighian corpuscles in the kidney are named after him.

McBurney, Charles (1845–1914): New York surgeon. McBurney's point (projection of the vermiform appendix to the abdominal surface) is named after him.

Meissner, Georg (1829–1905): Physiologist and zoologist at Basle, Freiburg, and Göttingen. The tactile corpuscles in the dermis are named after him.

Merkel, Friedrich S.M. (1845–1919: Göttingen anatomist. The tactile Merkel cells in the epidermis are named after him.

Monro, Alexander (Secundus) (1733–1817): Scottish anatomist and surgeon. The interventricular foramen of Monro is named after him.

Naegele, Franz (1777–1851): Heidelberg gynecologist. The probable date of delivery can be calculated using Naegele's rule.

Nissl, Franz (1860–1919): Heidelberg psychiatrist and neurohistologist. The Nissl granules in nerve cells are named after him.

Oddi, Ruggero (1864–1913): Italian physician. The sphincter of Oddi in the major duodenal papilla is named after him.

Pacchioni, Antoine (1665–1726): Physician in Tivoli and Rome. The pacchionian granulations (projections of the arachnoid into the venous sinuses) are named after him.

Pacini, Filippo (1812–1883): Florentine anatomist. The Vater–Pacini bodies (pressure receptors) derive their name from him.

Peyer, Johann Konrad (1653–1712): Schaffhausen physician. The Peyer's patches, collections of lymphoid follicles in the ileum, are named after him.

Purkinje, Johannes Evangelista (1787–1869): Anatomist and physiologist at Breslau and Prague. The Purkinje fibers in the conduction system of the heart are named after him.

Ranvier, Louis Antoine (1835–1922): Paris histologist. The constrictions of myelinated nerves are named after him.

Reissner, Ernst (1824–1878): Anatomist at Dorpat and Breslau. Reissner's membrane of the inner ear is named after him.

Schlemm, Friedrich (1795–1858): Berlin anatomist. The circular vein in the angle between iris and cornea is named after him.

Schwann, Theodor (1810–1882): Anatomist and physiologist at Leeuwen and Liege. The outer sheath of nerve fibers is named after him.

Sertoli, Enrico (1842–1910): Milan physiologist. The testicular Sertoli cells are named after him.

Sharpey, William (1802–1880): Anatomist at Edinburgh and London. Sharpey's fibers in the desmodontium are named after him.

Sylvius, Jacobus (1478–1555): Latinized form of Jacques Dubois, French anatomist at Paris. Probably the anatomist who described the cerebral aqueduct.

Tawara, K. Sunao (1873–1952): Pathologist in Fukuoka, Japan. The sinoatrial node and the branches of the ventricular conducting system are named after him.

Vater, Abraham (1684–1751): Anatomist and botanist at Wittenberg. The ampulla of Vater in the duodenum and the Vater–Pacini corpuscles in the skin are named after him.

Volkmann, Richard (1800–1877): German surgeon. He described Volkmann's canals in bone.

Waldeyer, Heinrich W.G (1836–1921): German anatomist who described the ring of lymphoid tissue in the throat.

Wernicke, Karl W. (1848–1905): Neurologist in Berlin, Breslau, and Halle. Wernicke's auditory association area in the superior temporal gyrus is named after him.

Westphal, Karl F.O. (1833–1890): German neurologist. His name is associated with the Edinger–Westphal nucleus, the parasympathetic nucleus of cranial nerve X (vagus nerve).

Willis, Thomas (1621–1675): English anatomist and physician. The circulus arteriosus of Willis is named after him.

Index

Page numbers in **bold type** refer to illustrations

H

W

X

Y

Z